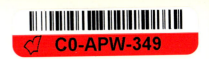

RECENT ADVANCES
IN RESPIRATORY MEDICINE

T. B. STRETTON

MB FRCP
*Consultant Physician,
Manchester Royal Infirmary;
Senior Lecturer in Medicine,
University of Manchester*

RECENT ADVANCES IN RESPIRATORY MEDICINE

EDITED BY

T. B. STRETTON

NUMBER ONE

CHURCHILL LIVINGSTONE
Edinburgh London and New York
1976

CHURCHILL LIVINGSTONE
Medical Division of Longman Group Limited

Distributed in the United States of America by
Longman Inc., 19 West 44th Street, New York,
N.Y. 10036, and by associated
companies, branches and representatives
throughout the world

First published 1976

ISBN 0 443 01458 2

Printed in Great Britain

PREFACE

There have been so many developments in respiratory medicine in the past decade it has been difficult to keep abreast of them, especially for those who do not work in specialist centres. It is hoped that the topics chosen for this volume will bring together some of these developments in a way that is helpful to all clinicians responsible for the care of patients with lung disease: to paediatricians and geriatricians as well as general physicians and those with a special interest in diseases of the chest.

An initial chapter dealing with the growing contribution of nuclear medicine is followed by a review of the current position of cytopathology in chest medicine and then a chapter which highlights some of the fascinating advances in respiratory pathology. Hypoxia is so often the ultimate pathophysiological problem facing our patients; already introduced in the section on pathology, and a recurring theme later in the book, the whole of the next chapter is devoted to this important subject. The notable progress that has been made in our knowledge of the morphology of the lungs is reviewed in Chapter 5. This is followed by a series of clinical reviews. The first of these deals with the common problem of airways obstruction and diseases causing this. The second looks at the broad spectrum of conditions which cause widespread damage to the gas-exchanging zone of the lungs. Diseases of the respiratory system are a major cause of illness and death in the newborn and in infancy. These are reviewed in the penultimate chapter. Finally, several topics of recent interest are considered in Chapter 9; one is purely technical (bronchoscopy) while the others share some ground in common with pulmonary oedema.

The mmHg has been retained throughout. Conversion to kPa is easy for those who are already familiar with SI units: divide by 7.5. The Ångstrom (10^{-10}) has also been kept; this is synonymous with 0.1 nanometre.

Finally, I should like to take the opportunity to thank the Jefferson librarians at Manchester Royal Infirmary for help in preparing this volume and Mrs June Lawson for her invaluable secretarial assistance.

Manchester, 1976   T. B. STRETTON

CONTRIBUTORS

D. M. ACKERY MA, MB, BChir, MSc
Consultant in Nuclear Medicine, Wessex Regional Department of Nuclear Medicine, Southampton University Hospitals

E. BLANCHE BUTLER MD, FRCOG
Senior Lecturer, Department of Pathology (Cytopathology), University of Manchester; Cytopathologist, St Mary's Hospital and Manchester Royal Infirmary

D. C. FLENLEY BSc PhD MB FRCP FRCPEd
Reader in Medicine, University of Edinburgh; Honorary Consultant Physician, Royal Infirmary, Edinburgh

DONALD HEATH PhD MD FRCP FRCPath
The George Holt Professor of Pathology, University of Liverpool

K. HORSFIELD PhD MD FRCP
Deputy Director, Midhurst Medical Research Institute, Midhurst, Sussex

J. B. L. HOWELL BSc PhD MB FRCP
Professor of Medicine, University of Southampton

A. L. MUIR MD FRCPEd
Senior Lecturer in Medicine, University of Edinburgh; Honorary Consultant Physician, Royal Infirmary, Edinburgh

N. R. C. ROBERTON MA MB MRCP
Consultant Paediatrician, Addenbrooke's Hospital, Cambridge

G. M. STERLING MD MRCP
Consultant Physician, Western Hospital, Oakley Road, Southampton

T. B. STRETTON MB FRCP
Consultant Physician, Manchester Royal Infirmary; Senior Lecturer in Medicine, University of Manchester

MARGARET TURNER-WARWICK MA DM PhD FRCP
Professor of Medicine (Thoracic Medicine), University of London; Brompton Hospital and Cardiothoracic Institute, London

CONTENTS

1
RADIOISOTOPES IN THE STUDY OF PULMONARY FUNCTION AND DISEASE

D. M. Ackery   G. M. Sterling

Since the early part of the twentieth century many tests have been devised to measure cardiac output and ventilatory function, but it was not until 1934 (Björkman, 1934) that attempts were made to measure the *regional* function of the lungs. Techniques for selective catheterisation of the bronchi were later developed by Martin, Cline and Marshall (1953), and Mattson and Carlens (1955), and these were used to measure lobar ventilation and blood flow. Radioisotopes were first used to assess pulmonary function by Knipping (Knipping et al, 1955). His results were extended and developed by groups at the Hammersmith Hospital, London, and in Montreal and Malmö, who undertook studies to establish the physiological basis for alterations of regional lung function which are observed in patients. Radioisotope investigations remained in the sphere of research until the early 1960s, when successful attempts were made to measure regional pulmonary blood perfusion by temporary blockade of small vessels with particles of macroaggregated human serum albumin labelled with iodine-131 (Taplin et al, 1964; Tow et al, 1966). These investigations were shown to be effective and safe, and have since been adopted as a routine procedure in many hospitals, particularly for the investigation of pulmonary vascular disorders. Measurements of the distribution of ventilation with radioactive gases are largely still limited to specialised pulmonary function departments (Milic-Emili, 1971), but with the increasing availability of scintillation cameras and data acquisition systems many centres should soon be able to offer these as a routine investigation.

Equipment

After intravenous administration or inhalation of a suitable radioactive pharmaceutical, regional blood flow in the pulmonary circulation, or gas flow in airways, is estimated by placing a radiation detector over the chest, to measure the amount of radioactivity in the underlying lung. Scintillation detectors are used for this purpose, and these consist of a crystal of sodium iodide, generally several inches in diameter, with which the gamma rays interact and lose their energy. Energy is then released by the crystal in the form of light, which is detected by a photocathode, and in turn the output of the latter is converted into a voltage pulse by a photomultiplier. The height of the final voltage pulse is proportional to the energy deposited by the gamma interaction in the crystal, and pulse height analysis is used to select particular energies and reject background radiation. This greatly enhances the accuracy of the measurement.

Two types of scintillation detector can be used. The first, called a scintillation probe, has a single crystal of sodium iodide. It can be employed as a static detector to measure changes in count-rate over a fixed region of the chest, or it can be driven mechanically, either as a profile scanner moving up the chest, or in two dimensions as a rectilinear scanner. The final output for each of these is, respectively, a numerical measurement of count-rate; a graph of change of count-rate against distance up the lung; a pictorial 'scan', or 'image', of distribution of count-rate in the chest.

A directional property is given to the probe by the attachment of a lead 'collimator', which excludes gamma radiation that arises from those parts of the chest not within the region of the measurement. The design of the collimator will fix the size of region to be examined, and thus determine the ability to detect small regions of absent activity, the 'spatial resolution' of the detector. For fixed scintillation probes, often used in groups of four or six either side of the chest, the collimator is a circular shield allowing a large region of lung activity to be measured; this gives a high count (sensitivity) but poor spatial resolution. The collimator of the rectilinear scanner has a focusing property, which measures activity only from a point directly beneath the detector and gives much better spatial resolution. As the probe is driven mechanically to and fro across the patient, the different count-rates are fed as an analogue signal either to a light source projected on to x-ray film (Photo-scan), or to a variable speed dotter printing on to paper (Dot-scan). Different activities in the chest are thus displayed as an image of relative optical density, or blackening, on the film, or as a colour contour display on paper. The scanner electronics allow adjustments of speed and density so that a good quality display is obtained under widely differing conditions from patient to patient. The collimator focuses preferentially on a slice of lung a few centimetres within the chest, so in order to establish the pattern of activity in all regions of the lung it is necessary to scan from anterior, posterior and both lateral aspects. Each scan takes 15 to 20 min, so the whole procedure may well last over 1 h. The process can be speeded up by the use of a rectilinear scanner which has two scanning heads viewing two aspects of the chest simultaneously.

The second type of detector is the scintillation camera, which consists of a single disc of sodium iodide approximately 30 cm diameter and 1 cm thick. A multihole lead collimator fitted in front of the crystal allows radiation to be detected from all regions simultaneously, the spatial position within the crystal of each gamma event being determined electronically. Since scanning is not involved, an image is accumulated in a much shorter time than for a rectilinear scanner. The image is displayed either on polaroid or x-ray film, or by a printer after suitable computer processing.

Most scintillation cameras do not give a direct digital output, and in order to quantify the display an analogue to digital converter and digital store must be added. This transposes the image into a digital matrix, usually of 64×64 lines, with 4096 intercept points, so that each image is composed of 4096 numbers which can be stored in a digital memory, for example on magnetic tape or disc. This system enables serial images to be stored during an investigation, for instance to show the temporal changes in ventilation during the wash-in and wash-out of xenon-133. Subsequent analysis of stored data gives a graphical display of changes of count-rate with time for each region of the lung. An on-line digital computer allows mathematical calculations, which are used for correction of non-uniformity of detection across the field of the scintillation camera, for statistical smoothing of the data, and for division of one matrix by another to give a relative ventilation-perfusion image.

The final display from the rectilinear scanner or scintillation camera is a pictorial representation of function and carries little anatomical information. It is essential that the image is compared carefully with the chest radiograph, so that function can be related to anatomical position. Apparent impairment of function may be simply explained by a large heart, a raised hemi-diaphragm, or other anatomical variations. The scintillation camera and rectilinear scanner relate the count-rate within each region of the chest to the maximum count-rate detected. Thus each image gives a display of *relative* function within the lung. Absolute measurements of pulmonary blood perfusion or ventilation are more difficult to obtain, and are rarely made in clinical applications of radioisotopes.

Perfusion Techniques

Two general methods are available for the measurement of regional pulmonary blood flow. Either intravenous radioactive labelled particles are administered which are filtered from the circulation by the pulmonary capillaries, or the distribution within the alveolar gas of radioactive xenon is measured after injection. Due to its low solubility, xenon is rapidly transferred from the plasma to alveolar gas, and its regional distribution is then proportional to the pulmonary blood flow of that region of the lung.

Particle method

Small particles of diameters of approximately 10 to 50 μm are prepared under aseptic conditions in the laboratory, or pharmacy, and labelled with a suitable gamma-emitting radioisotope. These are injected into a peripheral vein, usually in the arm, and mix randomly with the circulating red blood corpuscles during their passage through the heart and into the pulmonary circulation. On arrival at the pulmonary capillary bed the particles become trapped in a distribution which is proportional to the regional flow of blood to that part of the capillary network, and this can be displayed by external measurement with a scintillation detector. In fact the particles remain in situ in the capillaries for several hours so that a delayed measurement will still show the distribution of blood at the time of injection. This has been used to study the distribution of perfusion in antigravity situations in aircraft, the scans having been performed after landing (Wagner et al, 1966).

The proportion of capillaries which are blocked by the particles is small, and the procedure has been shown to be safe. In a typical procedure, less than a million particles are injected, while it has been estimated that there are about 280 billion pulmonary capillaries (Weibel, 1963). Experiments in animals show that the number of particles in a typical clinical injection must be greatly exceeded before any rise in pulmonary vascular pressure can be detected, even with a severely impaired pulmonary circulation, and this is supported by the very low reported mortality for the technique, which is now widely used.

A number of different types of particle have been proposed, but the most usual is human serum albumin. This is heat coagulated to give macro-aggregates of suitable particle size. Recently, commercial supplies of micro-spheres of human serum albumin have become available (Rhodes et al, 1969) which have a more predictable diameter than laboratory prepared macroaggregates. Technetium-99m is the usual radioactive label, with a photon energy of 140 kiloelectron volt (keV). It has the advantage over iodine-131, which may also be used, that its low patient radiation dose permits larger activities to be administered, and this gives an increased regional count rate and a technically superior result.

Inorganic particles such as ferric hydroxide labelled with indium-113m have also been used for blood flow imaging of the lung. Precipitation of the hydroxide from ferric chloride solution ensures a fairly uniform particle size, and gives technically good scans, but several reactions to this agent have been reported (see Toxicity and Hazards).

Gaseous methods

Radioactive gases offer an alternative to the particle technique. Xenon-133 was first used to study ventilation (Knipping et al, 1955) and is now commonly used for perfusion also. The elements of the principal respiratory gases, oxygen, nitrogen and carbon dioxide, all have radioisotopes with short physical half-lives and are therefore not readily available for routine clinical work except in special centres with ready access to a cyclotron. Xenon-133 is reactor-produced and has a half-life of 5.3 days. Its photon energy is 81 keV, which is rather low to be ideal for patient measurements, since many emitted gamma photons are scattered. In spite of its poor solubility, it has a partition coefficient between saline and air which permits intravenous injection of several millicuries for perfusion studies. Injected xenon in solution is carried by the circulating blood to the lungs, at which point the great majority is evolved into the alveolar gas. Distribution of activity within the alveolar gas can be measured with a scintillation camera, the regional distribution being proportional to the relative blood flow to that part of the lung. It is usual for the patient to take a full inspiration and then to breath-hold immediately after injection to minimise the redistribution of xenon within the lung during the measurement.

Choice of perfusion method

Although the use of xenon-133 provides a simple, rapid and safe method of obtaining an image of pulmonary perfusion, it ideally requires both a scintillation camera and cooperation from the patient (but see p. 15). It may not be easy for the breathless or anxious patient to breath-hold at total lung capacity for many seconds, which is essential if sufficient counts are to be collected for a good image of regional perfusion. Furthermore, only one aspect of the chest can be imaged for each breath-hold procedure and repeated views increase the patient's radiation dose. Since the lateral views are so important when evidence of pulmonary thromboembolic disease is looked for, it is preferable to use the particle technique. This has the advantage that once the macroaggregate injection is given, there is no great hurry to make a measurement, and either a rectilinear scanner or scintillation camera can be used to measure the distribution from all directions.

Quantitative analysis of the perfusion image

One advantage of radioisotope techniques is that data obtained from the patient can be easily expressed in quantitative terms. It is then possible to determine the functional loss of blood flow in an affected region of the lung, and to follow the changes from one perfusion study to the next during the course of an illness. This offers a distinct advantage, since it may be difficult for an observer to make a visual comparison between images taken at different times because the final quantitative display is influenced by a variety of technical factors.

The image may be quantified in a number of ways, the simplest of which integrates the total counts measured separately from each lung, and expresses those in the right lung as a percentage of the whole. This proportion has been shown to agree closely with the relative blood flow to each lung measured by differential bronchospirometry (Lopez-Majano et al, 1964; Miörner, 1968). This relative quantification is helpful in the follow-up of patients with discrete thromboembolism.

Toxicity and hazards

The potential risks associated with pulmonary artery blood flow studies may be separated into those due to the physical interruption of blood flow by the aggregate injection, and those due to absorbed radiation dose.

Three deaths have been reported following intravenous administration of macroaggregated human serum albumin. One patient had extensive infiltration of the pulmonary vascular bed with metastatic breast carcinoma and was acutely ill at the time of the scan. She reacted immediately to the injection of macroaggregates with profound dyspnoea and cyanosis, but regained her prescan condition after several hours. However, she died the following day (Dworkin, Smith and Bull, 1966). The second case, a child who had undergone ventriculovenous shunt for treatment of hydrocephalus and had severe pulmonary vascular occlusive disease, developed rapid respiratory and cardiac collapse following injection and died a few hours later (Vincent, Goldberg and Desilets, 1968). The third patient also had occlusion of the pulmonary vascular bed with pulmonary hypertension, and died a few hours after injection (Williams, 1974b).

In addition to the deaths associated with macroaggregated albumin injection, a further nine deaths are reported using ferric hydroxide particles (Robinowitz et al, 1973; Williams, 1974a). Ferric hydroxide has been shown to give a high incidence of adverse reaction after intravenous administration, and for this reason has been largely abandoned as a vehicle for radioisotope lung perfusion imaging. In relation to the large number of perfusion scans that have been performed, the mortality is extremely low, and apart from those associated with idiosyncrasy to ferric hydroxide, fatalities have only occurred in patients with already severely compromised pulmonary circulations. In less seriously ill subjects, the injection of particles for perfusion scanning has no detectable effect on pulmonary mechanics or gas exchange (Gold and McCormack, 1966) and the procedure appears to be very safe.

A dose of between 200 and 400 mrad is given to the lung by 1 mCi of $^{99}Tc^m$ labelled macroaggregates. An injection of about 3 to 4 mCi is given per test (ICRP publication 17, 1971). Injection of xenon-133 gas dissolved in saline gives up to 20 mrad/mCi, and several millicuries may be required for a good quality scintillation camera image. The radiation dose for these procedures is approximately the same as for standard radiographic procedures.

Ventilation Procedures

Although the perfusion scan alone can give useful anatomical information about the distribution of pulmonary blood flow, it is of limited use in the investigation of regional lung function unless supplemented by some measurement of the regional distribution of ventilation. An immediate difficulty in measuring ventilation is to retain sufficient radioactivity in the lung during the period of the measurement. This is solved in one of two ways; the first involves inhalation of radioactively labelled aerosol particles which remain for long enough in the lung to be counted by a rectilinear scanner. The second technique requires inhalation, or injection, of a radioactive gas and measurement of its emission over a short period of time by a bank of fixed counters or by a scintillation camera.

Aerosol methods

Small aerosol particles of albumin labelled with radioactive iodine or technetium can be generated in an ultrasonic nebuliser, and are thought, if 1 μm or less in diameter, to penetrate to the alveoli and to be distributed according to relative regional ventilation (Pircher et al, 1967). However, a number of factors, which include local turbulence of airflow, excessive mucus, and clumping of the particles, may lead to their preferential deposition in larger airways (Despas et al, 1970), with failure to penetrate to the periphery. The scan may therefore give information about particle deposition rather than distribution of ventilation, and this can be demonstrated by comparing the aerosol pattern with inhaled radioactive gas in the same subject (Shibel, Landis and Moser, 1969). In general, areas of lack of penetration of aerosol particles correlate well topographically with regions of decreased ventilation assessed by radioactive gas, but there are important exceptions. Aerosols tend to exaggerate the severity of defects and may suggest a false impression of lack of function since collateral ventilation of lung distal to a bronchial stenosis can sometimes be demonstrated with radioactive gas, when missed with aerosols (Siegel and Potchen, 1973). Indeed, gas may fail to detect obstruction of a bronchus since, especially in adults, collateral ventilation may be surprisingly fast and allow normal gaseous exchange in the lung distal to the obstruction.

One advantage of the aerosol method is that particles remain in the lungs for several hours which enables scans from different aspects of the chest to be made, without increase in radiation dose. A specific use of aerosol scans, deriving from retention of deposited particles, is for the study of mechanisms of regional clearance. Most particles are removed in the bronchial mucus and the rate of clearance indicates the local efficiency of the 'mucus escalator', impairment of which may be clinically important in reducing the lung defences against infection. Despite this specific use, and the fact that it may be complementary to the gas method in assessing regional anatomy and physiology, the aerosol method is not widely used in clinical practice and its value in the investigation of local lung lesions has not yet been adequately studied (Lin, Burke and Silverstein, 1973).

Gas methods

The most widely used gas for ventilation measurements is xenon-133, which, with a half-life of 5.3 days, is convenient for distribution and storage. Xenon is physiologically and chemically inert, and being relatively insoluble is not removed from the alveolar gas by the circulation to any great extent. However, a certain amount of activity does enter solution if a rebreathing technique is used, and a significant background count from circulating xenon-133 in the chest wall and other tissues can build up. Fortunately, the extent of this build-up can be estimated from the radioactivity remaining after subsequent wash-out and an appropriate correction made to the total count to allow for the tissue background. More detailed methodology of inhaled gas techniques will be described under specific uses in later sections. Recently, alternative radioisotopes of xenon have been considered for lung function; of these xenon-127 seems to show the greatest promise (Goddard and Ackery, 1975), but at present is too expensive for routine use. Continuous inhalation of krypton-81m has recently been shown to give good functional images of regional ventilation (Fazio and Jones, 1975). The basis of the technique is that radioactive krypton does not reach equilibrium within poorly ventilated regions of the lung since radioactive decay takes place (physical half-life 13 s) before equilibration is attained. Regions of poor gas turnover therefore show as 'cold' regions in the image. The major limitation of this elegant technique for routine purposes is the short half-life (4.5 h) of rubidium-81, the parent radioisotope for krypton-81m.

In assessing regional lung function, the ventilatory component can potenti- ally give information about (a) regional lung volumes, (b) regional ventilation, (c) effects of gravity upon regional ventilation, (d) physiological control of regional ventilation, and (e) regional ventilation/perfusion relationships. In practice, absolute values for the latter are hard to obtain since they depend on complex calculations and assumptions, and relative values are more commonly used. The application of the techniques can be considered under the broad heading of (i) physiological and (ii) clinical, though there is con- siderable overlap between these two fields.

Physiological Studies of Ventilation

Total and regional lung volumes

Estimation of lung volume was one of the first uses of inhaled isotopes, and the method has been developed by Ball and co-workers in Montreal (Ball et al, 1962) and latterly by Matthys in Germany (Matthys et al, 1972). In essence the technique is similar to other gas dilution methods, the subjects rebreathing a known quantity of xenon-133 from a spirometer until equili- brium is achieved. By knowing the starting volume and concentration in the spirometer, and applying a correction for xenon-133 taken up by the circula- tion, it is possible to calculate the total lung volume at the start of rebreathing from the concentration at equilibrium. By starting from different lung volumes it is possible to measure, for instance, residual volume, functional residual capacity and total lung capacity, with good agreement compared to values obtained by helium dilution or by use of a body plethysmograph (Matthys et al, 1972). Non-radioactive methods are, however, preferred on grounds of safety and repeatability, and the primary reason for validating the radioactive method against these is to provide a basis for estimating relative regional lung volumes. If the lung volume corresponding to the total counts is known, the proportionate volume of smaller lung regions can be derived simply from the number of counts in that region. In fact, knowledge of regional lung volume at equilibrium has little direct application in itself and is used mainly as a constant with which to compare the 'effective regional volume' of the same area after a single breath of radioactive gas, in an attempt to quantify regional gas distribution and hence ventilation.

Normal regional ventilation

Variants of this technique have been developed and applied to a large extent by Bates, Dollfuss, Milic-Emili and others in the physiological field, whilst investigating the effect of gravity on regional ventilation (Ball et al, 1962; Dollfuss, Milic-Emili and Bates, 1967; Milic-Emili et al, 1966). In the upright posture, during breathing at normal lung volumes, the alveoli towards the lung bases are smaller than those near the apices, lie on a steeper part of their volume–pressure curve and, therefore, would be expected to inflate more during inspiration. During a single breath inhalation of xenon-133, inspiration is halted at intervals while regional counts are made and these can then be compared with the same regional counts at total lung capacity (TLC) to give the relative regional volume at each stopping point through inspiration. This simple ratio of regional counts at intermediate volumes to regional counts at TLC is then plotted against percentage of whole lung TLC to give a graph similar to that shown in stylised form in Figure 1 (Bake et al, 1967). If different parts of the lung expand evenly, all regions should follow the line of identity shown in Figure 1. In fact it can be seen that at all volumes below TLC, the apical alveoli are relatively over-expanded, whereas those at the bases are relatively small. At very low lung volumes, the proportional change in regional volume over a given increase in whole lung volume is steeper at the apices than at the bases, which indicates greater inflation of the upper zones at this point in lung volumes, but as inspiration proceeds the slope of the basal line becomes steeper, indicating that over most of the usual respiratory range (i.e. above functional residual capacity) basal alveoli change more in size than those at the apex. This implies that under these semistatic conditions, ventilation of the lung will increase from the apices down to the bases, and with a fairly normal slow breathing pattern it is likely that the same pattern of ventilation pertains. A number of workers using similar techniques have confirmed these results (Dollfuss et al, 1967; Newhouse et al, 1968) and in the upright posture there appears to be a 20 to 30 per cent increase in ventilation from apex to base. Although this is in the same direction as the vertical differences in pulmonary perfusion, it is comparatively much less and does little to offset gravity-dependent ventilation/perfusion imbalance.

A more direct approach to regional ventilation is the dynamic one of measuring gas wash-out after rebreathing xenon-133 to equilibrium. This overcomes the objection that semistatic regional gas distribution may not accurately reflect regional ventilation, and has the advantage of simplicity, which has commended it for clinical purposes. However, unless some separate means of measuring total ventilation is used, the wash-out technique gives only qualitative information and attempts to obtain some quantitative estimate involve either complex computation or rather arbitrary assumptions. Nevertheless, the results broadly confirm that at normal lung volumes in the upright posture under quiet breathing conditions, the lung bases are better ventilated than the apices (Miller, Ali and Howe, 1970).

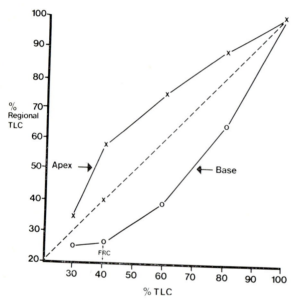

Figure 1 Stylised graph of regional expansion against total lung expansion (after Bake et al, 1967). At volumes above about functional residual capacity the relative expansion (and hence ventilation) of the bases is greater than that of the apices

The simplest approximate quantification of wash-out curves, and one which has been used quite widely in practice, is to regard them as a single exponential function and to use some point on this, for instance the $T_{\frac{1}{2}}$ (time to half wash-out) as an index of ventilation (MacIntyre et al, 1970; MacIntyre and Inkley, 1973). When this is done the pattern of increasing ventilation towards the lung bases is again apparent. By analogy with nitrogen wash-out curves, it has been suggested that a better guide to regional ventilation would be some index of 'turnover' that is to say of fall-off in radioactivity in relation to ventilation measured by other means, rather than in relation simply to time. One such index, which has been widely used in regional studies in patients with airways obstruction is derived from the formula:

$$\tilde{V} = 1/T_{\frac{1}{2}} \times \text{FRC}/\dot{V}_{\text{I}} \times 100$$

where $\dot{V}$ = 'regional ventilatory index'

$T_{\frac{1}{2}}$ = time to 50 per cent wash-out

FRC = functional residual capacity (approximate lung volume during quiet breathing)

$\dot{V}_I$ = inspired minute volume during wash-out

This method complicates the technique of measurement and is of limited clinical application though it is more 'physiological' than measurements simply of loss of activity against time.

Effect of gravity on regional ventilation

Although it is generally agreed that there is a vertical gradient of ventilation in the upright lung, the exact mechanism for this is uncertain. Some evidence points to inherent regional differences in lung elastic properties (Bake et al, 1967), while other workers claim that the regional differences in alveolar size can be explained entirely on the basis of a pleural pressure gradient which causes higher transpulmonary pressures at the apices than at the bases. In support of the latter possibility is the observation that the gradient can be reversed by inverting the subject, which suggests at least that gravitational effects on the lungs can outweigh inherent local lung elastic properties (Glaister, 1967; Clarke, Jones and Glaister, 1969). Effects of gravity on the lung are also thought to underly the currently popular concept of 'closing volume' which states that owing to the smaller transpulmonary pressure in the lower part of the chest there is less lung elastic recoil available to keep small airways in dependent parts of the lungs open on full expiration, so that the first gas inhaled during an inspiration from residual volume will tend to enter the upper lobes through their permanently patent bronchi. If, at residual volume, a bolus of marker gas is inhaled, followed by a chaser of air to total lung capacity, and the lungs are then slowly emptied again, the bolus should enter the upper lobes preferentially, and at the end of the following expiration will show a sharp increase in concentration as the lower lobe airways close off and no longer contribute diluting non-marker gas to the exhaled mixture (Fig. 2).

This pattern of exhaled marker concentration can be shown by measurement of radioactivity at the mouth after inhalation of a bolus of xenon-133. Other non-radioactive gases are now commonly used for clinical purposes since this permits the test to be repeated frequently; nevertheless the radioactive gas method had the important initial advantage of confirming that a bolus of gas taken in at residual volume actually ended up mainly in the upper lobes (Fig. 3). After rebreathing to equilibrium the gas distribution becomes uniform and proportional to lung volume, so that the ratio of counts after a single breath to counts after equilibration gives an index of the effects of gravity on the regional distribution of a bolus of gas taken in at low lung volume (Fig. 4).

Control of regional ventilation

Inhaled radioactive gases have also been used to investigate the effects of the pulmonary circulation on the distribution of ventilation. It has been found using physiological methods of measurement, that total unilateral pulmonary artery occlusion with a balloon catheter in either the left or right pulmonary artery causes, both in the dog and in man, an ipselateral increase in airflow resistance and slight decrease in lung compliance (Severinghaus et al, 1961; Swenson, Finley and Guzman, 1961). This has the effect of diverting ventilation to the opposite lung and thus reduces the amount of 'wasted ventilation', or increase in physiological dead space, that would

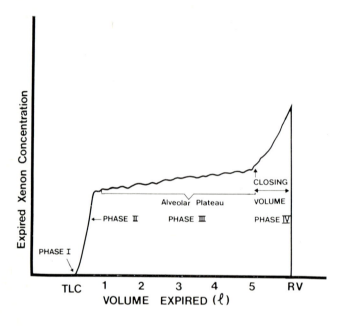

Figure 2 Xenon count-rates at the mouth during slow expiration after prior inhalation of a bolus of xenon-133 at residual volume, to show closing volume, or phase IV

otherwise follow unilateral vascular occlusion. These measurements involved not only right heart catheterisation, but also anaesthesia and differential bronchospirometry which might have interfered with the bronchial responses being studied, and other workers have used a radioactive aerosol instead. Although this is non-specific in terms of the precise physiological changes which cause redistribution of ventilation it has the great advantage of involving no mechanical interference with the tracheobronchial tree, and using it, a shift of ventilation away from the occluded side in dogs has been confirmed (Allgood et al, 1968). This response was still present after excision and re-implantation of the lung to interrupt nervous pathways and was prevented by ventilation of the occluded lung with 6 per cent CO_2, suggesting that it was due to a direct local action of hypocapnia. In addition to avoiding the need for intubation, radioactive methods allow the study of much smaller regions than can be achieved with bronchospirometry, which is limited to effects on a whole lung. As yet, rather little use has been made of radio-isotope techniques in this field though changes in regional ventilation and ventilation/perfusion ratios after inhalation of a bronchodilator aerosol have been reported, using radioactive xenon (Matthys et al, 1972).

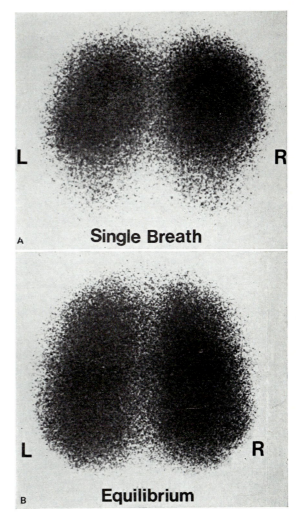

Figure 3 Distribution of inspired gas in normal erect subject: a bolus of xenon-133 was inhaled at residual volume followed by slow inspiration of air to total lung capacity, at which volume (3A) counts were made during breath-holding. The bolus gas is mainly in the upper zones, compared with more even distribution (3B) after re-breathing to equilibrium. (Reproduced by kind permission of Pitman Publishing)

Ventilation/Perfusion Ratios

The matching of ventilation and perfusion to ensure efficient gas exchange is an important property of the ideal lung, but in practice is impossible to achieve, largely because of the effects of gravity on the distribution of pulmonary blood flow, the consequences of which have been widely studied in both healthy and diseased lungs (West and Dollery, 1960; West, 1962; Milic-Emili et al, 1966; West, 1967). In normal subjects in the erect posture, the gradient of pulmonary perfusion leads to over-perfusion of the lung bases relative to their ventilation (low ventilation/perfusion ratio) and the reverse at the apices. The former causes a tendency to arterial hypoxaemia due to venous admixture or effective right-to-left 'shunting' of blood through the lung bases, while the latter leads to 'wasted ventilation' of poorly perfused alveoli, which is an inefficient use of ventilatory energy. The gradient of decreasing ventilation/perfusion ratios as one moves down from the lung apices has been estimated by a variety of physiological and radioactive methods (Martin and Young, 1957; West, 1963) and there is general agreement that these ratios range from more than two at the apices to less than

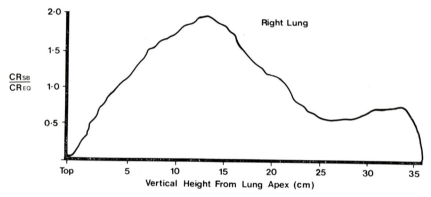

Figure 4 Distribution of inspired gas (data taken from Fig. 3): ratio of counts after single breath to counts at equilibrium down a sagittal slice of lung. This gives a more quantitative assessment of the preferential distribution of the bolus of gas to the upper zones in Figure 3. (Reproduced by kind permission of Pitman Publishing)

unity at the bases. Early radioisotope measurements involved the use of short-lived isotopes of normal respiratory gases, and it has proved difficult to obtain absolute values for ventilation/perfusion ratios using more convenient gases such as xenon-133. Separate measurements of ventilation and perfusion have been made during breath-holding at total lung capacity (Dollery and Gillam, 1963), but these are not very physiological conditions and may give a false impression of ventilation/perfusion relationships during normal tidal breathing (Hughes et al, 1968; Matthys et al, 1972). In an attempt to overcome this criticism, regional 'steady-state' ventilation/perfusion ratios have been measured by means of constant infusion of xenon and rebreathing of the same gas to equilibrium; in four normal subjects, the results were similar to those obtained by single breath methods, though there were some small unexplained discrepancies (Anthonisen, Dolovich and Bates, 1966). However, in another attempt to estimate regional ventilation/perfusion ratios under physiological conditions Inkley and MacIntyre (1973) measured wash-out of injected xenon-133 during normal tidal breathing after breath-holding at functional residual capacity. They also measured total ventilation directly and cardiac output by a radioisotope technique and somewhat surprisingly found no gradient of ventilation/perfusion ratios in the upright posture. Other workers, using similar dynamic techniques but no absolute measurements of ventilation or cardiac output, calculated regional ventilation/perfusion indices rather than true ratios and found a decrease from apex to base as with single breath methods, but the range of these indices during normal breathing was narrower than the range of ventilation/perfusion ratios at total lung capacity (Inkley and MacIntyre, 1973). The above techniques are rather laborious and the calculations are not only complex, but entail certain assumptions which makes them unsuitable for patients with any severity of local lung disease. Moreover, patients with lung disease may have ventilation/perfusion abnormalities which cause marked hypoxaemia but which cannot be demonstrated at a regional level because they are too diffuse, and beyond the spatial resolution of present radioisotope techniques (Anthonisen et al, 1968).

Although these difficulties severely limit the application of measurements of absolute ventilation/perfusion ratios to disease states, a number of simpler relative indices have been developed, which do at least allow comparison of one lung region with another. These indices are based on the injection of dissolved xenon-133 which when released on reaching air-filled alveoli gives a measure of relative regional perfusion: subsequent wash-out of this gas by ventilation yields relative regional ventilation indices, which are then combined with the perfusion findings to obtain an estimate of the regional ventilation/perfusion ratio relative either to other regions or to the whole lung. These techniques involve some simplifying assumption about the pattern of wash-out, and the usual one is that at least over the first 60 per cent (MacIntyre and Inkley, 1973), wash-out can be described by a single exponential function of the form:

$$Q_t = Q_0 e^{-\lambda t}$$

where Q_t = count-rate at time t after start of wash-out

Q_0 = original count-rate

λ = turnover or clearance constant, analogous to regional minute ventilation divided by resting lung volume (cf. 'ventilation index', p. 10).

The entire measurement can be made during tidal breathing, thus avoiding the problem of subject cooperation in breath-holding (Heckscher, Larsen and Lassen, 1966) and the technique has recently been extended to the study of regional lung function in infants and children, using nitrogen-13 (Godfrey et al, 1975). These methods give valuable information about regional relative ventilation/perfusion ratios and being relatively easy to apply, are finding increasing clinical use, but it must be emphasised that they do not measure absolute ventilation/perfusion ratios in the physiological sense.

CLINICAL STUDIES

The Normal Perfusion Image

With the thorax in the upright position blood flow within the pulmonary circulation shows a gradient down the lung, with relatively less perfusion

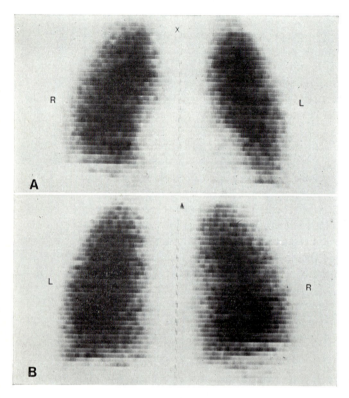

Figure 5   Normal distribution of perfusion measured by a rectilinear scanner. (A) Anterior and (B) posterior views

per unit lung volume in the upper zones, and greater in the lower (West and Dollery, 1960). A more even distribution of flow is obtained with the patient supine, and this position is preferred if pathological changes of blood flow are to be observed in all parts of the lung. For this reason radioactive microspheres or xenon injections are usually administered with the patient supine. Measurement of the normal perfusion pattern by a rectilinear scanner is shown in Figure 5.

Allowing for some line to line variation due to technical factors, the borders of the image should appear well defined and convex, although diaphragmatic movement gives an irregular appearance to the lower borders. The anterior scan shows clearly the cardiac borders, which may give poor definition of the lower zone of the left lung, particularly if the heart is enlarged. In the posterior view the lungs appear symmetrical, with straight and parallel medial borders. The cardiac impression is often seen as a region of low count rate at the medial lower zone of the left lung. Mediastinal or hilar enlargement appears as a concave impression at the medial border of either lung image. The lateral views are particularly important since they can show the segmental pattern of perfusion impairment.

Both lateral views should have a roughly triangular appearance (Fig. 6), with smooth borders. The inferior anterior surface on the left may show a reduced count-rate due to the left ventricle, which may give difficulties in

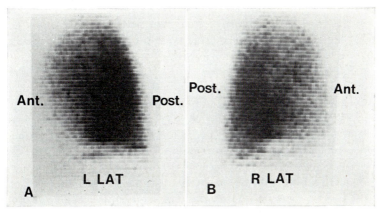

Figure 6 Normal distribution of perfusion measured by a rectilinear scanner. (A) Left lateral and (B) right lateral views

interpreting perfusion losses in the lingula. Although perfusion should be fairly uniform throughout the image, quite often the lower lobe can be distinguished as a region of increased activity. In obese patients, or when the breasts are large, the anterior or posterior images show rounded lateral contours at the base due to increased attenuation of low energy photons. The count-rate given by the 140 keV photons of $^{99}Tc^m$ is reduced to half by 5 cm of tissue. Similarly fluid in the pleural cavity can attenuate the radiation and give a misleading impression of reduced perfusion in the underlying lung.

It is important that albumin microspheres or macroaggregates are well shaken before intravenous administration. If not, there is a risk of injecting larger aggregates, which may give localised regions of very high count-rate in the lungs, and show as 'hot spots' in the image. This gives a misleading image, which is difficult to interpret clinically. It has been shown however (Harding et al, 1973) that a single large particle of albumin in fact blocks less of the pulmonary capillary circulation than the same mass of albumin divided into smaller particles.

Pulmonary Embolism

An important role for lung imaging is in the diagnosis of pulmonary thromboembolism, and in the study of its response to therapy (Johnson, 1971). The condition is difficult to diagnose clinically, and most diagnostic aids are non-specific, and although electrocardiographic changes or serum enzyme measurements may be suggestive, the results can be misleading. Chest radiographic signs which increase the probability of diagnosis are an elevated diaphragm, pleural effusion, or pulmonary infiltration; but quite often the radiograph is normal. Pulmonary angiography will show the anatomy of the vascular bed, but this is a complex procedure with some morbidity, and it may not show up the smaller vessels of the pulmonary tree. Radio-isotope imaging of the pulmonary circulation pattern on the other hand is convenient and lacks significant morbidity, and repeated investigation allows the progress of the patient to be followed.

The radioactive particle technique is best used for this purpose. Particles are trapped on first transit in the capillary bed, and remain in situ for several hours, so that distribution images of blood flow can be made from anterior, posterior and lateral views of the chest without repeating the injection. Injection of the patient in the supine position lessens the normal pulmonary perfusion gradient in the lung due to gravity, and thus facilitates the recognition of perfusion losses in the upper lobes. The injection is given over several cycles of quiet tidal breathing, and the subsequent distribution of activity within the lung is measured by scanning or scintillation camera imaging.

The functional image in pulmonary embolism

The lung image is a measurement of pulmonary arterial blood flow, and it is the effect of an embolus on that flow pattern that is seen in the image. The embolus itself is not detected. With modern equipment perfusion losses of only greater than about 2 cm in diameter can be detected.

The clearest evidence of pulmonary embolism in the radioisotope image is loss of perfusion which shows a lobar or segmental distribution. Other causes for segmental infiltration must be excluded by the chest radiograph, but if this is normal or shows signs suggesting embolism, then a segmental loss in the image is likely to be due to thromboembolism. The segmental anatomy of the lung is best displayed by the lateral views, which should be taken whenever possible. In the anterior or posterior views segmental losses show as regions of low count-rate in the upper or lower zones, or, if the loss is in the mid-zone, as a concave defect in the lateral and medial borders of the image.

Other diseases, for example chronic obstructive airways disease (see p. 27), may also show perfusion abnormalities in the image when the x-ray is normal, and it is not uncommon for middle-aged heavy smokers to show patchy perfusion losses with a normal radiograph. These losses in blood flow in patients with chronic parenchymal lung disease are seldom segmental. Nevertheless, they may present a difficulty when scanning is used to confirm

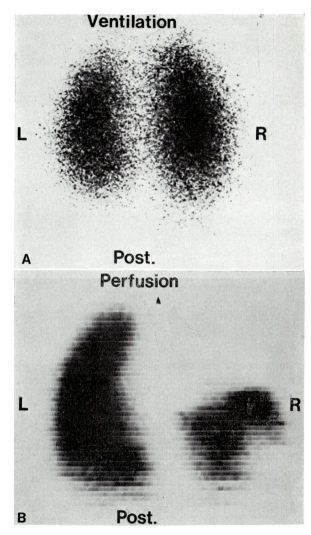

Figure 7 Pulmonary embolism. (A) Distribution of single inspiration of xenon-133 measured with a scintillation camera shows ventilation to be unaffected. (B) Microsphere study with a rectilinear scanner shows considerable perfusion loss in the right lung

a presumptive diagnosis of pulmonary embolism in the presence of pre-existing chronic lung disease. It has been suggested that pulmonary angiography may be necessary in this situation (Poulose et al, 1970).

It has been reported (Medina et al, 1969; De Nardo et al, 1970; Moser et al, 1971) that the regional ventilation is unaffected in those parts of the lung which show interruption of blood flow due to pulmonary embolism, whereas most parenchymal lung disease affects the regional ventilation and perfusion equally. The combination of a ventilation investigation can assist in interpretation of the perfusion image, particularly when this shows defects which are not clearly segmental. However, the place of the combined study in the investigation of pulmonary embolism is still not fully established, and

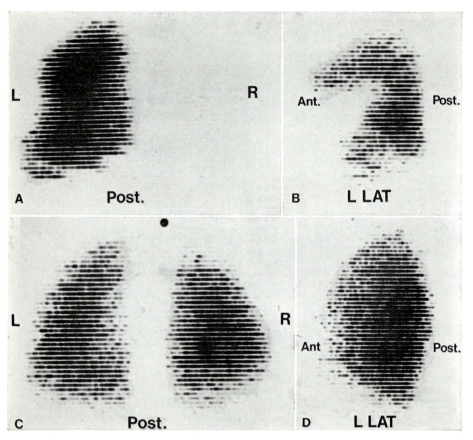

Figure 8   Pulmonary embolism: a young female postoperative patient. (A) Posterior recti-linear scan shows almost absent perfusion in right lung, and lateral edge defect in left lung. (B) Left lateral view shows lingular defect. (C) and (D). Restoration of blood flow one week later after thrombolytic therapy

at the present time it is not certain that the ventilation study can assist much in the difficult diagnostic situation of a patient with suspected pulmonary embolism who has poor lung perfusion due to pre-existing lung disease, pulmonary venous hypertension, or cardiac failure. Furthermore, not all patients who have regional perfusion losses due to embolism necessarily show normal ventilation in the affected regions (Kessler and McNeil, 1975).

An example of a patient with perfusion defects due to pulmonary embolism is shown in Figure 7. The radiograph was normal. Poorly perfused regions in the right lung are ventilated normally.

FOLLOW-UP OF PULMONARY EMBOLISM

One advantage of using radioisotope imaging methods in the study of thromboembolism is that the procedure may be repeated at regular intervals to monitor the course of the disease and its response to treatment. It is not always easy to obtain a technically identical result each time the patient is scanned, and for this reason quantification of the image (see p. 5) is useful. As long as changes are taking place in one lung alone, the changes in the relative blood flow to that lung can be used to confirm the impression gained from examination of the image.

Studies of the natural history of pulmonary thromboembolism suggest that blood flow is restored to the affected region in about one-third of patients within a week or so (Secker Walker, Jackson and Goodwin, 1970). Patients in the older age groups, or those with associated cardiac disease, have less likelihood of restoration to normal perfusion (Winebright, Gerdes and Nelp, 1970). Dramatic response to thrombolytic therapy can sometimes be seen after major embolic episodes, as shown in Figure 8. This young female patient had almost total loss of perfusion throughout the right lung, and also loss in the lingula on the left. Within 10 days of commencement of therapy the perfusion was normal.

Pulmonary Venous Hypertension

Pulmonary blood flow has been shown to decrease from the base to the apex of the lung in upright healthy subjects, but in patients with raised pulmonary venous pressure apical flow exceeds that at the base, so that a reversal of the normal gradient is seen (Fig. 9). It has been suggested (Hughes et al, 1969) that the relative increase in apical blood flow in these patients is related to increased perfusion pressures in that region of the pulmonary capillary bed, which are able to overcome the alveolar gas pressure, the controlling factor in blood flow in the apical region of the normal lung. The decrease in basal blood flow with raised pulmonary venous pressure is probably caused by increased pressure in the perivascular sheaths surrounding vessels due to interstitial oedema (West, Dollery and Heard, 1965). In patients with chronic pulmonary venous hypertension, for instance from long-standing mitral valve disease, increases in pulmonary blood flow to the apex relative to the base may persist after administration of acetylcholine, suggesting that after a time the reversed perfusion gradient becomes fixed, due to histological changes which supervene as a response to the prolonged rise in interstitial pressure (Glazier, Dollery and Hughes, 1968).

A number of authors have attempted to make use of the altered pulmonary blood flow gradient to predict the rise in pulmonary venous pressure. A simple method for obtaining a quantitative index from the scanner or scintillation camera is to divide the radioisotope image into upper and lower zones in the anterior and posterior views. The integrated counts in each zone are quantified, and upper–lower zone ratios determined. By this technique good correlation has been shown between zonal distribution of macroaggregated

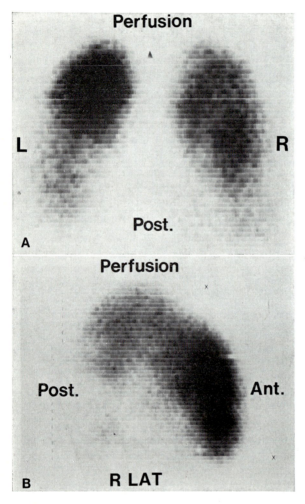

Figure 9 Pulmonary venous hypertension: male patient with mitral stenosis. (A) Posterior scan shows relative increase in blood flow to upper zones. (B) Right lateral view shows relative increase in blood flow to anterior regions of lungs (patient injected supine)

albumin injected with the patient in the upright position and mean left atrial pressure (Friedman and Braunwald, 1966). Although the technique estimates pulmonary hypertension pressures only indirectly it has the advantage of being simple and atraumatic and has been used in situations when repeated cardiac catheterisation was not justified, for instance following postoperative cardiac valve replacement (Krishnamurthy, Srinivasan and Blahd, 1972).

Carcinoma of Bronchus

There have been numerous reports showing the effect of bronchial carcinoma on regional blood-flow and ventilation when these are studied by radioactive methods. A review of the subject has been published recently (Fletcher, James and Holman, 1973). Although much interesting and sometimes useful information has been obtained, the place of these techniques in the investigation of patients with carcinoma is not yet clearly established. From a purely diagnostic point of view the perfusion scan is of limited value because it is non-specific and the size of the defect bears a variable relation to the radiological findings. In general, centrally placed tumours produce perfusion defects larger than expected from the x-ray and the radioactive method is therefore a sensitive indication of disease in such cases, and may suggest the presence of a lesion not clearly demonstrable radiologically (Fraser et al, 1970). On the other hand, up to 50 per cent of peripheral lesions may be missed by the perfusion scan basically because of the limited resolution of the technique (Maynard and Cowan, 1971).

Perfusion studies

There are several potential mechanisms by which carcinoma could lead to perfusion defects but pathological studies suggest that the most important is direct involvement of large pulmonary vessels. It is probably for this reason that relatively small central tumours may be associated with large perfusion defects, but it has also been suggested that local obstructive emphysema, due to incomplete bronchial occlusion, may lead to mechanical obstruction of part of the pulmonary circulation, or that local hypoxia due to underventilation may lead to local chemical pulmonary vasoconstriction, though no positive evidence exists to support these suggestions.

Despite the shortcomings of other methods such as bronchoscopy, sputum cytology and scalene node biopsy, which when combined give a pathological diagnosis in about 75 per cent of cases of carcinoma (Meyer and Umiker, 1961), standard perfusion scanning does not seem to add to diagnostic accuracy. This is mainly due to the non-specificity of perfusion defects which do not distinguish between benign and malignant tumours, inflammatory lesions (Secker Walker et al, 1971), or losses due to chronic airways obstruction which are commonly present in patients with carcinoma of the bronchus.

A more important potential use of the perfusion scan is in determining the extent and operability of a known carcinoma. A fairly good correlation has been reported between the degree of perfusion loss and the resectability of the tumour, and in general when more than two-thirds of the lung shows absent or diminished perfusion the tumour is inoperable (Secker Walker et al, 1971). The chances of resectability improve with decreasing perfusion loss so that when perfusion of the diseased lung relative to that for both lungs is 34 to 40 per cent, lobectomy is usually possible, and that when relative

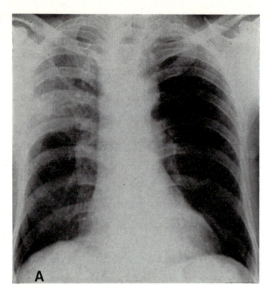

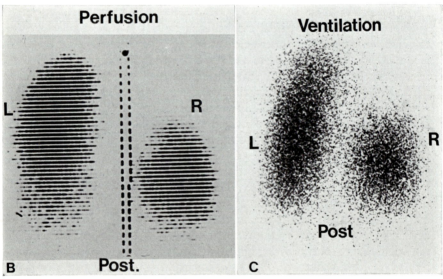

Figure 10   Bronchial carcinoma. (A) Chest radiograph shows lesion in right upper zone. (B) Perfusion and (C) ventilation are reduced in this region

perfusion is greater than 40 per cent pneumonectomy is possible. However, there are exceptions to all these findings and while the extent of perfusion loss may be a guide to resectability and help to influence the decision, it cannot be relied on alone to indicate whether a particular lesion is resectable.

In addition to studies of the affected lung which may suggest inoperability for technical reasons through involvement of major pulmonary vessels, perfusion scans may be useful in assessing the circulation to the opposite lung. This is important where major resection is proposed, in the presence of impaired overall lung function. In these circumstances operation would be undertaken more readily if the major perfusion defects were limited to the side of the tumour rather than involving both lungs. At present, such assessments are essentially subjective, but it is possible that more exact quantitative predictions of the postoperative reduction in the gas exchange function of the lungs will be achieved in the future. Already, the information gained from the scan may, when combined with tests of overall lung function, allow somewhat greater precision in the selection of patients fit for resection.

Combined ventilation and perfusion studies

Most emphasis has been given to the changes in perfusion associated with bronchial carcinoma, because perfusion scans are the most widely available, but a number of studies have also been made of regional ventilation (Fig. 10). In general, the distribution of decreased ventilation correlates well with bronchial invasion or occlusion by tumour, and may be evident before atelectasis makes radiographic localisation possible. In the early stages local ventilation may be reduced before perfusion, but the latter usually shows greater impairment in the long run and has been found to be more accurate in the preoperative assessment of resectability and in the prediction of survival (Svanberg, 1972). In a small proportion of patients vascular obstruction may precede occlusion of the airway by the tumour, and this results in the affected region of the lung showing an increase in the ventilation/perfusion ratio, more typically seen in pulmonary embolism (Grant and Ackery, 1975). Regional ventilation studies may reveal defects not suspected clinically or radiologically and may therefore help in predicting the function of the remaining lung after operation. As with perfusion scans, the ventilatory findings have not yet been placed on a quantitative basis and their predictive value is therefore limited.

Gallium-67

A very different use of radioisotopes in investigation of bronchial carcinoma involves the injection of the relatively long-lived isotope gallium-67 which is taken up by actively metabolising and dividing cells. If the lung is scanned 2 or 3 days later, after the clearance of normal tissue activity, cellular lesions which have taken up the isotope appear as regions of increased activity (Fig. 11). Studies have shown increased uptake of gallium in over 90 per cent of carcinomas (Langhammer et al, 1972). It was hoped that gallium concentration might prove specific for tumour localisation, but unfortunately positive uptake is found also in tuberculosis, sarcoidosis and other inflammatory conditions, and some tumours do not concentrate gallium (le Roux and Houlder, 1974). Although this has limited the diagnostic value of the investigation, it remains useful for detecting mediastinal tumours and lymph nodes

2

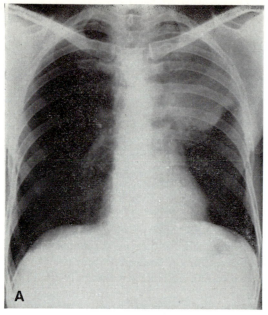

A

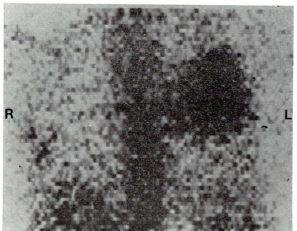

Ant.

Figure 11 Bronchial carcinoma. (A) Chest radio-
graph shows tumour in
left upper zone. (B) Gal-
lium-67: posterior recti-
linear scan shows marked
uptake of activity in
tumour. Mediastinal and
liver activity levels are
normal

which are radiologically invisible. It may also be helpful in assessing the
extent of neoplastic spread to the mediastinum, and thus avoid unnecessary
thoracic surgery. Gallium-67 is the best available tumour localising radio-
pharmaceutical, but its limited specificity, and its rather high cost, means
that it has little value in routine investigation. Its exact place in the investigation of bronchial carcinoma is yet to be determined.

Airways Obstruction

Asthma

The lung perfusion scan in asthma commonly shows patchy defects which may give the lung periphery a scalloped appearance or may closely resemble the segmental losses seen in pulmonary embolism. Ventilation techniques have proved useful in differentiating between the two conditions since in asthma there are usually regional ventilation defects which are more severe than those of perfusion in the same region (Wilson et al, 1970), and which consequently show local areas of low ventilation/perfusion ratio (Bentivoglio et al, 1963). As expected in such a variable condition as asthma, the pattern of abnormalities changes from time to time and the defects normally become more marked with increasing severity of bronchoconstriction (Heckscher et al, 1968). Some abnormalities, particularly those of ventilation, may however persist during periods when the patient is symptom free, and there has been recent interest in the use of radioisotope techniques as a sensitive way to detect lung dysfunction in the absence of radiological or physiological abnormalities (Alderson, Secker Walker and Forrest, 1974). In a study of 40 asthmatic subjects (Evans, 1974) it was found that 28 patients with symptoms had scattered abnormalities of ventilation and perfusion, shown as uniform retention of injected xenon-133 and this was interpreted as indicating either large airway obstruction or widespread peripheral airway narrowing. In 12 symptom-free subjects, retention of xenon was confined to the lower zones, implying peripheral airway narrowing chiefly in dependent parts of the lung. These particular patients had normal lung volumes and ventilatory capacities, so it appears that the radioactive xenon technique can detect minor degrees of regional impairment of function when conventional tests give normal results. That these changes in fact represent small airway disease is open to question, but the results do suggest that the technique could be added to other pulmonary function tests in assessing asthmatic subjects. In this study the methods used to assess overall lung function were not described in detail, and this is clearly of crucial importance if the relative sensitivity of different techniques is to be established. In another more detailed study of 10 symptom-free asthmatics (Heckscher et al, 1968) all were shown to have regional abnormalities of ventilation at a time when in only seven the FEV was reduced to below 70 per cent of predicted, but all 10 had reduction of maximum mid-expiratory flow rate to less than this level. It seems from these findings that radioactive methods add little to the sensitivity of mechanical tests for detecting minor abnormalities, but do give regional information which shows the distribution of abnormal lung function. Their application in the study of asthma has been largely experimental but the more frequent use, particularly of ventilation techniques, has already had the benefit of inducing greater caution in the interpretation of simple perfusion scans in cases of suspected pulmonary embolism.

Chronic bronchitis

One of the main problems in patients with chronic airways obstruction remains that of detecting early pathological changes. These are thought to occur chiefly in the small (less than 2 mm diameter) airways, which contribute less than 20 per cent of the total resistance to airflow in the normal lung, and therefore need to be severely diseased before tests of overall airway function, such as forced respiratory flow rates and airways resistance, show impairment (Hogg, Macklem and Thurlbeck, 1968). A number of studies of regional function in chronic bronchitis have been reported (Pain et al, 1967), which show beyond doubt that radioactive methods are more sensitive than standard radiology in detecting regional abnormalities (Alderson et al, 1974). It is well recognised, though, that the x-ray is a poor guide to function, and even relatively simple functional tests of lung mechanics such as the maximum mid-expiratory flow rate, thought to be more sensitive than the timed forced expiratory volume to narrowing of small airways, are usually abnormal by the time that regional reduction in ventilation is detected by the radioactive xenon-133 technique. In a detailed study of bronchitic patients from Montreal (Anthonisen et al, 1968), at least one aspect of lung mechanics was abnormal in all of 10 subjects, although some had only mild impairment of forced expiratory flow rates. Carbon monoxide extraction ratios were normal suggesting an absence of significant structural emphysema, and yet all 10 subjects showed abnormalities of regional ventilation, the lung bases being the worst affected. Xenon-133 was given both by inhalation and by intravenous injection, and local ventilation indices calculated from the half-time of wash-out and turnover of gas. Often the local ventilation index was seen to be lower after intravenous rather than inhaled xenon, indicating that intraregional areas of lower ventilation/perfusion ratios were present, in which gas was evolved from blood to alveolae, but not subsequently cleared from the lungs. These areas did not equilibrate during rebreathing of inhaled xenon and therefore contributed less to the wash-out gas than when the xenon was given by injection. Such intraregional inhomogeneity was not seen in asthmatic subjects (Heckscher et al, 1968) and could account for the greater impairment of gas exchange with relatively mild mechanical abnormalities in the bronchitics.

Although radioactive ventilation methods have thus given some further insight into regional and subregional function in chronic bronchitis, their use has remained largely experimental. They do not add greatly to the sensitivity of established mechanical tests in detecting mild functional defects, and the demonstration of the exact distribution of ventilatory defects has no therapeutic value at present.

Emphysema

GENERALISED

There has been relatively little experimental work on the effects of this condition on regional perfusion and ventilation, partly because of the difficulty of diagnosing generalised emphysema accurately during life. The observations that have been made confirm the expected patchy abnormalities, with ventilation generally being more affected than perfusion, though the defects usually correspond spatially (Bentivoglio et al, 1963; Lopez-Majano, Tow and Wagner, 1966). There may also be intraregional inhomogeneity below the resolution of the counters, but detected, as in chronic bronchitis, by the different wash-out time constants for inhaled and injected xenon-133 respectively. These findings are non-specific in terms of pathology, but may be useful in confirming local reduction in function in mild cases with little impairment of overall lung mechanics (Nairn, Prime and Simon, 1969).

LOCAL BULLOUS

Radioactive techniques are more applicable in this form of emphysema than in the generalised form, giving valuable information not only about the severity and extent of the local lesion, but also about the function of the remainder of the lungs, which may be of great importance if surgery is being considered. Prediction of the functional outcome of bullectomy is well known to be difficult (Pride et al, 1970), and a number of attempts have been made to assess the likely value of local lung resection by preoperative perfusion and ventilation studies. The results indicate that there is still some doubt as to the value of the techniques even in this situation. One drawback is that the usual posterior ventilation image gives topographical rather than anatomical information, which is of limited assistance to the surgeon. This limitation might be overcome by studying ventilation from the lateral aspect of the chest, but this would generally need to be done from both sides, entailing twice the radiation dose. It has been shown that xenon-133 measurements using a profile scanning probe add little to the information that can be gained by inspiratory and expiratory radiographs and tomography (Barter et al, 1973). However, experience with a scintillation camera suggests that isotope methods often reveal clinically unsuspected regions of impaired function and should be taken into account when deciding how much lung to resect (Macleod, personal communication). One useful feature in predicting a good response to surgery is the presence of compressed lung around the margin of a bullous area, and the perfusion scan has been claimed to be of considerable help in determining whether such compressed lung is well perfused and likely to function well when able to re-expand (Foreman et al, 1968; Lopez-Majano et al, 1969), but these patients commonly have a degree of generalised as well as localised emphysema and quantitative assessment of local function remains impossible in most cases. However, even qualitative results may be helpful in these circumstances and although the predictive value of perfusion and ventilation studies has yet to be proven, they undoubtedly yield some interesting preoperative information which could not be obtained by other means.

ALPHA$_1$-ANTITRYPSIN DEFICIENCY

Homozygous subjects for alpha$_1$-antitrypsin deficiency may show symptoms and signs of chronic obstructive airways disease, typically with preferential involvement of the lung bases by pan-acinar emphysema. Increase in chronic obstructive airways disease may also be more common in the heterozygous state (which occurs fairly commonly in the general population) but the severity of pulmonary symptoms is usually less than for the homozygote.

Studies in both homozygotes and heterozygotes suggest that radioisotope measurements of regional lung function are sensitive in detecting early signs of airways disease in this condition. Levine et al (1960) carried out perfusion and ventilation measurements with xenon-133 and scintillation probe detectors in seven homozygotes of various ages. Five of these displayed an altered distribution of pulmonary perfusion between the base and apex of the lung; one subject was aged 14 and had normal pulmonary physiology test results.

In another study xenon-133 and iodine-131 macroaggregated albumin were used with a scintillation camera to investigate 50 subjects with alpha$_1$-antitrypsin deficiency (Fallat et al, 1973). These subjects were compared with normal individuals or those with chronic obstructive disease who were not deficient for alpha$_1$-antitrypsin. The criteria used were delayed clearance of radioxenon from the lungs, or heterogeneity of pulmonary blood flow seen in the perfusion study. Retention of xenon at the lung bases was seen in seven out of nine homozygotes and seven out of eleven heterozygotes aged 34 years or over. The authors emphasise that none of the heterozygotes had previously suspected lung disease, and often spirometric measurements were normal. Patchy perfusion losses were also observed, and it was concluded that the radioisotope studies were a highly sensitive test of early pulmonary ventilatory dysfunction in patients with this condition.

Miscellaneous Conditions

Inflammation and infiltration

Surprisingly little use has been made of radioactive isotopes in investigation of inflammatory lung conditions, perhaps because these have been thought to be adequately delineated radiologically. Scattered cases of pneumonic consolidation have been studied and the scans usually show perfusion and ventilation defects corresponding topographically with areas of shadowing on the x-ray. The loss of perfusion can lead to confusion between infection and infarction, particularly since even in the latter condition local ventilation may be decreased in the presence of radiologically demonstrable lung damage. Angiography generally shows that in pneumonia the vessels are anatomically patent, which may give a false functional appearance, since presumably in vivo perfusion of the affected areas is reduced, in view of the perfusion scan defects. These findings emphasise the need for caution in interpreting perfusion scans, and in particular it should be realised that if there are radiological abnormalities, then there are likely to be corresponding perfusion defects, irrespective of the underlying pathology, and that such defects do not necessarily imply any structural abnormality of the pulmonary vessels. In tuberculosis, as in other lung infections, the perfusion scan may show marked defects, which are commonly more extensive than the x-ray would suggest.

Infiltrative lung diseases such as sarcoidosis and fibrosing alveolitis do not show any specific pattern of abnormality on the lung scan. With hilar lympha-denopathy, local defects corresponding to the enlarged nodes are seen, and there may also be patchy defects in perfusion in the lung fields when the x-ray is normal. With radiologically visible lung shadows, the scan commonly shows patchy perfusion defects, but it may appear normal in the presence of diffuse infiltration, since the ventilation/perfusion abnormalities demonstrated physiologically in this situation are often below the resolution of present radioactive techniques.

Hepatic cirrhosis

Arterial oxygen saturation is not uncommonly reduced in hepatic cirrhosis and this cannot be explained on the grounds of a shift of the oxygen–haemo-globin dissociation curve or by hypoventilation. Arteriovenous anastomoses such as pleural spider naevi may partially account for the desaturation, but ventilation/perfusion imbalance must also contribute significantly, since the hypoxaemia can be significantly reduced by the inhalation of high concentra-tions of oxygen (Mellemgaard et al, 1963). Radioisotope studies have shown that the main abnormality occurs in the lower regions of the lungs, which have low ventilation/perfusion ratios, and hence are a source of venous admixture (Ruff et al, 1971). The use of radioactive xenon has demonstrated that in these parts the regional residual volume to total lung capacity ratio is increased and may be greater than that near the apex of the lung, which is the reverse of the normal situation. The mechanism of this over-inflation and relative under-ventilation of the lower zones is probably premature closure of small airways during expiration, since closing volume, also measured with xenon-133, has been shown to be increased (Ruff et al, 1971), and in most of the subjects studied, exceeded functional residual capacity. This interesting work is an outstanding example of the combined experimental and clinical application of radioactive xenon to the solution of an important clinical problem, which again could not have been achieved by other methods.

Obesity

There has been considerable interest in the effects of obesity on lung mechanics and gas exchange since the original description of the 'Pick-wickian syndrome' of extreme obesity, hypoventilation and hypoxaemia (Burwell et al, 1956). One mechanical effect is a reduction in the expiratory reserve volume (ERV) so that the subject breathes at a lower lung volume than normal; the possibility that this might result in reduced ventilation of the lung bases with a low ventilation/perfusion ratio and hence hypoxaemia has been investigated in Montreal (Holley et al, 1967). In a group of 12 obese subjects, eight with a moderate decrease in ERV had fairly normal vertical distributions of perfusion and ventilation, but four others, with a more severe reduction in ERV to less than 0.4 litres, showed reversal of the normal gravitational gradient of ventilation. This leads to abnormally low ventilation/perfusion ratios at the lung bases with consequent hypoxaemia. In fact, the hypoxaemia in the subjects described was not severe, but this mechanism could explain the finding that patients with Pickwickian syndrome sometimes have hypoxaemia disproportionate to the severity of their hypoventilation.

Old age

With increasing age there is a gradual fall in arterial oxygen levels without any rise in carbon dioxide tension, and this takes place without marked change in lung mechanics apart from slight reduction in lung elastic recoil. The cause of this hypoxaemia appears to be ventilation/perfusion imbalance, since it can be corrected by inhalation of oxygen-rich gas mixtures. The site and mechanism of these regions of low ventilation/perfusion ratio have been investigated in six men between the ages of 65 and 70, using radioactive xenon by inhalation and injection (Holland et al, 1968). It was found that the normal vertical gradient of perfusion was only slightly less than that found in younger subjects, and that the vertical distribution of ventilation, in favour of the lung bases, was maintained during vital capacity manoeuvres. However, during tidal breathing at normal lung volumes, the gradient of ventilation was reversed, leading to regions of low ventilation/perfusion ratio at the lung bases. A similar effect is seen in younger subjects only when they breathe at a lung volume below FRC and has been attributed to airway closure during expiration at these low lung volumes. In elderly subjects closing volume (i.e. the volume above RV at which airways close during expiration) has been shown often to exceed FRC and hence will affect the normal tidal volume range, and this has been suggested as the mechanism for the low basal ventilation/perfusion ratios and tendency to hypoxaemia in old age.

Unilateral transradiancy of the lung

There are many causes for the radiographic appearance of unilateral transradiancy of the thorax but one of the more specific is that associated with diffuse obstruction of small bronchi in childhood, possibly due to infection, (Swyer and James, 1953; Macleod, 1954; Reid et al, 1967). This syndrome is characterised by a normal-sized or small lung with deficient vascular markings on the affected side on inspiration, and evidence of air trapping, leading to deviation of the mediastinum to the opposite side, on expiration. Overall lung mechanics may be little affected, but radioisotope investigations confirm the clinical and radiographic impressions of reduced ventilation and perfusion on the affected side, and it has been suggested that the pattern of radioactive gas trapping on ventilatory wash-out is more peripheral than that seen in obstruction of a main bronchus (Mishkin and Brashear, 1971).

Summary

From the 18 years' experience that has been gained from study of lung function with radioisotopes, it may be concluded that these measurements permit sensitive detection of impaired regional ventilation and perfusion, often when other investigations are normal. The procedures are simple and carry a minimal risk to the patient. They are therefore best used before proceeding to more complex investigation. Nevertheless, radioisotope imaging equipment and radiopharmaceuticals are costly, and it is seldom justified to employ them in studying total lung function when less expensive physiological testing can provide an adequate assessment for clinical purposes.

The pulmonary arterial blood flow study is of greatest value for the diagnosis and follow-up investigation of pulmonary embolism, since it has more sensitivity than conventional diagnostic procedures. It is particularly useful for the investigation of unexplained breathlessness in patients up to middle-age, when the relatively normal blood flow pattern allows embolic losses to be detected easily. In older patients the interpretation may be more difficult since impairment of pulmonary blood flow due to other causes is shown by the technique, and patchy perfusion losses due to chronic bronchitis or heart disease may obscure evidence of underlying pulmonary embolism. Results in such patients should be judged with prudence.

The role of radioisotope measurements in preoperative thoracic surgery is less certain. Although an assessment of regional function can be of value prior to thoracotomy, the precise benefit to a particular patient is difficult to quantify, and further study is required.

Similarly, in chronic airways disease the regional radioisotope study has provided interesting, rather than directly beneficial information. It may act as a reminder that an asthmatic patient in clinical remission still retains a considerable amount of regional dysfunction; it may assist in the detection of early airways disease; and it may help in the management of patients with chronic obstructive lung disease. Each of these aspects needs further examination before the place of radioisotope procedures can be established with certainty.

REFERENCES

General Reading and Reviews

Freeman, L. M. & Blaufox, M. D. (1973) Radionuclide studies of the lung. *Seminars in Nuclear Medicine*, **1**, 1–515.

Gilson, A. J. & Smoak, W. M. (1970) *Pulmonary Investigation with Radionuclides.* Springfield, Illinois: Thomas.

Holman, B. L. & Lindeman, J. F. (1973) *Progress in Nuclear Medicine*, **3**. Basel: Kargel.

Mishkin, F. S. & Brashear, R. E. (1971) *Use and Interpretation of the Lung Scan.* Springfield, Illinois: Thomas.

Wagner, H. N. (1968) *Principles of Nuclear Medicine.* Philadelphia: Saunders.

West, J. B. (1970) *Ventilation/Bloodflow and Gas Exchange*, 2nd edn. Oxford: Blackwell Scientific.

Original Articles

Alderson, P. O., Secker Walker, R. H. & Forrest, J. V. (1974) Detection of obstructive pulmonary disease. *Radiology*, **112**, 643–648.

Allgood, R. J., Wolfe, W. G., Ebert, P. A. & Sabiston, D. C. Jr (1968) Effects of carbon dioxide on bronchoconstriction after pulmonary artery occlusion. *American Journal of Physiology*, **214**, 772–775.

Anthonisen, N. R., Bass, H., Oriol, A., Place, R. E. G. & Bates, D. V. (1968) Regional lung function in patients with chronic bronchitis. *Clinical Science*, **35**, 495–511.

Anthonisen, N. R., Dolovich, M. B. & Bates, D. V. (1966) Steady state measurement of regional ventilation to perfusion ratios in normal man. *Journal of Clinical Investigation*, **45**, 1349–1356.

Bake, B., Bjure, J., Grimby, G., Milic-Emili, J. & Nilsson, N. J. (1967) Regional distribution of inspired gas in supine man. *Scandinavian Journal of Respiratory Diseases*, **48**, 189–196.

Ball, W. C. Jr, Stewart, P. B., Newsham, L. G. S. & Bates, D. V. (1962) Regional pulmonary function studied with xenon-133. *Journal of Clinical Investigation*, **41**, 519–531.

Barter, C. E., Hugh-Jones, P., Laws, J. W. & Crosbie, W. A. (1973) Radiology compared with xenon-133 scanning and bronchoscopic lobar sampling as methods for assessing regional lung function in patients with emphysema. *Thorax*, **28**, 29–40.

Bentivoglio, L. G., Beerel, F., Stewart, P. B., Bryan, A. C., Ball, W. C. Jr & Bates, D. V. (1963) Studies of regional ventilation and perfusion in pulmonary emphysema using xenon-133. *American Review of Respiratory Disease*, **88**, 315–329.

Björkman, S. (1934) Bronchospirometrie: eine klinische methode, die funktion der menschlichen lungen getrennt und gleichzeitig zu untersuchen. *Acta Medica Scandinavica*, Suppl. 56, 1–199.

Burwell, C. S., Robin, E. D., Whaley, R. D. & Bickelmann, A. G. (1956) Extreme obesity associated with alveolar hypoventilation—a Pickwickian syndrome. *American Journal of Medicine*, **21**, 811–818.

Clarke, S. W., Jones, J. G. & Glaister, D. H. (1969) Change in pulmonary ventilation in different postures. *Clinical Science*, **37**, 357–369.

De Nardo, G. L., Goodwin, D. A., Ravasini, R. & Dietrich, P. A. (1970) The ventilatory lung scan in the diagnosis of pulmonary embolism. *New England Journal of Medicine*, **282**, 1334–1336.

Despas, P., Walker, A., McRae, J. & Read, J. (1970) Inhalation and perfusion lung scans in bronchial asthma. *Australasian Annals of Medicine*, **19**, 304–309.

Dollery, C. T. & Gillam, P. M. S. (1963) The distribution of blood and gas within the lungs measured by scanning after administration of xenon-133. *Thorax*, **18**, 316–325.

Dollfuss, R. E., Milic-Emili, J. & Bates, D. V. (1967) Regional ventilation of the lung studied with boluses of xenon-133. *Respiration Physiology*, **2**, 234–246.

Dworkin, H. J., Smith, J. R. & Bull, F. E. (1966) A reaction following administration of macroaggregated albumin (MAA) for a lung scan. *American Journal of Roentgenology*, **98**, 427–433.

Evans, C. C. (1974) Regional lung function in bronchial asthma. *Thorax*, **29**, 611.

Fallat, R. J., Powell, M. R., Kueppers, F. & Lilker, E. (1973) Xenon-133 ventilatory studies in alpha$_1$-antitrypsin deficiency. *Journal of Nuclear Medicine*, **14**, 5–13.

Fazio, F. & Jones, T. (1975) Assessment of regional ventilation by continuous inhalation of krypton-81m. *British Medical Journal*, **3**, 673–676.

Fletcher, J. W., James, A. E. & Holman, B. L. (1973) Regional lung function in cancer. In: *Progress in Nuclear Medicine*, **3**, ed. Holman, B. L. & Lindeman, J. F., pp. 135–148. Basel: Kargel.

Foreman, S., Weill, H., Duke, R., George, R. & Ziskind, M. (1968) Bullous disease of the lung: physiologic improvement after surgery. *Annals of Internal Medicine*, **69**, 757–767.

Fraser, H. S., Macleod, W. M., Garnett, E. S. & Goddard, B. A. (1970) Lung scanning in the preoperative assessment of carcinoma of the bronchus. *American Review of Respiratory Disease*, **101**, 349–358.

Friedman, W. F. & Braunwald, E. (1966) Alterations in regional pulmonary blood flow in mitral valve disease studied by radioisotope scanning. *Circulation*, **34**, 363–376.

Glaister, D. H. (1967) The effect of posture on the distribution of ventilation and blood flow in the normal lung. *Clinical Science*, **33**, 391–398.

Glazier, J. B., Dollery, C. T. & Hughes, J. M. B. (1968) Effects of acetylcholine on regional pulmonary blood flow in patients with mitral stenosis. *Journal of the American Heart Association*, **38**, 136–143.

Goddard, B. A. & Ackery, D. M. (1975) Xenon-133, ^{127}Xe and ^{125}Xe for lung function investigations: a dosimetric comparison. *Journal of Nuclear Medicine*, **16**, 780–786.

Godfrey, S., Freedman, N. M. T., Glass, H. I., Winlove, C. P. & Ronchetti, R. (1975) Regional lung function studies in infants and children using $^{13}N_2$. *Clinical Science*, **48**, 17–18P.

Gold, W. M. & McCormack, K. R. (1966) Pulmonary-function response to radioisotope scanning of the lungs. *Journal of the American Medical Association*, **197**, 146–148.

Grant, R. W. & Ackery, D. M. (1975) Radioisotope measurements of regional lung function in bronchogenic carcinoma. *British Journal of Radiology*, **48**, 843–845.

Harding, L. K., Horsfield, K., Singhal, S. S. & Cumming, G. (1973) The proportion of lung vessels blocked by albumin microspheres. *Journal of Nuclear Medicine*, **14**, 579–581.

Heckscher, T., Bass, H., Oriol, A., Rose, B., Anthonisen, N. R. & Bates, D. V. (1968) Regional lung function in patients with bronchial asthma. *Journal of Clinical Investigation*, **47**, 1063–1070.

Heckscher, T., Larsen, O. A. & Lassen, N. A. (1966) A clinical method for determination of regional lung function using intravenous injection of xenon-133. *Scandinavian Journal of Respiratory Diseases*, Suppl. 62, 31–39.

Hogg, J. C., Macklem, P. T. & Thurlbeck, W. M. (1968) Site and nature of airway obstruction in chronic obstructive lung disease. *New England Journal of Medicine*, **278**, 1355–1360.

Holland, J., Milic-Emili, J., Macklem, P. T. & Bates, D. V. (1968) Regional distribution of pulmonary ventilation and perfusion in elderly subjects. *Journal of Clinical Investigation*, **47**, 81–92.

Holley, H. S., Milic-Emili, J., Becklake, M. R. & Bates, D. V. (1967) Regional distribution of pulmonary ventilation and perfusion in obesity. *Journal of Clinical Investigation*, **46**, 475–481.

Hughes, J. M. B., Glazier, J. B., Maloney, J. E. & West, J. B. (1968) Effect of lung volume on the distribution of pulmonary blood flow in man. *Respiration Physiology*, **4**, 58–72.

Hughes, J. M. B., Glazier, J. B., Rosenzweig, D. Y. & West, J. B. (1969) Factors determining the distribution of pulmonary blood flow in patients with raised pulmonary venous pressure. *Clinical Science*, **37**, 847–858.

Inkley, S. R. & MacIntyre, W. J. (1973) Dynamic measurement of ventilation–perfusion with xenon-133 at resting lung volumes. *American Review of Respiratory Disease*, **107**, 429–441.

International Commission on Radiological Protection (1971) *Protection of the Patient in Radionuclide Investigations*, ICRP Pub. 17. Oxford, New York, Toronto, Sydney, Braunschweig: Pergamon Press.

Johnson, P. M. (1971) The role of lung scanning in pulmonary embolism. *Seminars in Nuclear Medicine*, **1**, 171–184.

Kessler, R. M. & McNeil, B. J. (1975) Impaired ventilation in a patient with angiographically demonstrated pulmonary emboli. *Radiology*, **114**, 111–112.

Knipping, H. W., Bolt, W., Venrath, H., Valentin, H., Ludes, H. & Endler, P. (1955) Eine neue Methode zur Prüfung der Herz-und Lungen-funktion: die regionale Funktions-analyse in der Lungen- und Herzklinik mit Hilfe des radioaktiven Edelgases xenon-133 (Istopen-Thorakographie). *Deutsche Medizinische Wochenschrift*, **80**, 1146–1147.

Krishnamurthy, G. T., Srinivasan, N. V. & Blahd, W. H. (1972) Pulmonary hypertension in acquired valvular cardiac disease: evaluation by a scintillation camera technique. *Journal of Nuclear Medicine*, **13**, 604–611.

Langhammer, H., Glaubitt, G., Grebe, S. F., Hampe, J. F., Haubold, U., Hör, G., Kaul, A., Koeppe, P., Koppenhagen, J., Roedler, H. D. & van der Schoot, J. B. (1972) Gallium-67 for tumour scanning. *Journal of Nuclear Medicine*, **13**, 25–30.

Levine, B. W., Talamo, R. C., Shannon, D. C. & Kazemi, H. (1970) Alteration in distribution of pulmonary blood flow. An early manifestation of alpha$_1$-antitrypsin deficiency. *Annals of Internal Medicine*, **73**, 397–401.

Lin, M. S., Burke, G. & Silverstein, G. E. (1973) A radioaerosol technique for 113m In lung scintigraphy. *Radiology*, **107**, 449–451.

Lopez-Majano, V., Chernick, V., Wagner, H. N. & Dutton, R. E. (1964) Comparison of radioisotope scanning and differential oxygen uptake of the lungs. *Radiology*, **83**, 697–698.

Lopez-Majano, V., Kieffer, R. F., Marine, D. N., Garcia, D. A. & Wagner, H. N. (1969) Pulmonary resection in bullous disease. *American Review of Respiratory Disease*, **99**, 554–564.

Lopez-Majano, V., Tow, D. E. & Wagner, H. N. (1966) Regional distribution of pulmonary arterial blood flow in emphysema. *Journal of the American Medical Association*, **197**, 81–84.

MacIntyre, W. J. & Inkley, S. R. (1973) Evaluation of regional lung function with xenon-133. In *Radioactive Isotopes in Clinical Medicine and Research*, **X**, 321–334. Munich: Urban and Schwarzenberg.

MacIntyre, W. J., Inkley, S. R., Roth, E., Drescher, W. P. & Ishii, Y. (1970) Spatial recording of disappearance constants of xenon-133 wash-out from the lung. *Journal of Laboratory and Clinical Medicine*, **76**, 701–712.

Macleod, W. M. (1954) Abnormal transradiancy of one lung. *Thorax*, **9**, 147–153.

Martin, C. J., Cline, F. & Marshall, H. (1953) Lobar alveolar gas concentrations: effect of body position. *Journal of Clinical Investigation*, **32**, 617–621.

Martin, C. J. & Young, A. C. (1957) Ventilation–perfusion variations within the lung. *Journal of Applied Physiology*, **11**, 371–376.

Mattson, S. B. & Carlens, E. (1955) Lobar ventilation and oxygen uptake in man; influence of body position. *Journal of Thoracic Surgery*, **30**, 676–682.

Matthys, H., Rühle, K. H., Schlehe, H., Konietzko, N. & Adam, W. E. (1972) Ventilation–perfusion relationships studied with xenon-133 before and after bronchodilating drugs in patients with obstructuve lung disease. *Bulletin de Physio-Pathologie Respiratoire*, **8**, 599–610.

Maynard, C. D. & Cowan, R. J. (1971) Role of the scan in bronchogenic carcinoma. *Seminars in Nuclear Medicine*, **1**, 195–205.

Medina, J. R., L'Heureux, P., Lillehei, J. P. & Loken, M. K. (1969) Regional ventilation in the differential diagnosis of pulmonary embolism. *Circulation*, **39**, 831–835.

Mellemgaard, K., Winkler, K., Tygstrup, N. & Georg, J. (1963) Sources of venoarterial admixture in portal hypertension. *Journal of Clinical Investigation*, **42**, 1399–1405.

Meyer, J. A. & Umiker, W. O. (1961) A review of problems relating the 'diagnostic triad' in lung cancer: bronchoscopy, scalene lymph node biopsy, and cytopathology of bronchial excretions. *Surgical Clinics of North America*, **41**, 1233–1244.

Milic-Emili, J. (1971) Radioactive xenon in the evaluation of regional lung function. *Seminars in Nuclear Medicine*, **1**, 246–262.

Milic-Emili, J., Henderson, J. A. M., Dolovich, M. B., Trop, D. & Kaneko, K. (1966) Regional distribution of inspired gas in the lung. *Journal of Applied Physiology*, **21**, 749–759.

Miller, J. M., Ali, M. K. & Howe, C. D. (1970) Clinical determination of regional pulmonary function during normal breathing using xenon-133. *American Review of Respiratory Disease*, **101**, 218–229.

Miörner, G. (1968) ^{133}Xe-radiospirometry. A clinical method for studying regional lung function. *Scandinavian Journal of Respiratory Diseases*, Suppl. 64, 1–84.

Moser, K. M., Guisan, M., Cuomo, A. & Ashburn, W. L. (1971) Differentiation of pulmonary vascular from parenchymal diseases by ventilation/perfusion scintiphotography. *Annals of Internal Medicine*, **75**, 597–605.

Nairn, J. R., Prime, F. J. & Simon, G. (1969) Association between radiological findings and total and regional function in emphysema. *Thorax*, **24**, 218–227.

Newhouse, M. T., Wright, F. J., Ingham, G. K., Archer, N. P., Hughes, L. B. & Hopkins, O. L. (1968) Use of scintillation camera and ^{135}Xenon for study of topographic pulmonary function. *Respiration Physiology*, **4**, 141–153.

Pain, M. C. F., Glazier, J. B., Simon, H. & West, J. B. (1967) Regional and overall inequality of ventilation and blood flow in patients with chronic airflow obstruction. *Thorax*, **22**, 453–461.

Pircher, F. J., Knight, C. M., Barry, W. F., Temple, J. R. & Kirsch, W. J. (1967) Retention, distribution and absorption of inhaled albumin aerosol and absorbed dose estimates from its I^{131} and Tc^{99m} labels. *American Journal of Roentgenology, Radium Therapy and Nuclear Medicine*, **100**, 813–821.

Poulose, K. P., Reba, R. C., Gilday, D. L., Deland, F. H. & Wagner, H. N. Jr (1970) Diagnosis of pulmonary embolism. A correlative study of the clinical, scan and angiographic findings. *British Medical Journal*, **3**, 67–71.

Pride, N. B., Hugh-Jones, P., O'Brien, E. N. & Smith, L. A. (1970) Changes in lung function following the surgical treatment of bullous emphysema. *Quarterly Journal of Medicine*, **39**, 49–69.

Reid, L., Simon, G., Zorab, P. A. & Seidelin, R. (1967) The development of unilateral hypertransradiancy of the lung. *British Journal of Diseases of the Chest*, **61**, 190–192.

Rhodes, B. A., Zolle, I., Buchanan, J. W. & Wagner, H. N. (1969) Radioactive albumin microspheres for studies of the pulmonary circulation. *Radiology*, **92**, 1453–1460.

Robinowitz, M., Mathew, J., Eckelman, W. & Harbert, J. C. (1973) Fatal reactions following $99mTc$-ferrous hydroxide lung scans. *Journal of Nuclear Medicine*, **14**, 445–446.

le Roux, B. T. & Houlder, A. E. (1974) Gallium-67 as a diagnostic tool in the evaluation of peripheral pulmonary lesions. *Thorax*, **29**, 355–358.

Ruff, F., Hughes, J. M. B., Stanley, N., McCarthy, D., Greene, R., Aronoff, A., Clayton, L. & Milic-Emili, J. (1971) Regional lung function in patients with hepatic cirrhosis. *Journal of Clinical Investigation*, **50**, 2403–2413.

Secker Walker, R. H., Jackson, J. A. & Goodwin, J. (1970) Resolution of pulmonary embolism. *British Medical Journal*, **4**, 135–139.

Secker Walker, R. H., Provan, J. L., Jackson, J. A. & Goodwin, J. (1971) Lung scanning in carcinoma of the bronchus. *Thorax*, **26**, 23–32.

Severinghaus, J. W., Swenson, E. W., Finley, T. N., Lategola, M. T. & Williams, J. (1961) Unilateral hypoventilation produced in dogs by occluding one pulmonary artery. *Journal of Applied Physiology*, **16**, 53–60.

Shibel, E. M., Landis, G. A. & Moser, K. M. (1969) Inhalation lung scanning evaluation—radioaerosol versus radioxenon techniques. *Diseases of the Chest*, **56**, 284–289.

Siegel, B. A. & Potchen, E. J. (1973) Radionuclide studies of pulmonary function: anatomic and physiologic considerations. In: *Progress in Nuclear Medicine*, **3**, 49–66, ed. Holman, B. L. & Lindeman, J. F. Basel: Karger.

Svanberg, L. (1972) Regional functional decrease in bronchial carcinoma. *Annals of Thoracic Surgery*, **13**, 170–180.

Swenson, E. W., Finley, T. N. & Guzman, S. V. (1961) Unilateral hypoventilation in man during temporary occlusion of one pulmonary artery. *Journal of Clinical Investigation*, **40**, 828–835.

Swyer, P. R. & James, G. C. W. (1953) A case of unilateral pulmonary emphysema. *Thorax*, **8**, 133–136.

Taplin, G. V., Johnson, D. E., Dore, E. K. & Kaplan, H. S. (1964) Lung photoscans with macroaggregates of human serum radioalbumin. Experimental basis and initial clinical trials. *Health Physics*, **10**, 1219–1227.

Tow, D. E., Wagner, H. N., Lopez-Majano, V., Smith, E. M. & Migita, T. (1966) Validity of measuring regional pulmonary arterial blood flow with macroaggregates of human serum albumin. *American Journal of Roentgenology, Radium Therapy and Nuclear Medicine*, **96**, 664–676.

Vincent, W. R., Goldberg, S. J. & Desilets, D. (1968) Fatality immediately following rapid infusion of macroaggregates of $99mTc$ albumin (MAA) for lung scan. *Radiology*, **91**, 1180–1184.

Wagner, H. N., Tow, D. E., Lopez-Majano, V., Chernick, V. & Twining, R. (1966) Factors influencing regional pulmonary blood in man. *Scandinavian Journal of Respiratory Diseases*, Suppl. 62, 59–72.

Weibel, E. R. (1963) *Morphometry of the Human Lung*. Berlin: Springer-Verlag.

West, J. B. (1962) Regional differences in gas exchange in the lung of erect man. *Journal of Applied Physiology*, **17**, 893–898.

West, J. B. (1963) Distribution of gas and blood in the normal lungs. *British Medical Bulletin*, **19**, 53–58.

West, J. B. (1967) Pulmonary function studies with radioactive gases. *Annual Review of Medicine*, **18**, 459–470.

West, J. B. & Dollery, C. T. (1960) Distribution of blood flow and ventilation–perfusion ratio in the lung, measured with radioactive CO_2. *Journal of Applied Physiology*, **15**, 405–410.

West, J. B., Dollery, C. T. & Heard, B. E. (1965) Increased pulmonary vascular resistance in the dependent zone of the isolated dog lung caused by perivascular edema. *Circulation Research*, **17**, 191–206.

Williams, E. S. (1974a) Adverse reactions to radio-pharmaceuticals: a preliminary survey in the United Kingdom. *British Journal of Radiology*, **47**, 54–59.

Williams, J. O. (1974b) Death following injection of lung scanning agent in a case of pulmonary hypertension. *British Journal of Radiology*, **47**, 61–63.

Wilson, A. F., Surprenant, E. L., Beall, G. N., Siegel, S. C., Simmons, D. H. & Bennett, L. R. (1970) The significance of regional pulmonary function changes in bronchial asthma. *American Journal of Medicine*, **48**, 416–423.

Winebright, J. W., Gerdes, A. J. & Nelp, W. B. (1970) Restoration of blood flow after pulmonary embolism. *Archives of Internal Medicine*, **125**, 241–247.

2
THE CYTOLOGY OF RESPIRATORY SECRETIONS

E. Blanche Butler

Microscopic examination of respiratory secretions has been practised for more than a century. One of the earliest descriptions of malignant cells in sputum was by Beale (1861) who examined material sent by Mr S. Newham of Bury St Edmunds and the first recorded diagnosis of a primary tumour of the pleura, by examination of pleural fluid, was made by Warthin in 1897. Warthin also referred to the work of Quincke (1882) in which he established the principle that it is possible to distinguish between malignant cells and mesothelial cells in pleural fluid. The work of Widal and Ravaut (1900) is of interest as these workers studied benign pleural effusions and in particular tuberculous pleural fluid. It is perhaps surprising that needle puncture of the lung preceded sputum examination as a routine investigation in the diagnosis of pulmonary disease. Needle puncture was reported by Hellendall (1899) to obtain material for histological diagnosis and by Horder (1909) for bacterial examination. Professor L. S. Dudgeon at St Thomas's Hospital was the first to make use of sputum cytology as a routine investigation in cases of suspected carcinoma of bronchus (Bamforth, 1966). With Wrigley (Dudgeon and Wrigley, 1935) he showed that sputum cytology could yield 68 per cent of positive results in cases later proved to be malignant.

At first cytological examinations were made using fresh unfixed material but in 1880 Ehrlich introduced the use of air-dried stained preparations. Slightly later, cell blocks were made from concentrated cellular material and processed for histological examination; this method was described by Bahrenberg in 1896. In 1927 Dudgeon and Patrick described the advantages of wet fixation of cytological material and used Mayer's haemalum and eosin to stain the smears. Papanicolaou also recognised the advantages of wet fixation in the preservation of good nuclear detail and this forms an important part of the staining technique which is associated with his name. In many laboratories Papanicolaou's stain is used for all types of cytological material, butsome workers prefer haematoxylin and eosin while others find that the Romanowsky stains have advantages (Lopes Cardozo et al, 1967). Cell blocks are also still used, so each of these methods of preparation has something to contribute to the cytological examination of respiratory secretions.

SPUTUM

Cytological examination of sputum is an investigation used in most cases of suspected carcinoma of bronchus. Collection of specimens is simple and causes no inconvenience to the patient. Cancer detection rates improve with the examination of multiple specimens. Erozan and Frost (1970) found that in their series only 42 per cent of cases with cancer had a positive report on the first sputum examination while by the third specimen 73 per cent of the group had a positive result and by the fifth specimen 84 per cent. Additional specimens improved the detection rate by only 3 per cent. Similarly Oswald et al (1971) report a detection rate of 41 per cent when one specimen of sputum was examined, 69 per cent with three specimens and 85 per cent with four or more specimens. The number of specimens examined will depend on locally available facilities though these figures indicate that there should be a minimum of three and that there is little advantage in examining more than five specimens at any one time if these are all completely negative. Specimens should be collected in the morning as soon as the patient wakes and it is important that he is instructed to cough deeply to produce material from the lungs.

Preparation of specimens

When sputum samples can be sent to the laboratory within 2 h of collection, fixation is not necessary, but when there is likely to be delay before processing, it is better to collect the sputum into 50 per cent alcohol. On reaching the laboratory various methods of processing are available but it is usual to select any opaque or blood-stained fragments to make direct smears. A common procedure is to make three smears which are fixed in 95 per cent alcohol for staining by Papanicolaou's method or haematoxylin and eosin, while one is air-dried for staining by one of the Romanowsky stains. Some workers recommend the use of mucolytic agents and a simple way to lyse mucus is to use 8 per cent hydrochloric acid as described by Taplin (1966). After liquefaction, material that remains after making three or four smears can be filtered on to a suitable membrane filter, such as a Millipore or Nucleopore filter, or can be concentrated to make a cell block. The addition of a drop of nutrient agar to the cell deposit prevents crumbling, and the block can be processed and sectioned by the usual techniques to prepare material for histological examination. Unfixed material received in a cytology laboratory is handled with the same precautions to prevent infection that are used in departments of bacteriology, but it is helpful if a note is made on the request card in cases where tuberculosis is suspected.

Cellular Content of Sputum

Aerosol induced sputum in normal subjects contains squamous cells (mainly from the mouth), mucus, a few neutrophils and lymphocytes, and carbon containing macrophages. A few ciliated columnar cells may be found;

these may be shed from the nasopharynx or the bronchial tree. The presence of carbon containing macrophages is of importance as this is generally accepted as certain evidence that the material is sputum and not saliva. In the presence of disease other cell types are seen and these will be considered individually.

Bronchial columnar epithelium

Chodosh and Medici (1971) made quantitative and qualitative determinations of bronchial epithelial cells exfoliated into sputum in the presence of acute infection superimposed on stable chronic bronchitis. They found an increase in the total number of these cells over and above the increased exfoliation which occurs in most types of pulmonary disease. The normal bronchial columnar cell is tall with a basal nucleus which has a regular, finely granular chromatin pattern and one or more small nucleoli. These cells

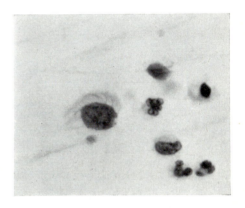

Figure 1   Ciliocytophthoria. A fragment of degenerate chromophilic cytoplasm (with inclusions) which bears cilia. Sputum. Papanicolaou's stain, × 800

are usually ciliated and an end plate can be recognised. Occasionally a goblet cell with a large vacuole is found but this usually reflects bronchial irritation from whatever cause as do degenerative changes in columnar cells. The most obvious of these is ciliocytophthoria, first described by Papanicolaou in 1956. He recognised the association with lung cancer (Papanicolaou, 1958) and also with virus infections (Papanicolaou, Bridges and Railey, 1961). The nuclear changes in ciliocytophthoria include pyknosis, hyperchromasia and chromatin-clumping at the nuclear membrane. Eosinophilic cytoplasmic inclusions may be present but the most characteristic feature is fragmentation of the cell so that it consists of a non-ciliated part with a nucleus and a ciliated fragment with no nucleus (Fig. 1).

In the presence of infection the nuclei of bronchial columnar cells show separation of chromatin and prominent nucleoli. These can cause problems in diagnosis when the epithelium exfoliates in fragments which twist into spirals because of the loss of applied tension. Such fragments are found in postbronchoscopy specimens of sputum and also in patients with asthma

(Naylor and Railey, 1964). When degeneration is present as well, these fragments can be confused with those from an adenocarcinoma, but careful examination (in some cases with the ×100 objective) will demonstrate the presence of cilia, which are not found on malignant cells (Figs. 2, 3).

Squamous metaplasia

Groups of immature squamous cells of the parabasal type are found in many specimens of sputum (Fig. 4). The appearance of these cells is very

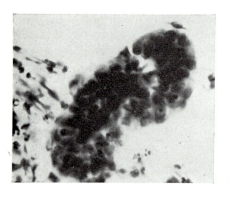

Figure 2   A fragment of bronchial columnar epithelium with hyperchromatic nuclei which looks like a papillary fragment. Sputum. Papanicolaou's stain, ×400

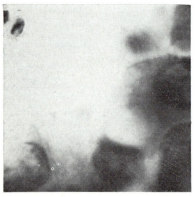

Figure 3   The surface of the same fragment as in Figure 2 which shows cilia and an end plate on the cell at the top right hand corner. Sputum. Papanicolaou's stain, ×2000

similar to that seen in smears from the cervix uteri in the presence of squamous metaplasia. Histological examination of the bronchial tree has shown that replacement of respiratory columnar epithelium by squamous epithelium occurs in cases where there has been chronic irritation of the respiratory tract. The presence of squamous metaplasia is of importance because of its relationship to the development of cancer. Nasiell (1966) found squamous metaplasia in bronchial epithelium in 88 per cent of patients with squamous cell or undifferentiated cancer compared with 34 per cent in a control series. In a parallel series in which cytological examination was made on sputum the figures were 80 per cent and 36 per cent. Evidence of squamous metaplasia is found in the sputum of heavy smokers, and Fullmer et al (1969) report regression of these changes within one to three years after giving up the habit. Other workers are less convinced that metaplastic epithelium can revert to normal ciliated columnar epithelium (Grunze, 1958). Metaplasia also occurs in chronic disease such as bronchiectasis and in the presence of long-standing infection, particularly tuberculosis.

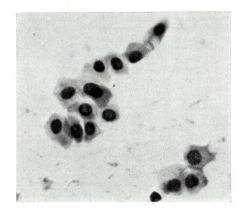

Figure 4 A group of immature squamous cells (parabasal type), shed from an area of sqamous metaplasia. Sputum. Papanicolaou's stain, ×400

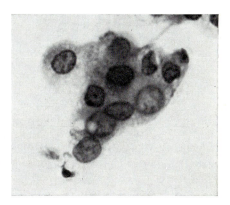

Figure 5 A group of atypical squamous cells consistent with being shed from an area of atypical squamous metaplasia (dysplasia). Sputum. Papanicolaou's stain, ×800

Atypical metaplasia and carcinoma in situ

Premalignant changes occurring in metaplastic epithelium of the cervix uteri are well documented (Langley and Crompton, 1973) and observations have been made on a similar progression in the development of bronchial cancer (Nasiell, 1966; Fullmer et al, 1969; Saccomanno et al, 1974). Atypical immature squamous cells, similar to the cells seen in cervical smears in the presence of dysplasia and carcinoma in situ, are sometimes seen in sputum (Fig. 5). The relationship of such findings to the development of squamous cell carcinoma and small cell undifferentiated carcinoma is particularly well shown by Saccomanno and his colleagues (1974) who studied sputum collected from uranium miners at intervals since 1957 and found a definite progression from minor atypia to invasive cancer in 17 cases. When features that suggest pre-invasive cancer are present in sputum there are problems of management which will be considered later.

Respiratory macrophages

The origin of these cells is not certain but it seems probable that they exfoliate from the alveolar epithelium and become phagocytic. They usually appear as round or oval cells measuring 10 to 25 μm in diameter and their cytoplasm contains carbon particles. In cases of cardiac failure they appear as 'heart failure cells', and the inclusions are yellow-brown in colour and give a positive stain for haemosiderin. Similar cells without dust particles do occur and they are present in relatively large numbers in cases of pneumonia. In these cases the cells can be large and grouped together, and as

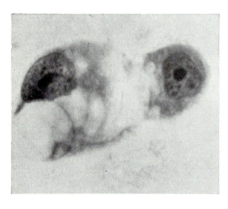

Figure 6 Atypical respiratory macrophages present in the sputum of a patient found to have pulmonary infarction at necropsy. Papanicolaou's stain, $\times 800$

they have prominent nucleoli they may be confused with cells shed from an adenocarcinoma. However, the nuclei do not show features characteristic of malignancy and comparison with morphologically similar cells which contain dust particles should prevent wrong diagnoses. Greater problems of diagnosis arise in cases of pulmonary infarction when these cells may exfoliate as small tissue fragments of two or three cells, sometimes with vacuolation, but again the nuclear chromatin pattern appears bland (Fig. 6).

Curshman's spirals

Curshman's spirals (Fig. 7) are formed in the finer bronchioles and were described in the sputum of asthma patients by Curshman in 1884 (Walker and Fullmer, 1970). While investigating the possibility of early cancer detection in heavy smokers Walker and Fullmer (1970) found that Curshman's spirals were present in 94 per cent of their cases. Frost et al (1973) suggested that spirals were formed because of an alteration in the chemistry of the mucus produced by the respiratory epithelium in chronic cigarette smokers and patients with chronic bronchitis. The mucus becomes rubbery, thick and tenacious, and forms a cast of fine bronchioles. This is the core of the spiral. In its passage through the bronchial tree the spiral acquires a mantle which reflects the condition of the bronchial epithelium. Thus, these authors found that in asthmatics the mantle was packed with neutrophils, in heavy smokers there was no cellular content and in cases of carcinoma they noted the presence of haemosiderin and serum.

Cell changes in the presence of virus infection

The cytopathic effect of virus infections has long been noted in histological and cytological material. Among the earlier reports is that of Warthin (1931) who observed the presence of giant cells in the tonsils during the prodromal stage of measles. Naib et al (1968) described the cell changes seen in tracheal aspirates collected from children with clinical respiratory infection and also

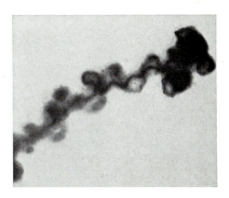

Figure 7 Curshman's spiral. Sputum. Papanicolaou's stain, ×400

correlated their findings with virus isolation and identification. Cellular changes were present in 31 of the 50 patients from whom a virus was isolated or in whom there was a fourfold or greater rise in antibody titre. The changes included multinucleation and intranuclear and intracytoplasmic inclusions, as well as the ciliocytophthoria which has already been described. The appearances associated with herpes simplex infection are perhaps the most specific and easily recognised (Fig. 8). Multinucleated giant cells are seen with their nuclei tightly moulded together. The intranuclear inclusions may be large homogeneous inclusions that almost fill the nucleus or discrete hyperchromatic inclusions surrounded by a halo. Naib et al (1968) were able to recognise specific changes in the presence of parainfluenza virus, adenovirus, cytomegalic virus and measles, but this degree of precision requires considerable experience with virus infected material.

Malignant cells

As with other specimens, when sputum is examined to detect the presence of cancer the first object is to recognise malignant cells and the second is to classify the tumour in terms of its predominant histological type. The diagnosis of malignancy depends mainly on changes seen in the nucleus, such as an irregular chromatin pattern, prominent and irregular nucleoli and irregularities in the relationship of nucleus to cytoplasm. The cytoplasmic differentiation and the pattern of exfoliation give information which helps in the classification of the type of tumour.

SQUAMOUS CELL CARCINOMA

Although most primary tumours of the lung arise in bronchial epithelium a high proportion are squamous in type and the association with squamous metaplasia has been discussed already. The carcinoma may be well differentiated and shed cells which resemble squamous cells though they do show characteristic abnormalities. The cytoplasm is often keratinised and this is shown by a clear orange staining reaction when Papanicolaou's stain is used.

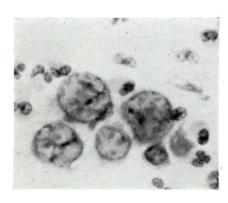

Figure 8   Cells showing homogeneous intranuclear inclusions. Virus pneumonia confirmed at necropsy; herpes simplex virus isolated. Sputum. Papanicolaou's stain, × 800

Bizarre cell forms such as 'fibre cells' and 'tadpole cells' may be seen and there is great variation in the size of cells. Nuclei can disappear so that keratinised ghost cells result or the nuclei can be degenerate and pyknotic. A high nuclear/cytoplasmic ratio is not a feature of these well-differentiated cells and similar cells can be found in cases where there has been long-standing infection such as tuberculosis, bronchiectasis and lung abscess. It is, however, usually possible to find less well-differentiated cells in which the sharp outline of the cytoplasm indicates squamous differentiation whilst the nucleus is sufficiently well preserved to show nuclear patterns characteristic of malignancy (Fig. 9).

Squamous cell carcinomas exfoliate as single cells, but with the less well-differentiated forms of the tumour, cells may exfoliate in small clusters or sheets. In these cases the cytoplasm may have a soft or hazy outline and squamous cell differentiation is not obvious, so that it is only possible to report such cells as being shed from a large cell undifferentiated carcinoma.

SMALL CELL UNDIFFERENTIATED CARCINOMA (OAT CELL CARCINOMA)

The cytological presentation of this tumour is characteristic but exfoliation is often scanty. Meticulous screening of the smears is therefore essential. The tumour cells are shed in small groups often strung out in a stream of mucus. They are small cells with apparently bare nuclei but in most cases a very narrow rim of basophilic cytoplasm is present, although it may be necessary to use the × 100 objective to identify this. The nuclei may be

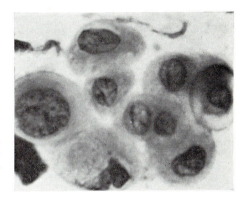

Figure 9 Cells shed from a squamous cell carcinoma. The chromatin pattern is irregular and abnormal keratinisation can be seen in one cell. Sputum. Papanicolaou's stain, × 800

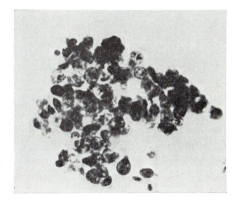

Figure 10 Cells shed from an oat cell carcinoma. Sputum. Papanicolaou's stain, × 400

superimposed on each other or moulded loosely together like pieces in a mosaic. It is usually possible to recognise an irregular nuclear chromatin pattern and sometimes prominent nucleoli are seen. Groups of lymphocytes and macrophages can sometimes be mistaken for groups of oat cells though lymphocyte nuclei are usually smaller. When in doubt it is useful to compare the nuclear size with that of neutrophil nuclei and nuclei in normal inter-mediate squamous cells. When this is done it is apparent that the nuclei of cells shed from an oat cell carcinoma are appreciably larger than the nuclei of lymphocytes (Fig. 10). The Romanowsky stains are particularly useful in distinguishing between oat cells and large lymphocytes because the staining reaction is quite different. Oat cells can be recognised by their relatively large pink staining nuclei and rim of blue cytoplasm; the mosaic effect is usually more pronounced than in smears wet-fixed and stained by Papanicolaou's method (Spriggs and Boddington, 1968).

ADENOCARCINOMA

Adenocarcinoma may arise from the bronchial tree and have a 'central' origin or it may be a terminal bronchiolar carcinoma which arises in the periphery of the lung. A peripheral carcinoma is less likely to exfoliate cells into the bronchial secretion and so there is a lower detection rate for adeno-carcinoma by cytological examination of the sputum. It is not usually possible to distinguish the two types of adenocarcinoma from the cytological appearances. Cells from an adenocarcinoma most often exfoliate in well-demarcated clusters or tissue fragments (Fig. 11) but single cells, which are larger than

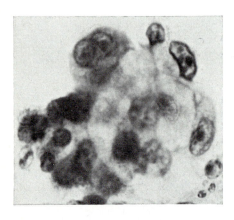

Figure 11 An acinar fragment shed from an adenocarcinoma. Sputum. Papanicolaou's stain, × 800

the cells in the clusters, may be seen. The nuclear chromatin can have a 'ground glass' appearance with a denser rim of chromatin at the nuclear membrane. Prominent, often irregularly shaped nucleoli are common and there is moulding of nuclei in the tissue fragments. Cytoplasm is scanty and not well demarcated, the cells may be vacuolated but this is not common. The problems of differential diagnosis are, perhaps, greater in cases of adenocarcinoma than with other lung tumours. Fragments of hyperplastic epithelium are shed in the presence of infection or asthma and can be difficult to distinguish from an adenocarcinoma, particularly if the tumour is well differentiated. Features characteristic of an adenocarcinoma are the absence of cilia, the tendency of cells to be superimposed on each other and the absence of a palisade of columnar cells at the periphery of the cluster. In addition, postbronchoscopy specimens usually contain fragments of bronchial epithelium and it is useful if these specimens are identified as such. Atypical respiratory macrophages as seen in pneumonia and pulmonary infarction also give rise to difficulties in differential diagnosis.

METASTATIC CARCINOMA

Many tumours in the body metastasise to the lungs but it must be remembered that a primary tumour elsewhere does not exclude the possibility of a second primary in the lung. In addition, x-ray appearances which suggest a secondary tumour in the lung may be due to benign lesions and so it is useful if the diagnosis can be confirmed by cytological examination. Koss (1968) considers that approximately 50 per cent of metastatic lung tumours can be detected cytologically but this is only possible if the secondary deposit is within the bronchial wall. Many of the secondary tumours are adenocarcinomas and it is seldom possible to identify the site of the primary tumour unless there are distinguishing features such as the presence of melanin in metastatic malignant melanoma or the multinucleation seen in choriocarcinoma.

The Accuracy of Cytology in Typing Lung Cancer

Discrepancies are found when cytological typing is compared with the histology report on resected or necropsy specimens. The cytological diagnosis is more likely to be the one that is accurate when the histological diagnosis depends on necropsy material which has undergone postmortem autolysis or in cases where death has followed radiotherapy. In other cases poor differentiation of the tumour can cause difficulties in distinguishing between cells shed from an adenocarcinoma or from a squamous cell carcinoma and it is wiser to admit the uncertainty in cytological reports. Discrepancies also occur when there is more than one tumour type in the primary growth and an insufficient number of tissue blocks are taken to make the histological diagnosis.

The accuracy of cytological typing is similar in most published reports. Oswald et al (1971) made correct diagnoses of squamous cell carcinoma in 89 per cent of cases, of adenocarcinoma in 97 per cent and of oat cell carcinoma in 79 per cent. The comparable figures given by Lange and Høeg (1972) were 91, 100 and 86 per cent.

THE DIAGNOSIS OF LUNG CANCER

In expert hands it is possible to diagnose lung cancer by means of sputum cytology in as many as 90 per cent of cases (Nasiell, 1967). This involves the meticulous examination of multiple specimens and in an average laboratory a 70 per cent detection rate would be more realistic. Sputum examination is convenient for the patient but when a suspicious lesion can be seen on x-ray and sputum cytology and bronchoscopy are negative other methods of obtaining cytological material have to be introduced.

Bronchial aspiration and bronchial washing

In the course of bronchoscopic examination secretion may be aspirated from the trachea or main bronchi. Some workers prefer to instil a small amount of sterile saline which washes the bronchus and is then reaspirated.

The aspirated material may be used to make direct smears or it can be filtered on to a membrane filter such as a Millipore or Nucleopore filter. Another method is to concentrate the material to make a cell block which is processed for histological examination. Diagnostic accuracy is again in the range of 70 to 80 per cent though Nasiell (1965) found that the detection rate using this method was 20 per cent lower than the detection rate when sputum was examined.

Bronchial brush or swab
Duguid and Huish (1963) reported improved diagnostic accuracy when smears were made directly from bronchial swabbings. Kuper et al (1966) extended this work by introducing a swab made of acetone soluble material which could be dissolved away leaving the remaining cells to be concentrated to make a cell block; this was processed for histological examination and cut

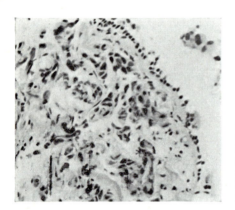

Figure 12   A fragment of bronchial columnar epithelium infiltrated by tumour. The specimen was collected by bronchial swab (Kuper's swab) and concentrated to make a cell block which was processed for histological examination. Haematoxylin and eosin, × 200

at three levels (Fig. 12). These methods, although useful, did not overcome the problem of collecting material from areas which were beyond vision using a standard bronchoscope. The late Dr S. W. A. Kuper of the Brompton Hospital overcame this problem by bonding acetone soluble material on wire in the form of a 'pipe cleaner' (personal communication). Suitable lengths of 'pipe cleaner' can be introduced into the mouth of the relevant bronchus under bronchoscopic control and advanced as far as possible. After removal the swab is placed in formol saline and processed in the manner described by Butler, Monahan and Warrell (1971). A similar technique using cores cut from an acrylic baby sponge was described by Smith and Warrack (1972).

Other workers have introduced more sophisticated techniques in methods designed to bring a brush into contact with peripheral lesions. Fennessy (1968) devised a method based on the methods used in selective arteriography. He used a radiopaque catheter which was positioned under fluoroscopy, a nylon bristle brush or a steel bristle brush was passed through the catheter and the material collected was used for bacteriology as well as to make smears for cytological examination. Forrest (1973) described a similar technique but he entered the bronchial tree through a transcricothyroid membrane puncture.

The introduction of fibreoptic bronchoscopy has been of great assistance in the diagnosis of malignancy and Ikeda (1970) was among the first to describe its use in collecting cytological material from the more peripheral lesions. Endoscopically visible lesions can be brushed under direct vision and more peripheral lesions under fluoroscopic control (Richardson et al, 1974). A nylon brush is used and the material collected can be processed by any of the standard methods.

Needle aspiration biopsy of the lung

In recent years there has been a renewed interest in the use of needle aspiration biopsy to obtain material for cytological diagnosis. Dahlgren and Nordenström (1966) and Nasiell (1967) describe the use of transthoracic needle aspiration biopsy while Lopes Cardozo et al (1967) and Grunze (1973) have found transtracheal and transbronchial needle aspiration biopsies of value. The introduction of fine needles (less than 1 mm in external diameter) for this work, as developed by Dr Sixten Franzen at the Radiumhemmet, Stockholm, and Dr Paul Lopes Cardozo in Leiden, has been an important factor in the increased use of this technique. The risk of implanting metastases along the needle tract is thought to be negligible and the possibility of complications such as pneumothorax, haemorrhage or air embolism is greatly reduced. Improved radiological methods for localising peripheral lesions with accuracy have also been important. The material obtained is of good quality and the cell degeneration, which can cause difficulties in sputum diagnosis, is seldom a problem. A needle of suitable length is used with a disposable 10 to 20 ml syringe. It is an advantage to use the syringe holder developed at the Radiumhemmet, Stockholm, as this allows easier control during aspiration. The puncture is made into the tumour under fluoroscopic control and material is aspirated into the needle. Smears are made and can be fixed at once in 95 per cent alcohol for staining by Papanicolaou's method, or air dried and one of the Romanowsky stains used.

The method is of particular value in cases where there is a small peripheral lesion on x-ray and sputum cytology is negative. Hayata et al (1973) found transthoracic puncture more accurate than bronchial brushing under fluoroscopy for lesions smaller than 2 cm in diameter. Dahlgren and Lind (1972) found the method to be of value in distinguishing between malignant and benign lesions, particularly in cases of tuberculosis. Transthoracic puncture has also been used in cases with metastatic tumour in the lung when it may be possible to identify the site of the primary tumour by examining aspirated material. In the same way needle aspiration of enlarged lymph nodes can be used in the assessment of lung cancer.

Population screening

The Registrar General's Statistical Review for England and Wales for 1971 gives the death rate per million of the female population for carcinoma of the cervix uteri as 92. The comparable figure for women dying of carcinoma of the trachea, bronchus and lung is 224 and for men 1060. Population screening to detect cancer of the cervix is well established and these figures would seem to suggest that a similar programme for early detection of lung cancer might be of even greater value. There are a number of reports in the literature describing the results of screening programmes conducted on groups particularly at risk for lung cancer, either because they are heavy smokers or by reason of their occupation (Fullmer and Parrish, 1969; Grzybowski and Coy, 1970; Frost et al, 1973; Saccomanno et al, 1974). Aerosol induced and spontaneously produced sputum has been used and individuals have been found with malignant cells in the sputum but with negative findings on x-ray; in some cases the cell changes are consistent with a diagnosis of dysplasia or carcinoma in situ (Fullmer et al, 1969; Saccomanno et al, 1974). If it were possible to locate the lesion in these cases, surgery might be expected to result in greatly increased survival rates. The difficulty is to localise the lesion. Differential aspirations from the main lobar bronchi have been used with success in some cases. But after resection of the appropriate lobe it has occasionally not been possible to demonstrate tumour in the resected lung tissue. In one such case reported by Oswald et al (1971) the carcinoma appeared in the opposite lung a year later. Grzybowski and Coy (1970) screened 2112 male patients and found 17 cases of lung cancer (seven by cytology alone) but at the time of diagnosis only six patients were fit for surgery, and three of these were inoperable at thoracotomy. These workers also screened their subjects radiographically and eight had positive x-ray findings but negative cytology. In addition, when Grzybowski and Coy reviewed a group which had been negative on screening in 1965 they found that in the meantime nine had died of lung cancer, and they concluded that five of these cases must have had the disease at the time of first screening. Such findings are of evident importance to any consideration of the cost-effectiveness of screening groups at risk for lung cancer.

PLEURAL FLUID

Pleural effusions can occur as a manifestation of systemic disease. They also occur in the presence of benign or malignant disease of the lung or mesothelium. Cytological examination of the aspirated fluid can give useful information which is of assistance in reaching a final diagnosis.

Preparations of specimens

Serous fluids usually clot and it is advisable to collect them into an anticoagulant. Some of the anticoagulants in common use distort or destroy cells but 3.8 per cent sodium citrate (1 ml/10 ml of pleural fluid) is satisfactory. If immediate processing is not possible it is better to use a carrying medium. Using a heparin–dextran mixture (20 000 units freeze dried heparin in 40 ml dextran; 5 ml of this mixture per 100 ml of fluid) cell preservation remains good for two or three days at room temperature. When possible at least 100 ml of the fluid removed should be sent to the laboratory.

The fluid can be processed in various ways. Some workers prefer to use a Millipore or Nucleopore filter while others centrifuge the specimen and make direct smears from the deposit. Most laboratories use Papanicolaou's stain or haematoxylin and eosin but it is very useful to make at least one air-dried Romanowsky stained smear. Any clot which is present and any deposit which remains can be fixed in formol saline and a cell block made using a drop of nutrient agar. This is processed by the usual technique and sections are cut at three levels.

The introduction of the Shandon cytocentrifuge has been of importance in processing serous fluids as it has become possible to centrifuge a monolayer of cells directly on to the slide. When using this technique it is necessary to adjust the cellularity and this may mean that aliquots of the original fluid need to be diluted with saline. Conversely the scanty cell content of a large volume of fluid can be concentrated to make one cytocentrifuge preparation.

When fluid is heavily blood-stained, better results are obtained if red cells are removed. Flotation techniques have been described and also methods to lyse red cells. A simple procedure is to centrifuge a large volume of fluid in several containers and to combine the layers pipetted from the interface between the supernate and the red cells in a Wintrobe tube. After further centrifugation it is usually possible to recognise a deep 'buffy' layer which can be removed with a pipette and resuspended in saline to make cytocentrifuge preparations.

Pleural Fluid in Systemic Conditions

Transudates

Conditions such as cardiac failure and renal diseases which produce oedema also produce effusions of oedema fluid in serous cavities, including the pleura. Cardiac failure is often accompanied by pulmonary disease so that 'true' pleural transudates occur most often in patients with renal disease. The cell count is usually very low so that a large volume of fluid has to be concentrated to make a smear. Occasionally the cellular deposit is relatively heavy but Spriggs and Boddington (1968) found that in these cases there was evidence of a pulmonary infarct or the possibility of one. These workers doubted whether a high cell count could occur in a pure transudate.

Systemic lupus erythematosus

Pleural effusions are common in these cases and in a few of them typical LE cells can be seen but otherwise the cytological picture has been thought to be variable and non-specific (Spriggs and Boddington, 1968). However, Kelley, McGarry and Hutson (1971) describe large cells which they also identified in sections of the inflammatory infiltrate of the pleura. They considered these cells to be characteristic of the disease.

Rheumatoid arthritis

Nosanchuk and Naylor (1968) reported a characteristic cytological picture in rheumatoid effusions. This consists of a background of amorphous material and the presence of large multinucleated epitheloid cells which are often elongated or with tails (Fig. 13). Boddington et al (1971) reviewed 20 cases of rheumatoid arthritis in which pleural effusions (in one case a pericardial effusion) were also present. They found that the cellular picture described by Nosanchuk and Naylor was reliable in distinguishing rheumatoid effusions

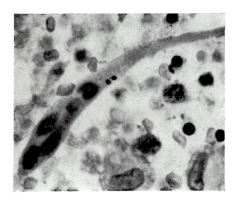

Figure 13 An elongated multinucleated epithelioid cell as seen in a rheumatoid effusion. The typical background of amorphous debris is also seen. Pleural fluid. Papanicolaou's stain, × 800

from effusions which were not due to the disease. These multinucleated epithelioid cells should not be confused with the 'RA' cells or 'ragocytes', sometimes seen in rheumatoid effusions (Carmichael and Golding, 1967), which are leucocytes containing inclusions and are non-specific.

Leukaemias and reticuloses (lymphoma)

Pleural and ascitic effusions complicate the clinical course of about 20 to 30 per cent of malignant lymphomas and in a few cases an effusion is the first manifestation of the disease (Melamed, 1963). The cytological appearance seen in the various forms of this group of diseases are described in detail by Melamed (1963) and also by Spriggs and Boddington (1968). The classification of lymphomas is based on their cellular features and the cytological morphology is well known to haematologists; it is therefore not surprising that malignancies of this type can be distinguished from epithelial tumours on the appearances of cells exfoliated into pleural fluid, and sometimes the type of lymphoma can be identified. Examination of air-dried Romanowsky stained smears is very helpful in such cases, particularly as these can be discussed with colleagues who are experienced in haematology.

Pleural Fluid in Benign Lesions of the Lung

Acute infection

Acute inflammatory effusions are seen commonly with pneumonia and may occur in patients with lobar collapse of the lung. The cellular exudate is pleomorphic: neutrophils, lymphocytes and macrophages predominate but mesothelial cells are also seen and in some cases eosinophils and basophils (Fig. 14). The neutrophils are well preserved. Lymphocytes are always present in moderate numbers and in the later stages may predominate. Eosinophils occur in some cases of postpneumonic effusions in relatively large numbers, particularly in cases of viral pneumonia. When an empyema

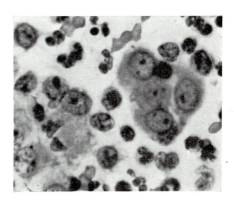

Figure 14 The cytological picture in a postpneumonic effusion. Benign active mesothelial cells are present which show prominent nucleoli. Pleural fluid. Papanicolaou's stain, × 800

is present almost all of the cells present are neutrophils and these show the typical degenerative changes seen in pus.

Tuberculous effusions

Tuberculous effusions are predominantly lymphocytic except in the earliest stages when neutrophil counts of 10 to 40 per cent may be found (Spriggs and Boddington, 1968). Absence of mesothelial cells is almost always a feature of tuberculous effusions because the mesothelium is destroyed, though the finding is not specifically restricted to tuberculosis. Lymphocytic effusions are also seen in cases with metastatic cancer but in these cases there is more likely to be profuse exfoliation of mesothelial cells. There is too much individual variation for this difference to be diagnostic but it can be useful in indicating the probable cause of an effusion.

Pulmonary infarction

The pleural effusion is often blood-stained and contains a high proportion of mesothelial cells. These can be present singly, in sheets, or in clusters and as they have prominent nucleoli and separation of nuclear chromatin they can cause difficulty in the differential diagnosis of cancer, particularly malignant mesothelioma (see below). The cytological picture in other respects resembles that seen in postpneumonic effusions.

Malignant Effusions

Primary carcinoma of lung

Bronchogenic carcinoma can cause obstruction and collapse of a lobe of the lung resulting in an inflammatory effusion. This is not strictly a malignant effusion although its primary cause is a neoplasm; in these cases malignant cells are not seen. A lung cancer which lies close to the pleura can produce a reactive effusion characterised by abundant exfoliation of mesothelial cells and lymphocytes. In some cases the lymphocytic reaction is very pronounced

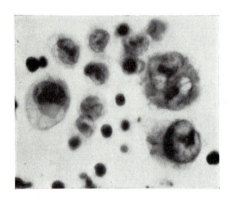

Figure 15   Single cells shed from squamous cell carcinoma. Primary tumour in the lung. Pleural fluid. Papanicolaou's stain, × 800

and immature forms are present which must be distinguished from blast cells in cases with lymphoma. A few malignant epithelial cells may be found as the tumour begins to ulcerate through the mesothelial lining. In other cases the lung tumour metastasises to the pleura and there may be a profuse exfoliation of malignant cells.

SQUAMOUS CELL CARCINOMA

It is seldom that pleural metastases from a squamous cell carcinoma exfoliate well differentiated keratinised squamous cells. It is more usual to see single cells with a central nucleus and a prominent nucleolus. The cytoplasm is basophilic with a sharp edge which may have a ring of small vacuoles at the periphery (Fig. 15). These cells must be distinguished from the very active mesothelial cells seen in cases with a pulmonary infarct and also from malignant mesothelial cells. The malignant features seen in the nucleus and the appearances of the cytoplasm help in the differential diagnosis; and in some cases the squamoid morphology can be recognised in tissue fragments seen on section of the cell block.

OAT CELL CARCINOMA

Spriggs (1954) found that this was the most common malignant cell to be seen in pleural effusions due to primary carcinoma of lung. When Papanicolaou's stain is used the cells appear as clusters of small cells with very scanty cytoplasm. The nuclei are usually larger than the nuclei of lymphocytes but the difference is very obvious when Romanowsky stained smears are examined. The large pink staining nuclei and the mosaic like effect are characteristic and quite unlike the appearance of lymphocytes (Fig. 16).

ADENOCARCINOMA

It is seldom possible to distinguish between a primary adenocarcinoma of lung which has metastasised to the pleura and metastatic adenocarcinoma

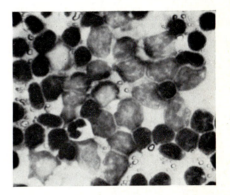

Figure 16 The central group of cells with paler nuclei are shed from an oat cell carcinoma and contrast well with the surrounding lymphocytes. Pleural fluid. Jenner Giemsa stain, × 800

from some other site when the exfoliated malignant cells are seen in pleural fluid. The appearances will be considered in the next section.

Pleural metastases from sites other than lung

Pleural metastases from other sites are much more frequent than pleural metastases from primary lung tumour. Ovary, uterus, breast and gastro-intestinal tract are common sources for the primary tumour and in all of these the lesion is most likely to be an adenocarcinoma; the exception is a squamous cell carcinoma of the cervix uteri. The cytological pattern is variable and includes acinar fragments (which may be vacuolated), papillary fragments and single cells. Occasionally there are features which give some indication of the primary tumour and the cell block may include tissue fragments which, on section, have a characteristic appearance seen in tissue morphology. Pleural metastases also occur from other tumours such as malignant melanoma, carcinoma of bladder and kidney, prostate gland, etc. For detailed descriptions reference should be made to *The Cytology of Effusions* by Spriggs and Boddington (1968).

3

Diffuse mesotheliomas

The association of malignant mesothelioma with exposure to asbestos was reported by Wagner, Sleggs and Marchand in 1960 and since then the International Agency for Research on Cancer has sponsored a Working Group which has studied this condition as well as the other biological effects of asbestos. Details of this work will be found in the Report and Recommendations of a Working Group on Asbestos and Cancer (1965) and Bogovski et al (1974).

Diagnosis by means of exfoliative cytology has been developed because of the poor results with needle core biopsy of the pleura and the frequency with which cases deteriorate after open biopsy. Koss (1968) describes the cytological findings in 43 cases but in none of them was the unequivocal primary diagnosis made on these grounds. Klempman (1962) considered that the diagnosis could be made on cell morphology and Naylor (1963) was of the same opinion. Butler and Berry (1974) compared the cytology of fluid from 48 cases of mesothelioma (collected in Britain and South Africa) with the cytology in cases of mesothelial reaction and metastatic carcinoma.

CYTOLOGICAL PATTERNS

Papillary pleomorphic: tissue fragments are seen with many rounded into morulae together with cells and groups of cells. There is considerable variation in cell size.

Papillary non-pleomorphic: there is profuse exfoliation of uniform small cells in tissue fragments and morulae with few single cells. This is the pattern which is usually described as characteristic of malignant mesothelioma.

A mixed pattern consisting of mesothelial type cells in sheets, chains, groups and as single cells.

Single cells: in these cases predominantly single cells are present with or without pleomorphism.

However, various forms of metastatic cancer can present with any of these patterns and mesothelial reaction can show a surprising degree of pleomorphism as well as exhibiting sheets of cells or morulae in addition to the more usual single cell pattern. Consequently the diagnosis is dependent on the morphological features of single cells.

BENIGN MESOTHELIAL CELLS

These are round or oval cells with one or more nuclei which can also be round or oval and centrally or almost centrally placed. The nuclear outline is regular and the nuclear chromatin is finely granular. Nucleoli are usually seen and these are also round or oval and regular in shape; they can be large and single or small and multiple. The cytoplasm is opaque and fades away at the periphery of the cell (Fig. 14).

MALIGNANT MESOTHELIAL CELLS

The nuclei show features characteristic of malignancy. The nuclear chromatin is irregular and coarsely granular. Nucleoli can be irregular in shape and large single nucleoli are often seen. The cytoplasmic differentiation is similar to that seen in the benign cell but the fading away at the periphery of the cell is exaggerated to a fine lace like vacuolation (Fig. 17).

DIFFERENTIAL DIAGNOSIS

The wide range of appearances which can be seen in cases with mesothelial reaction present the greatest diagnostic problem. Mesothelial reaction associated with pulmonary infarction can present with quite marked atypia of the mesothelial cells and the differential diagnosis depends on the presence or absence of malignant changes in the nucleus. It is unwise to make a diagnosis of malignant mesothelioma unless these are quite unequivocal

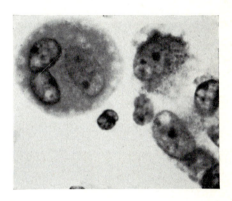

Figure 17   Malignant mesothelial cells. Compare with Figure 14. Papanicolaou's stain, × 800

Most cases of adenocarcinoma do not present a problem as they are characterised by vacuolated cytoplasm, obviously eccentric nuclei, or bizarrely shaped nuclei or macronucleoli, which are all features not seen in cells exfoliated from mesotheliomas. Difficulties are found with metastases from some ovarian carcinomas particularly papillary serous cystadenocarcinoma and mesonephroid carcinoma. Carcinoma of breast and some cases of squamous cell carcinoma can also present in fluid with patterns which resemble those seen in some cases of mesothelioma. Air-dried smears stained by the Romanowsky method can be useful in making the differential diagnosis as the cytoplasmic staining reaction in cell groups from a carcinoma does not usually have the clear deep blue colour seen in benign and malignant mesothelial cells. Examination of the cell block can also help as sections of tissue fragments may show characteristic morphology which can be more easily related to the tumour's histological appearances. Mucopolysaccharide and enzyme reactions are of little value in making a diagnosis of mesothelioma when cytological material is examined.

NON-EXFOLIATION

The histological pattern of mesotheliomas is so very variable it is not surprising that there is a range of exfoliative patterns. It seems probable that when there is a profuse exfoliation, the epithelial component of the tumour predominates, while a mainly stromal tumour will show poor exfoliation. It is very seldom that malignant stromal cells can be recognised in pleural fluid.

Failure of exfoliation also occurs in advanced cases as the tumour obliterates the pleural space.

REFERENCES

Bahrenburg, L. P. H. (1896) On the diagnostic results of the microscopical examination of the ascitic fluid in two cases of carcinoma of the peritoneum. *Cleveland Medical Gazette* **11**, 274 (quoted by Luse & Reagan, 1954).

Bamforth, J. (1966) *Cytological Diagnosis in Medical Practice*, p. 19. London: Churchill.

Beale, L. S. (1861) Examination of sputum from a case of cancer of the pharynx and adjacent parts. *Archives of Medicine*, **2**, 44–46.

Boddington, M. M., Spriggs, A. I., Morton, J. A. & Mowat, A. G. (1971) Cytodiagnosis of rheumatoid pleural effusions. *Journal of Clinical Pathology*, **24**, 95–106.

Bogovski, P., Gilson, J. C., Timbrell, V. & Wagner, J. C. (Ed.) (1974) *Biological Effects of Asbestos.* Lyons I.A.R.C. Scientific Publications No. 8.

Butler, E. B., Monahan, P. B. & Warrell, D. W. (1971) Kuper brush in the diagnosis of endometrial lesions. *Lancet*, **2**, 1390–1392.

Butler, E. B. & Berry, A. V. (1974) Diffuse mesotheliomas; diagnostic criteria using exfoliative cytology. In *Biological Effects of Asbestos*, ed. Bogovski, P. et al. Lyons I.A.R.C. Scientific Publications No. 8.

Carmichael, D. S. & Golding, D. N. (1967) Rheumatoid pleural effusion with 'R.A. cells' in the pleural fluid. *British Medical Journal*, **2**, 814.

Chodosh, S. & Medici, T. C. (1971) The bronchial epithelium in chronic bronchitis. I. Exfoliative cytology during stable, acute bacterial infection and recovery phases. *American Review of Respiratory Disease*, **104**, 888–898.

Dahlgren, S. E. & Nordenström, B. (1966) *Transthoracic Needle Biopsy*. Stockholm: Almqvist and Wiksell/Gebers Förlag AB; and Chicago: Year Book Medical Publications Inc.

Dahlgren, S. E. & Lind, B. (1972) Comparison between diagnostic results obtained by transthoracic needle biopsy and by sputum cytology. *Acta Cytologica*, **16**, 53–58.

Dudgeon, L. S. & Patrick, C. V. (1927) New method for rapid microscopical diagnosis of tumours with an account of 200 cases so examined. *British Journal of Surgery*, **15**, 250–261.

Dudgeon, L. S. & Wrigley, C. H. (1935) On demonstration of particles of malignant growth in sputum by means of wet-film method. *Journal of Laryngology and Otology*, **50**, 752–762.

Duguid, H. L. D. & Huish, D. W. (1963) Clinical evaluation of cytodiagnosis in bronchial carcinoma. *British Medical Journal*, **2**, 287–291.

Ehrlich, P. (1880) Beiträge zur Atiologie und Histologie pleuritischer Exsudate. *Charité-Annln*, **7**, 199 (quoted by Spriggs and Boddington (1968), p. 1).

Erozan, Y. S. & Frost, J. K. (1970) Cytopathologic diagnosis of cancer in pulmonary material: a critical histopathologic correlation. *Acta Cytologica*, **14**, 560–565.

Fennessy, J. J. (1968) Bronchial brushing and transbronchial forceps biopsy in the diagnosis of pulmonary lesions. *Diseases of the Chest*, **53**, 377–389.

Forrest, J. V. (1973) Bronchial brush biopsy in lung cavities. *Diagnostic Radiology*, **106**, 69–72.

Frost, J. K., Gupta, P. K., Erozan, Y. S., Carter, D., Hollander, D. H., Levin, M. L. & Ball, W. C. (1973) Pulmonary cytologic alterations in toxic environmental inhalation. *Human Pathology*, **4**, 521–536.

Fullmer, C. D. & Parrish, C. M. (1969) Pulmonary cytology. A diagnostic method for occult carcinoma. *Acta Cytologica*, **13**, 645–651.

Fullmer, C. D., Short, J. G., Allen, A. & Walker, K. (1969) Proposed classification for bronchial epithelial cell abnormalities in the category of dyskaryosis. *Acta Cytologica*, **13**, 459–471.

Grunze, H. (1958) Long-term cytology study of squamous metaplasia of bronchial mucosa. In *Transactions of the 6th Annual Meeting of the Inter-Society Cytology Council*, pp. 153–156 (quoted by Koss (1968) p. 311).

Grunze, H. (1973) Cytologic diagnosis of tumours of the chest. *Acta Cytologica*, **17**, 148–159.

Grzybowski, S. & Coy, P. (1970) Early diagnosis of carcinoma of the lung: simultaneous screening with chest x-ray and sputum cytology. *Cancer*, **25**, 113–120.

Hayata, Y., Oho, K., Ichiba, M., Goya, Y. & Hayashi, T. (1973) Percutaneous pulmonary puncture for cytologic diagnosis—its diagnostic value for small peripheral pulmonary carcinoma. *Acta Cytologica*, **17**, 469–475.

Hellendall, H. (1899) Ein Beitrag zur Diagnostik dur lungengeschwälste. *Zeitschrift für klinische Medizin*, **37**, 435–455.

Horder, T. J. (1909) Lung puncture: a new application of clinical pathology. *Lancet*, **2**, 1345–1346.

Ikeda, S. (1970) Flexible bronchofiberscope. *Annals of Otology, Rhinology and Laryngology*, **79**, 916–923.

Kelley, S., McGarry, P. & Hutson, Y. (1971) Atypical cells in pleural fluid characteristic of systemic lupus erythematosus. *Acta Cytologica*, **15**, 357–362.

Klempman, S. (1962) The exfoliative cytology of diffuse pleural mesothelioma. *Cancer*, **15**, 691–704.

Koss, L. G. (1968) *Diagnostic Cytology and its Histopathologic Bases*, 2nd edn, pp. 505–510. Philadelphia and Toronto: Lippincott.

Kuper, S. W. A., Stradling, P., Davis, J. & Shortridge, D. (1966) The use of soluble swabs in exfoliative cytology of the bronchus and hollow viscera. *Lancet*, **2**, 680–681.

Lange, E. & Høeg, K. (1972) Cytologic typing of lung cancer. *Acta Cytologica*, **16**, 327–330.

Langley, F. A. & Crompton, A. C. (1973) *Recent Results in Cancer Research*, **40**. *Epithelial Abnormalities of the Cervix Uteri*. Berlin: Springer-Verlag.

Lopes Cardozo, P., De Graaf, S., De Boer, M. J., Doesburg, N. & Kapsenberg, P. D. (1967) The results of cytology in 1000 patients with pulmonary malignancy. *Acta Cytologica*, **11**, 120–131.

Luse, S. A. & Reagan, J. W. (1954) A histological study of effusions. *Cancer*, **7**, 1155–1181.

Melamed, M. R. (1963) The cytological presentation of malignant lymphomas and related disease in effusions. *Cancer*, **16**, 413–431.

Naib, Z. M., Stewart, J. A., Dowdle, W. R., Casey, H. C., Marine, W. R. & Nahmias, A. J. (1968) Cytological features of viral respiratory tract infection. *Acta Cytologica*, **12**, 162–171.

Nasiell, M. (1965) Exfoliativ cytodiagnostik av lung cancer med särskild känsyn till tidy diagnos. *Särtryck ur Nordisk Medicin*, **74**, 740–742.

Nasiell, M. (1966) Metaplasia and atypical metaplasia in the bronchial epithelium: a histo-pathologic and cytopathologic study. *Acta Cytology*, **10**, 421–427.

Nasiell, M. (1967) Diagnosis of lung cancer by aspiration biopsy and a comparison between the method and exfoliative cytology. *Acta Cytologica*, **11**, 114–119.

Naylor, B. (1963) The exfoliative cytology of diffuse malignant mesothelioma. *Journal of Pathology and Bacteriology*, **86**, 293–298.

Naylor, B. & Railey, C. (1964) A pitfall in the cytodiagnosis of sputum in asthmatics. *Journal of Clinical Pathology*, **17**, 84–89.

Nosanchuk, J. S. & Naylor, B. (1968) A unique cytological picture in pleural fluid from patients with rheumatoid arthritis. *American Journal of Clinical Pathology*, **50**, 330–335.

Oswald, N. C., Hinson, K. F. W., Canti, G. & Miller, A. B. (1971) The diagnosis of primary lung cancer with special reference to sputum cytology. *Thorax*, **26**, 623–631.

Papanicolaou, G. N. (1956) Degenerative changes in ciliated cells exfoliating from the bronchial epithelium as a cytological criterion in the diagnosis of diseases of the lung. *New York State Journal of Medicine*, **56**, 2647–2650.

Papanicolaou, G. N. (1958) Cellular changes in the development of pulmonary cancer as revealed by cytology: a case report. *Acta unio internationalis contra cancrum (Louvain)*, **4**, 479–484.

Papanicolaou, G. N., Bridges, E. L. & Railey, C. (1961) Degeneration of the ciliated cells of bronchial epithelium (ciliocytophthoria) in its relation to pulmonary disease. *American Review of Respiratory Disease*, **83**, 641–659.

Quincke, H. (1882) Über die geformten Bestandteile von Transudaten. *Deutsches Archiv für Klinische Medizin*, **30**, 58 (quoted by Warthin (1897)).

Registrar General's Statistical Review, Pt. 1. Medical Tables, 1971.

Richardson, R. H., Zavala, D. C., Mukerjee, P. K. & Bedell, G. N. (1974) The use of fiberoptic bronchoscopy and brush biopsy in the diagnosis of suspected pulmonary malignancy. *American Review of Respiratory Disease*, **109**, 63–66.

Saccomanno, G., Archer, V. E., Auerbach, O., Saunders, R. P. & Brennan, L. M. (1974) Development of carcinoma of the lung as reflected in exfoliated cells. *Cancer*, **33**, 256–270

Smith, G. H., & Warrack, A. J. N. (1972) An evaluation of brush biopsy in the diagnosis of peripheral pulmonary lesions. *Thorax*, **27**, 631–635.

Spriggs, A. I. (1954) Malignant cells in serous effusions complicating bronchial carcinoma. *Thorax*, **9**, 26–34.

Spriggs, A. I. & Boddington, M. M. (1968) *The Cytology of Effusions*, 2nd edn. London: Heineman Medical Books.

Taplin, D. J. (1966) Malignant cells in sputum: a simple method of liquefying sputum. *Journal of Medical Laboratory Technology*, **23**, 252–255.

Wagner, J. C., Sleggs, C. A. & Marchand, P. (1960) Diffuse pleural mesothelioma and asbestos exposure in the North Western Cape Province. *British Journal of Industrial Medicine*, **17**, 260–271.

Walker, K. R. & Fullmer, C. D. (1970) Progress report on the study of respiratory spirals. *Acta Cytologica*, **14**, 396–398.

Warthin, A. S. (1897) The diagnosis of primary sarcoma of the pleura from cells found in the pleuritic exudate. *Medical News (New York)*, **71**, 489–494.

Warthin, A. S. (1931) Occurrence of numerous large giant cells in the tonsils and pharyngeal mucosa in the prodromal stage of measles. Report of four cases. *Archives of Pathology*, **11**, 864–874.

Widal & Ravaut (1900) Applications cliniques de l'étude histologique des épanchements séro-fibrineux de la plèvre. *Compte rendu des séances de la Societé de Biologie*, **52**, 648, 651, 653 (quoted by Spriggs and Boddington (1968), p. 1).

Working Group on Asbestos and Cancer. Convened under the auspices of the Geographical Pathology Section of the International Union Against Cancer (1965) *Annals of New York Academy of Science*, 132.

3

PATHOLOGY OF THE LUNG

Donald Heath

During the past decade there have been several advances that have greatly influenced our approach to pulmonary pathology. I shall try to show how some have furthered our understanding of cardiorespiratory disease.

ELECTRON MICROSCOPY

In only a few years the electron microscope has changed from being a novelty into an essential item of equipment for the comprehensive assessment of the morbid anatomy of many disease processes. Chest diseases are no exception to this and studies of the ultrastructure of the lung have given a new insight into many cardiorespiratory disorders. Not so long ago it was still possible to debate whether the lung has an epithelial lining at all. Now it has become clear that there is a whole group of hitherto unfamiliar types of cell that line the alveolar spaces and the bronchial tree which have their role to play in various disease states. They may be identified with precision by means of electron microscopy and in some instances they may be recognised on light microscopy too. Already we know a great deal about the ultrastructure of these various types of cell but there is still much to be learned about their function. Increasingly it becomes necessary to review the pathology of different chest diseases in terms of the activity and behaviour of these newly prominent cells. Thus an up to date appreciation of much pulmonary disease demands familiarity with the membranous pneumocyte, the granular pneumocyte, the alveolar brush cell, the Feyrter cell, the Clara cell and the pulmonary mast cell. It is no longer adequate to regard all cells with copious cytoplasm lying free in alveolar spaces as 'pulmonary macrophages' and, as we shall see below, apparently uninteresting amorphous eosinophilic material in alveoli may yield fascinating information on electron microscopy.

The membranous pneumocyte
Most of the normal alveolar wall is covered by smooth, ultrathin extensions of membranous (type I) pneumocytes (Fig. 1). The nuclei of these cells are commonly situated in the corners and angles of alveoli with scanty small mitochondria and a little endoplasmic reticulum around them. Because of their large area and paucity of organelles, the squamous cytoplasmic exten-

sions of membranous pneumocytes seem to be metabolically dependent on the central perinuclear portion of the cells where the organelles are located, and thus quite vulnerable to a variety of injuries. The membranous pneumocyte appears to react in one of two ways in pathological processes. First, it may be destroyed by toxic substances such as paraquat, the weed-killer.

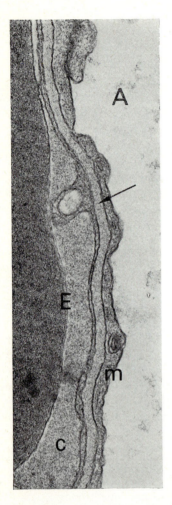

Figure 1   Electron micrograph of an alveolar wall in a Wistar albino rat. Its fused basement membrane (arrow) is covered on its alveolar aspect (A) by the thin cytoplasmic extension of a membranous pneumocyte (m). The inner aspect of the basement membrane is lined by the thin cytoplasm of an endothelial cell, lining a pulmonary capillary (c). The capillary contains an erythrocyte (E). Glutaraldehyde-osmic acid, × 45 000

Second, it may show intracytoplasmic oedema due to toxic or haemodynamic effects on the lung. Within 4 h of the administration of paraquat to rats there is an increase in the thickness of the cytoplasmic extensions of membranous pneumocytes (Smith and Heath, 1974a). Intracytoplasmic oedema becomes obvious within 8 h and 10 h later the membranous pneumocytes show a remarkable appearance with grossly cystic, oedematous cytoplasm which bulges into the alveolar space (Fig. 2). Two days after administration the

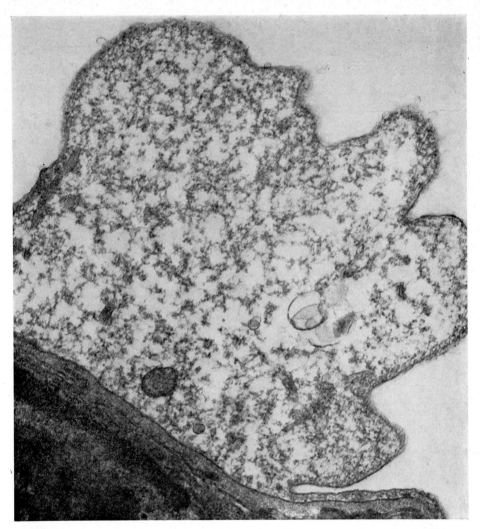

Figure 2 Electron micrograph of a membranous (type I) pneumocyte from a female Wistar albino rat showing gross intracytoplasmic oedema causing the cell to bulge into the alveolar space. The animal had been given a single intraperitoneal injection of 40 mg paraquat ion per kilogram body weight. Glutaraldehyde-osmic acid, × 33 750

cells have been destroyed leaving only small islands of surviving membranous pneumocytes to be engulfed by the subsequent progressive fibrosis.

Membranous pneumocytes normally show a certain degree of micropino-cytosis ('cell drinking' in which globules appear to be transported through the cytoplasm of the cell from one cell border). This micropinocytotic activity in membranous pneumocytes may be increased when the lung becomes oedematous irrespective of the basis for the oedema. Hence it occurs in rats

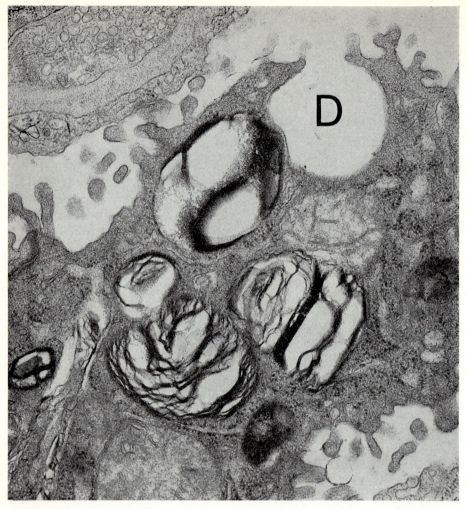

Figure 3 Granular (type II) pneumocyte of a rat exposed to a reduced barometric pressure of 265 mmHg for 12 h. The cell has a convex surface covered by short microvilli which project into the alveolar space. Prominent lamellar bodies are present within the cytoplasm. There is a flask-shaped depression (D) in the cell surface which marks the probable point of discharge of pulmonary surfactant into the alveolar space. Glutaraldehyde-osmic acid, × 33 750

poisoned with *Crotalaria spectabilis* seeds (Kay, Smith and Heath, 1969), in patients with mitral stenosis (Kay and Edwards, 1973), and in high altitude pulmonary oedema (Heath, Moosavi and Smith, 1973).

The granular pneumocyte

In striking contrast to the relatively quiescent membranous pneumocytes are the granular pneumocytes which undergo the most pronounced hyperplasia and shedding into the alveolar spaces under a variety of conditions. The granular (type II) pneumocytes are interposed between the flat membranous pneumocytes and unlike them do not have squamous extensions. The flat basal portion of the cell is attached to the underlying basement membrane of the blood–air barrier while the free convex surface of the cell projects into the alveolar space (Fig. 3). This free, curved surface of the granular pneumocyte is covered by microvilli which are short, straight and fairly regular. Within the abundant cytoplasm are prominent lamellar bodies which are considered by some to be the source of pulmonary surfactant (Fig. 3). Big mitochondria are present and they have branched and sharply kinked cristae. A well-developed rough endoplasmic reticulum is present. Granular pneumocytes have a much greater capacity for division and a shorter turnover time than membranous pneumocytes, and probably represent the reserve cells of the alveolar lining epithelium. They proliferate and replace membranous pneumocytes when the latter are destroyed. Thus, hyperplasia of granular pneumocytes can occur in a wide variety of circumstances and appears to be a basic mechanism of repair (Kapanci et al, 1969).

DESQUAMATIVE INTERSTITIAL PNEUMONIA

The granular pneumocyte made a prominent entrance into the field of thoracic pathology with the description of 'desquamative interstitial pneumonia' by Liebow, Steer and Billingsley in 1965. On the basis of 18 cases these authors described what they regarded as a distinctive type of interstitial pneumonia. It was characterised by an extensive desquamation of masses of 'large alveolar cells' which proliferated actively both in the walls and lumens of alveoli (Fig. 4). These cells contained brown granules which gave a positive staining reaction with the periodic acid Schiff technique but not for iron. Minute lymphoid follicles accumulated in the periphery of the lung. Necrosis, hyaline membranes and exudates of fibrin were absent. Most of the alveolar spaces were packed with the large cells so that the histological picture was uniform and monotonous. Giant cells were occasionally seen in alveoli (Fig. 5). Liebow and his colleagues believed that this condition of 'DIP', as it has come to be called, was characterised by an apparently good response to steroid therapy, usually with stabilisation, and sometimes by remission of clinical symptoms and radiological changes. We had the opportunity of studying the electron microscopy of a case of desquamative interstitial pneumonia and found the intra-alveolar cells to consist of granular pneumocytes and macrophages (Brewer, Heath and Asquith, 1969). The same combination of cells was reported by Shortland, Darke and Crane (1969).

There is no doubt that 'DIP' presents a striking histological picture that merits its recognition by the histopathologist. However, there seems to be little evidence to support the view of Liebow and his colleagues that it represents a distinct pathological entity (see also Chapter 7). From the outset Scadding and Hinson (1967) were very sceptical about recognising 'DIP' as such. In their view it was premature to conclude that because a recognisable variant of the basic histological pattern of interstitial pneumonia shows some correlation with clinical and radiological features it characterises a pathogenetically distinct subgroup. They regarded 'DIP' as a desquamative type of fibrosing alveolitis, representing the cellular extreme of the spectrum of histological changes to be found in this disease. The contrasting situation of classical diffuse interstitial fibrosis represents the other and commoner extreme, which Scadding and Hinson (1967) called the mural type of fibrosing alveolitis.

Sufficient time has now elapsed to follow up the subsequent course of patients diagnosed as having 'desquamative interstitial pneumonia' soon after

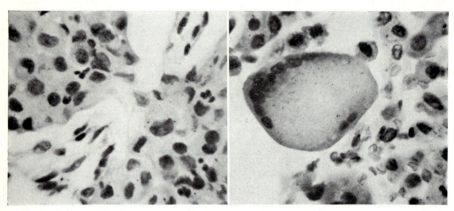

Figure 4   *Figure 5*

Figure 4   Intra-alveolar cells in a case of desquamative interstitial pneumonia in a man of 34 years. They form a syncytium in the alveoli and in this instance effect communication through a Cohn's pore. Haematoxylin and eosin

Figure 5   A giant cell, probably formed by the fusion of intra-alveolar cells from the same case of 'desquamative interstitial pneumonia' illustrated in Figure 4. Haematoxylin and eosin

the condition was described by Liebow and his associates. The man whose case we reported in 1969 (Brewer et al) died and at necropsy was found to have fibrosing alveolitis which had progressed to honeycomb lung (McCann and Brewer, 1974). This course of events supports the view of Scadding and Hinson (1967) that DIP is merely the early cellular stage of fibrosing alveolitis. The same view is now accepted by Patchefsky et al (1973) after a follow-up of cases they originally diagnosed as having desquamative interstitial pneumonia. Some of these patients subsequently developed honeycomb lung.

Alveolar brush cell

This cell, also called the type III pneumocyte, is infrequently seen because it comprises only 5 per cent of the total pneumocyte number (Meyrick and

Reid, 1970). It is shaped like a truncated pyramid, the base situated on the basement membrane and the tip protruding above the surrounding epithelial surface: the lateral aspects are covered by adjacent membranous or granular pneumocytes. Its most striking feature is the large regular microvilli which clothe its relatively small free surface. These microvilli are twice as thick as those of the granular pneumocyte, have a flat end, and contain numerous fine filaments which extend down into the cell body, below the nucleus, to the basement membrane. The alveolar brush cell is unique among the pneumocytes because it contains abundant glycogen granules, suggesting that metabolism can occur at low oxygen tensions (Meyrick and Reid, 1970). Glycogen is abundant in all fetal cells; the alveolar brush cell is not identified until the eighth week of postnatal life. This cell resembles brush cells found in the epithelium of conducting airways and in many other epithelia such as the gall bladder which have been shown to have neuronal connections. The existence of such neuronal connections has been suspected but not definitely established in alveolar brush cells (Weibel, 1973). Further research is needed before a function can be ascribed to this cell, but it is tempting to postulate that it may serve as a receptor because its ultrastructural features are similar to those of the chemoreceptor cell in taste buds (Meyrick and Reid, 1968; Weibel, 1973).

Hypoxia and the Chemoreceptor System

One of the common serious complications of respiratory disease is hypoxia and since this is monitored by the chemoreceptor tissues one would imagine that those interested in respiratory pathology would be very knowledgeable on the histopathology of the chemoreceptor system especially the carotid bodies. In fact morbid anatomists have largely ignored the carotid bodies, restricting their attention to the tumour of chemoreceptor tissue, the chemo-dectoma. This is unsatisfactory since, if an important functional disturbance produced by chest disease exerts one of its major effects outside the anatomical confines of the thorax it is there that the pathologist interested in respiratory disease must look. Advances in thoracic pathology are not confined to the thorax.

In fact one of the most interesting observations in morbid anatomy relating to thoracic disease of the last 10 years was made by Arias-Stella in 1969 when he reported that the carotid bodies of Quechua Indians born and living at high altitudes in the Peruvian Andes (Fig. 6) were larger than those of mestizos living on the coastal plain (Figs. 7, 8). Presumably the enlargement was a response to the chronic hypoxia produced by the diminished barometric pressure. Subsequent studies showed that the carotid bodies of animals indigenous to high altitudes were also enlarged and that the increase in size was due to a hyperplasia of the light variant of chief cell (Edwards et al, 1971). Interestingly enough a similar enlargement of the carotid bodies occurs in patients with emphysema complicated by hypoxia and right ventricular hypertrophy (Edwards, Heath and Harris, 1971). Characteristic ultrastructural changes occur in the carotid bodies of animals living at high altitude and exposed to chronic hypoxia on this account. They consist of vacuolation of the so-called catecholamine bodies within the cytoplasm of the chief cells so that the central osmiophilic core becomes smaller, less dense and excentric (Edwards, Heath and Harris, 1972). The functional significance of this ultrastructural change is as yet unknown. It may represent the damag-

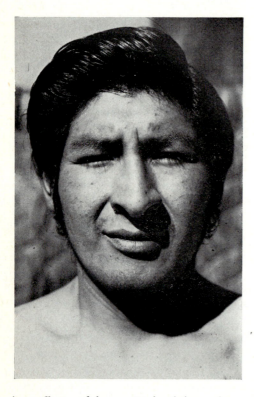

Figure 6 A young Peruvian Indian, Fernando, who was born and lived all his life at Cerro de Pasco, a mining town situated 14 250 ft above sea level in the Andes

ing effects of long-sustained hypoxia on chemoreceptor cells or even the secretion of some hormone from the carotid body under the hypoxic stimulus.

Not all chemoreceptor tissue lies outside the lung. There is a nodule of glomic tissue situated in the adventitia of the bifurcation of the pulmonary trunk (Edwards and Heath, 1969). This is regarded by Krahl (1960) as the true chemoreceptor of the sixth branchial arch, the 'glomus pulmonale' being supplied by, and monitoring blood from, the pulmonary trunk. We disagree with his view for our findings in rats and human newborns (Edwards and Heath, 1970) support the alternative opinion of Becker (1966) that this nodule of glomic tissue is merely one of the aorticopulmonary bodies supplied by blood from an intertruncal branch of a coronary artery. In other words we believe the 'glomus pulmonale' to be topographically but not functionally related to the pulmonary trunk.

Glomic tissue is also to be found occasionally around small pulmonary venules (Korn et al, 1960; Edwards and Heath, 1972) but its functional importance is not yet established. There have been no studies so far as I am aware of the reaction of the 'glomus pulmonale' and pulmonary venous glomic tissue to chronic hypoxia.

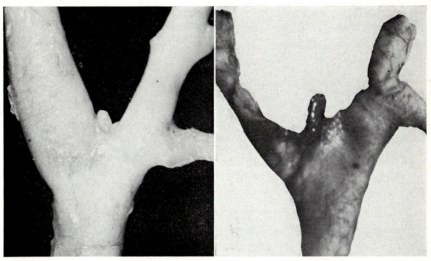

Figure 7   *Figure 8*

Figure 7   Normal left carotid body in a man of 50 years with polycystic disease of the kidneys who was born and lived all his life at sea level. The carotid body is situated at the bifurcation of the common carotid artery . It was normal in size and weight (6.9 mg). × 2.4

Figure 8   Enlarged left carotid body in a Quechua Indian who was born and lived all his life at Cerro de Pasco, a mining town situated 14 250 ft above sea level in the Peruvian Andes. × 2.4. (From a slide kindly provided by Professor Javier Arias-Stella)

The Feyrter cell

In addition to these chemoreceptor cells in the lung there are argyrophilic cells within the bronchial epithelium which bear a close ultrastructural resemblance to the chief cell of the carotid body (Lauweryns and Peuskens, 1969; Lauweryns, Peuskens and Cokelaere, 1970) (Fig. 9). In rats these so-called Feyrter cells moreover show the same ultrastructural changes in their intracytoplasmic vesicles on exposure to chronic hypoxia (Moosavi, Smith and Heath, 1973) (Fig. 10). It is conceivable that these cells act as airway chemoreceptors. On electron microscopy they have all the features of APUD (*a*mine *p*recursor *u*ptake and *d*ecarboxylation) cells, many of which are associated with the secretion of polypeptide hormones. It is conceivable that they too may have an endocrine function. Pearse (1969) has

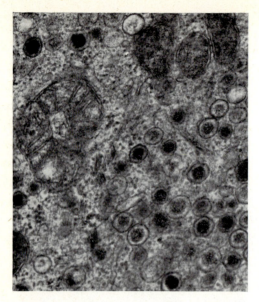

Figure 9   Catecholamine bodies within a bronchial argyrophilic (Feyrter) cell from a neonatal rat five days old. Each body consists of a central osmiophilic core, a narrow surrounding lighter halo, and an outer limiting membrane. Glutaraldehyde-osmic acid, × 45 000

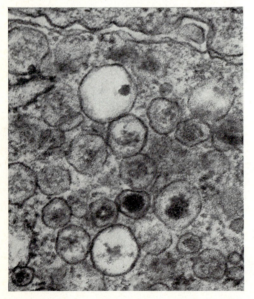

Figure 10   Catecholamine bodies within a bronchial argyrophilic (Feyrter) cell from a hypoxic rat subject to simulated high altitude in a hypobaric chamber for five days. The bodies show the same changes as are found in the chief cells of the carotid body in states of chronic hypoxia. The central core becomes small and excentric in some catecholamine bodies. In others it becomes less dense and granular and is eventually lost so that a microvacuole results. Glutaraldehyde-osmic acid, × 67 500. (By permission of the Editor of *Thorax*)

tentatively named this hypothetical hormone 'pneumokinin' but does not advance any view as to its possible action. It has been postulated that bronchial argyrophilic cells like argentaffin cells may produce amines such as histamine, catecholamines and the kinin-generating system (Lauweryns and Peuskens, 1969). These authors believe that such compounds might be of importance in dilating the pulmonary arterial musculature of the fetus, thus aiding adaptation to neonatal life. Certainly the number of Feyrter cells in bronchial epithelium falls away rapidly in the neonatal period. It is clear from what has been said that we have barely started to understand the role played by the Feyrter cell in cardiorespiratory disease.

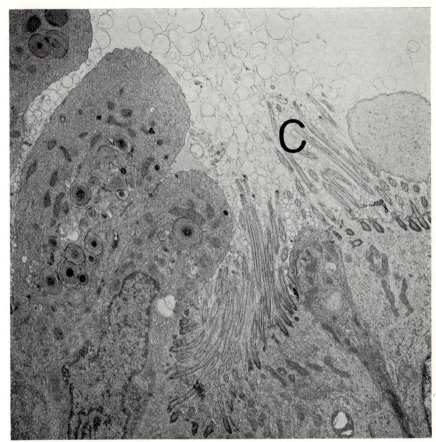

Figure 11 Electron micrograph of bronchiolar cells from a Sprague Dawley rat treated with chlorphentermine. Those to the right are respiratory epithelial cells and have cilia (C) projecting from their luminal surface. The cells to the left are Clara cells and contain lamellar inclusions. This figure illustrates the value of electron microscopy in the study of respiratory disease processes by precise identification of the cells involved and of the processes within their cytoplasm. Glutaraldehyde-osmic acid, × 6750. (By permission of the Editor of *Thorax*)

The Clara cell

Scattered among the familiar ciliated respiratory epithelial cells in the bronchi and especially in the respiratory bronchioles are the non-ciliated Clara cells (Fig. 11). The Clara cell has all the features of a secretory cell, the product of secretion accumulating within smooth cisternae at the apex of the cell (Smith, Heath and Moosavi, 1974). The apical region is then extruded into the bronchiolar lumen in a process of apocrine secretion. Acute hypoxia accelerates this secretion in adult rats but has little effect upon neonatal rats. Administration of chlorphentermine induces a hyperplasia of

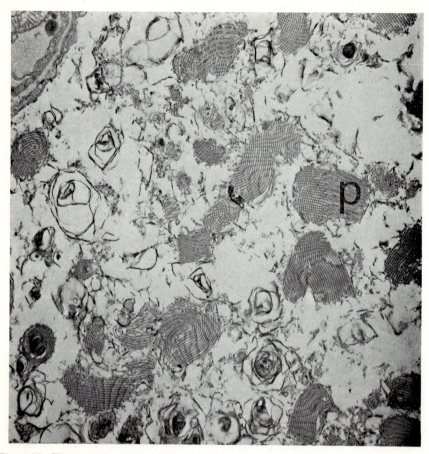

Figure 12 Electron micrograph of alveolar debris from a Sprague Dawley rat treated with chlorphentermine. It consists of lamellar material derived from Clara cells and granular pneumocytes, and phospholipid lattices (p). This figure illustrates how the ultrastructure of alveolar contents, apparently amorphous and featureless on light microscopy, may reveal components which help to elucidate the nature of the disease under investigation. Glutaraldehyde-osmic acid, ×11 250. (By permission of the Editor of *Thorax*)

Clara cells which is associated with the presence of large quantities of phospholipid within the alveolar spaces (Fig. 12) and in macrophages (Smith et al, 1974). The Clara cells also contain accumulations of what appear to be phospholipid (Fig. 11). This suggests the possibility that these cells secrete a phospholipid pulmonary surfactant. The granular pneumocyte may also produce pulmonary surfactant, perhaps of a different chemical nature, since like the Clara cell it will take up labelled palmitic acid, a precursor of the phospholipid pulmonary surfactant.

Lung mast cells and hypoxic pulmonary hypertension

In 1946 von Euler and Liljestrand suggested that the pulmonary vasculature constricts in response to hypoxia. Although these workers concluded that the effect was due to a direct action of hypoxia on the vessel walls, the local mechanism of hypoxic pulmonary hypertension has been the subject of considerable debate, and continues to be elusive. The greater pulmonary vasoconstrictor activity of extravascular alveolar hypoxia as contrasted with intravascular hypoxaemia favours an indirect mechanism of hypoxic pulmonary vasoconstriction (Reeves et al, 1962), and recent evidence suggests that

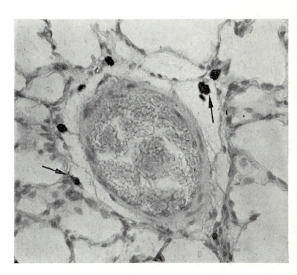

Figure 13 Transverse section of muscular pulmonary artery of rat. The vessel is entirely surrounded by alveoli. Portions of seven darkly stained mast cells (two indicated by arrows) are shown in perivascular tissue between alveolar walls and muscular media of pulmonary artery. Note the close relation of mast cells to both alveolar air and vascular smooth muscle. Metachromatic blue stain, × 340

histamine may act as a chemical mediator in this reaction (Hauge, 1968; Hauge and Melmon, 1968). In the lung, most of the histamine is stored in mast cells which are located predominantly in the perivascular and peribronchial connective tissues. Data showing that alveolar hypoxia is a more potent vasoconstrictor stimulus than pulmonary arterial hypoxaemia are consistent with the idea that there is a peripheral chemoreceptor located in close proximity to both pulmonary blood vessels and distal airways. Bergofsky (1969) has suggested that this chemoreceptor could be the perivascular lung mast cell (Fig. 13) which is an ideal anatomical situation to monitor alveolar oxygen tension and respond to hypoxia by releasing histamine which could then mediate pulmonary vasoconstriction. In support of this hypothesis, Haas and Bergofsky (1972) have shown that pulmonary arteries 50 to 500 μm in diameter in the rat have a predictable distribution of perivascular mast cells, and that such mast cells are degranulated in vivo during acute alveolar hypoxia. They also showed that hypoxia releases histamine from mast cells isolated from the peritoneal cavity without injuring them. It was further demonstrated that histamine is released from the lungs of intact guinea-pigs during alveolar hypoxia, and that the increase in pulmonary vascular resistance was proportional to the amount of histamine released. Further support for this hypothesis has been provided by Grover and Kay (1972) who investigated the effect of sodium cromoglycate (SCG) on acute hypoxic pulmonary hypertension in dogs. SCG has the unusual property of inhibiting the release of histamine from mast cells which is basis for its clinical use in the treatment of asthma and other allergic conditions (Cox, 1971). It was found that if suitably reactive dogs were premedicated with SCG, they failed to increase their pulmonary vascular resistance while spontaneously breathing a hypoxic gas mixture which diminished their systemic arterial oxygen tension to less than 40 mmHg.

Kay, Waymire and Grover (1974) have studied the role of lung mast cells and histamine in chronic hypoxic pulmonary hypertension in rats. Histamine is present in the lung in a preformed state, but it can also be produced as needed by enzyme induction of specific histidine decarboxylase leading to an increase in the histamine-forming capacity (HFC) of the tissue. In the case of acute hypoxic pulmonary vasoconstriction, the time course is rapid and compatible with the time course expected for the release of histamine stored in mast cells. If prolonged histamine release played a part in the development of chronic hypoxic pulmonary hypertension, it might be expected that this would necessitate an increase in the HFC of lung tissue. If the source of the released histamine were mast cells, then an increase in the HFC might be achieved either by enzyme induction in each individual mast cell, their number in the lung remaining unchanged, or by a proliferation of perivascular mast cells. The lung mast cell density was measured in the right lung and the HFC determined in the left lung of a group of eight rats confined for 20 days in a decompression chamber evacuated to a pressure of 380 mmHg. The results were compared with those obtained from a group of nine untreated control animals. A proliferation of mast cells occurred in the lungs of the chronically hypoxic rats so that in six of the eight animals the total lung mast cell count either equalled or greatly exceeded the highest figure in the control rats. The mean lung mast cell density in the hypoxic rats was $7.65 \pm 1.23/mm^2$ compared with a figure of $2.97 \pm 0.48/mm^2$ in the controls. There was a linear logarithmic relation between the right ventricular weight and lung mast cell density in the control and hypoxic rats (Fig. 14). These results are consistent with the hypothesis that lung mast cell proliferation is concerned with the development of chronic hypoxic pulmonary hypertension. However, the mean pulmonary HFC in the hypoxic rats did not differ significantly from that in the controls, and there was no apparent relation between the mast cell density in the right lung and the HFC of the left lung. These findings suggest that the major component of the total pulmonary HFC is located outside mast cells. Even though the number of mast cells in the hypoxic group of animals was doubled, any resultant increase in HFC attributable to these cells was masked by the predominant extramast cell component and was insufficient to produce a measurable change in the total lung HFC.

The present state of knowledge may be summarised by saying that alveolar hypoxia probably elicits pulmonary vasoconstriction through the mediation of a humoral substance released from the lung parenchyma. The available evidence suggests that this chemical mediator is histamine, and that it is released from perivascular mast cells which function as chemoreceptors and monitor oxygen tension in the distal airways. Thus mast cells and histamine may have important effects on the local regulation of blood flow in the lung

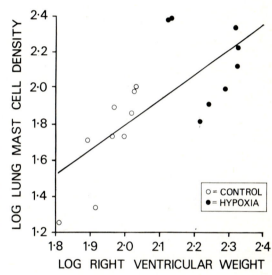

Figure 14 The relation between the logarithm of the total number of mast cells counted in 20.48 mm² lung, and the logarithm of the right ventricular weight (mg) in control and chronically hypoxic rats. $r=0.8716$, $P<0.001$. (By permission of the Editor of *The Journal of Physiology*)

where there is alveolar hypoxia. Consideration of the implication of these ideas may suggest new therapeutic approaches to the treatment of patients with pulmonary hypertension and cardiac failure complicating chronic bronchitis and emphysema.

The alveolar–capillary wall and pulmonary oedema

In the past, conventional teaching based on light microscopy has described pulmonary oedema in terms of an extravasation of plasma filtrate from the pulmonary capillaries directly across a simple membrane into the alveolar spaces. However, recent ultrastructural studies have revealed that the barrier between pulmonary capillary blood and alveolar gas is more complicated than histologists suspected, and that alveolar oedema is a late and not invariable manifestation of the excessive accumulation of water and plasma solutes in the lung.

The ultrastructural appearance of the alveolar septum in man is shown in Figure 15. The capillary blood is separated from alveolar air by three distinct anatomical layers: capillary endothelium; a narrow interstitial zone; and alveolar epithelium. The alveolar capillaries are lined by the thin cytoplasmic extensions of endothelial cells which contain few organelles apart from numerous small pinocytic vesicles bounded by a membrane identical to the cell membrane. Some of these vesicles communicate with the surfaces of the endothelial cell to form small flask-shaped indentations or caveolae. Normal alveolar capillary endothelial cells are not fenestrated. They abut bluntly or overlap so that a narrow cleft of variable size exists between adjacent cells. In the narrowest portion of the cleft, the adjacent cell membranes fuse

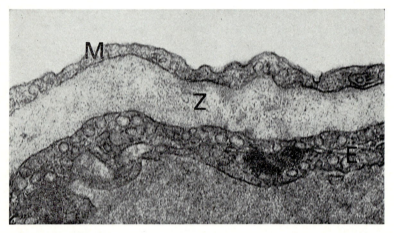

Figure 15   The thinnest portion of the alveolar–capillary wall in a normal human lung. The capillary endothelial cell (E) is separated from the membranous pneumocyte (M) by an amorphous granular zone (Z) consisting of their fused basement membranes. Glutaraldehyde-osmic acid, ×45 000. (By permission of the Editor of *The Journal of Pathology*)

(maculae occludentes) except for small slits 40 Å wide which allow communication between the capillary lumen and extravascular space (Schneeberger-Keeley and Karnovsky, 1968). Sandwiched between the capillary endothelium and alveolar epithelium is an interstitial zone of variable width. Over the convexities of the capillaries protruding into the alveoli, there is no true interstitial space because the contact surface between the endothelium and epithelium is formed exclusively by the fused basement membranes of these two cell layers. In other regions, the epithelial and endothelial basement membranes are separated by an interstitial space containing fine elastic fibres, bundles of collagen fibrils, fibroblasts and macrophages. The alveolar septa are devoid of lymphatics which first appear in the interstitial space surrounding terminal bronchioles, small arteries and veins. Over 95 per cent of the area of the alveolar walls is lined by the thin, extensive membranous pneumocytes. The cytoplasm of these epithelial cells closely resemble that of the subjacent endothelial cells: small membrane-bound vesicles are present, but other organelles are very scanty. The margins of adjacent membranous or granular pneumocytes abut bluntly or overlap with the formation of narrow clefts. However, unlike the endothelial cell junctions which allow some continuity of intravascular and extravascular spaces, the clefts between adjacent epithelial cells are obliterated by fusion of opposing cell membranes forming tight junctions or zonulae occludentes.

A great difference in the permeability of the epithelial and endothelial cell components of the alveolar–capillary wall has been demonstrated in ultrastructural studies using the electron-dense markers horseradish peroxidase (molecular weight 40 000; diameter 40 Å) and haemoglobin (molecular weight 64 500; diameter 65 Å). When Schneeberger-Keeley and Karnovsky (1968) injected the enzyme into mice intravenously, it passed through the endothelial cell junctions into the underlying basement membrane, but was prevented from entering the alveolar space by zonulae occludentes between membranous pneumocytes. Horseradish peroxidase was demonstrated in pinocytic vesicles of both endothelial and epithelial cells, but the role of these vesicles in net protein transport appeared to be minimal. Szidon, Pietra and Fishman (1972) examined the influence of capillary intraluminal pressure on the movement of macromolecules across the alveolar–capillary wall in an isolated dog lung preparation perfused in vivo with solutions of horseradish peroxidase or haemoglobin. When perfusion pressure was kept at near-normal levels (15–20 mmHg), neither horseradish peroxidase nor haemoglobin escaped from the capillaries. When the perfusion pressures were raised (peroxidase 30, and haemoglobin 40 mmHg) to induce pulmonary oedema, both tracers escaped through interendothelial junctions to enter the interstitial space of the alveolar septum. The tight junctions between the membranous pneumocytes prevented the entrance of tracers into the alveolar space. Only when the perfusion pressure exceeded 50 mmHg did leakage occur through epithelial cell junctions. These experiments showed that the permeability of interendothelial junctions is dependent on intraluminal pressure and that alveolar epithelium rather than capillary endothelium is the critical barrier to the entry of water and solutes into the alveolar spaces. Increased intravascular pressures seemed to widen the calibre of the pores between the endothelial cells and thus increase capillary permeability.

The distribution of interstitial oedema fluid in the alveolar septum appears to depend on whether pulmonary oedema is produced by haemodynamic changes or by the action of toxic substances on the alveolar–capillary wall (Cottrell et al, 1967). In haemodynamic pulmonary oedema, such as may occur in patients with mitral stenosis, the fluid is restricted to the collagen-containing portions of the alveolar wall (Fig. 16). It does not accumulate in the thinnest portions of the blood–air pathway over the convexities of the alveolar capillaries where there is fusion of the basement membranes of

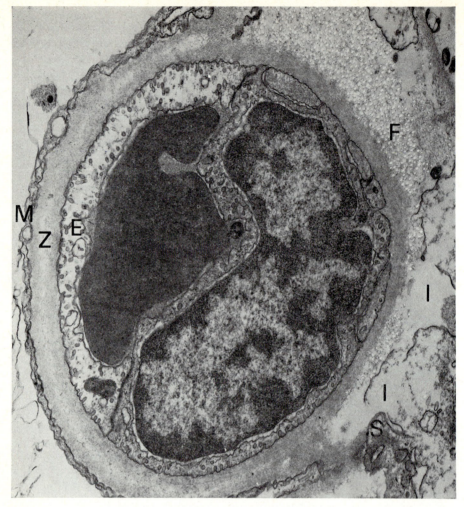

Figure 16 Interstitial oedema of the collagen-containing portion of the alveolar wall in mitral stenosis. Lucent areas of oedema (l), separate septal cell (S), and connective tissue fibrils (F). The thin granular, non-collagen-containing amorphous zone (Z), which separates membranous pneumocyte (M) from endothelial cell (E) over convexity of capillary, is not oedematous. Glutaraldehyde-osmic acid, ×16 875. (By permission of the Editor of *The Journal of Pathology*)

membranous pneumocytes and subjacent endothelial cells (Kay and Edwards, 1973). Toxic pulmonary oedema may be produced experimentally by the systemic administration of toxic substances such as monocrotaline (Kay et al, 1969), ammonium sulphate (Hayes and Shiga, 1970), and alpha-naphthyl-thiourea (Meyrick, Miller and Reid, 1972). It may also occur after the inhalation of ether (Finlay-Jones, Robertson and Walters, 1971) and in the acid pulmonary aspiration (Mendelson's) syndrome (Alexander, 1968). In toxic pulmonary oedema, there may be degeneration of both membranous pneumocytes and capillary endothelial cells. Fluid accumulates in the thinnest convex portion of the alveolar–capillary wall leading to detachment of the endothelial cell from the basement membrane. This causes the formation of endothelial blebs or vesicles which protrude into the capillary lumen and partially occlude it (Fig. 17). Haemodynamic pulmonary oedema appears to result from an accentuation of the normal process of fluid exchange within the lung whereas toxic pulmonary oedema is a purely pathological process.

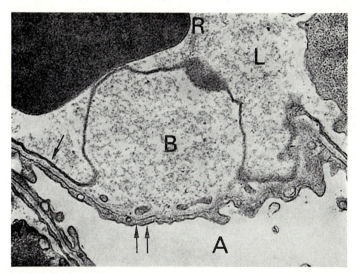

Figure 17 Toxic interstitial pulmonary oedema in a rat with pulmonary hypertension induced by feeding *Crotalaria spectabilis* seeds which contain the pyrrolizidine alkaloid monocrotaline. The endothelial cell (arrow) has been elevated from the basement membrane by interstitial oedema to form a bleb (B) which protrudes into the capillary lumen (L) containing an erythrocyte (R). The alveolar space (A) is lined by a membranous pneumocyte (two arrows). Glutaraldehyde-osmic acid, ×16 875

Ultrastructural studies of the early phases of haemodynamic pulmonary oedema in dogs have shown that fluid first accumulates in the collagen-containing portions of the alveolar septum, and that this stage of interstitial oedema is undetectable with conventional light microscopy (Cottrell et al, 1967). The earliest histological evidence of pulmonary oedema is seen in the connective tissue surrounding small bronchioles and blood vessels. Widening of the alveolar walls as visualised with the light microscope is a late and severe manifestation of excess water in the lungs. During the early phase of pulmonary oedema, excess water is rapidly transferred from the collagen-containing portion of the alveolar septa to the lymphatic channels surrounding small blood vessels and bronchioles. The classical histological picture of eosinophilic coagulum in the alveolar spaces is a late sequel to excess water accumulation in the lungs. Unfortunately, the early interstitial phase of pulmonary oedema is difficult to recognise both histologically and clinically. Abnormalities in gaseous exchange are insignificant in early haemodynamic interstitial pulmonary oedema because fluid accumulates in the collagen-containing part of the alveolar walls leaving the thin, convex portions of the blood–air pathway intact, so that systemic arterial hypoxaemia does not occur.

MENSURATION

One of the most important developments that have taken place over the past few years in the field of thoracic pathology has been the move to express data in quantitative as well as in qualitative terms. It is no longer regarded as satisfactory to describe a case as showing 'slight emphysema with moderate right ventricular hypertrophy'. Methods of tissue morphometry, many applicable to the lung, have been introduced largely by Weibel (1963) and applied and popularised in Great Britain by Dunnill (1962) in a series of outstanding papers. Some of these methods, especially those concerned with histology or electron microscopy, are advanced and capable of yielding a great deal of valuable information about respiratory diseases. Their application to randomly selected blocks of lung, fixed adequately as described below, transforms every 'routine necropsy' on a case of respiratory disease into a research investigation.

Cardiac Hypertrophy

The detection of hypertrophy of one or other cardiac ventricles is important in many cardiorespiratory diseases. Little reliance can be placed upon the measurement of the thickness of some arbitrary spot on the wall of the ventricle by a ruler often in an indifferent state of repair and yet this is the method still widely used today in Great Britain. This is in spite of the fact that rapid and satisfactory methods for the weighing of individual cardiac ventricles exist and can be applied with the minimum of time and trouble at necropsy. In the Department of Pathology at the University of Liverpool we use routinely the method introduced by Fulton, Hutchinson and Jones (1952). In this the free wall of the right ventricle, unfixed and trimmed of fat, is weighed while the interventricular septum is counted as part of the left ventricle. The normal right ventricle weighs less than 65 g while the unequivocally hypertrophied right ventricle exceeds 80 g in weight. The normal left ventricle weighs less than 185 g while the hypertrophied left ventricle weighs more than 200 g. In the normal heart the ratio of left to right ventricular weight lies in the range of 2.5 to 3.5. Isolated right ventricular hypertrophy which is the ventricular abnormality most likely to be encountered in respiratory disease is present when the left to right ventricular ratio is less than 2.0.

Lung preparation

In the same way disease processes involving the lung can be quantified but an essential preliminary to this is adequate fixation. The importance of this can hardly be over-emphasised. The customary practice of cutting lungs at postmortem could hardly be better designed to hide small cystic spaces by blood and collapse. Lungs for examination should be first distended with 10 per cent formol saline until the pleural surfaces are smooth and then left for two to three days before sectioning. If more modern techniques of morphometry on histological sections are to be carried out the lung should be fixed in inflation by the formalin steam method of Weibel and Vidone (1961). Sections of lung fixed by this method present a new world to the pathologist who sees the detail of the lung with the naked eye as never before. When adequate fixation of this type is introduced, strange things immediately begin to happen to the incidence of various classes of disease seen in the postmortem room. For example, the incidence of centrilobular emphysema is likely to increase rapidly from near zero once the pathologist rejects collapsed, blood-covered lungs for those properly fixed.

Point counting

Once a lung is adequately fixed, whole sections of it can be used for point counting to estimate the distribution and severity of disease. Use of points situated at the corners of equilateral triangles on a perspex sheet will enable one to determine the percentage of lung involved by a disease process. Once this is done one is in a position to understand better a given lung pathology. A postmortem report stating that the right ventricle weighed 100 g in a case of centrilobular emphysema involving 35 per cent of the lung substance is more valuable than one stating that a case of moderate emphysema had right ventricular hypertrophy.

AN APPLICATION OF POINT COUNTING

Armed with quantitative data on the heart and lungs in cardiorespiratory disease one can examine critically the relation between the two. Once one embarks on this exercise surprising facts begin to emerge. For example in one investigation we undertook (Hicken, Heath and Brewer, 1966) we found that in pulmonary emphysema there is no relation between the amount of lung destroyed by emphysema and the weight of the right ventricle. This is in conflict with the traditional misconception that mere loss of lung substance with included pulmonary capillary bed is capable of bringing about right ventricular hypertrophy. In spite of objective findings to the contrary this view is still reiterated in recently published papers (White, 1973).

Histological morphometry

More advanced techniques employing special eye pieces are available for study of histological sections of randomly selected blocks for the assessment of the internal surface area of the lungs and for the numbers of surviving alveolar spaces. We have employed such techniques as the mean linear intercept method for the determination of such values and find once again that in emphysema there is no relation between the amount of loss of internal surface area of lung or numbers of alveolar spaces on the one hand and the tendency to develop right ventricular hypertrophy on the other (Hicken, Brewer and Heath, 1966). There seems little doubt that we shall gain a great deal of information about cardiorespiratory disease in the near future from the applications of tissue morphometry not only at histological but also at ultrastructural level.

Hasleton (1973) found that there was no significant difference in right ventricular weight in panacinar and centrilobular emphysema, although less destruction of lung tissue was required to produce the same degree of right ventricular hypertrophy in the latter form. There is a close correlation between the percentage of emphysema as determined by the rapid method of macroscopic point-counting and the internal surface area of the lung as determined by the more complicated and time-consuming techniques of morphometry on histological sections (Hasleton, 1971). Thus the use of graphs prepared to correlate these values allows one to estimate the internal surface of the lung reasonably accurately from data quickly obtained by point-counting.

DRUGS AND THE LUNG

An interesting fact to have emerged over the past few years is that drugs may have profound pathological effects on the lungs producing structural changes in the lung parenchyma or the pulmonary circulation. We may briefly consider some of these drugs now.

Paraquat

In recent years there have been many fatalities following accidental, or sometimes deliberate, ingestion of the herbicide paraquat. They are of considerable interest on account of the unusual pulmonary pathology and the rapid and inexorable course of the disease. The clinical aspects of paraquat poisoning have been well documented elsewhere (Bullivant, 1966; Almog and Tal, 1967; British Medical Journal, 1967; Campbell, 1968; Fennelly, Gallagher and Carroll, 1968; Matthew et al, 1968; Oreopoulos et al, 1968; Lancet, 1971; Carson, 1972; Cooke, Flenley and Matthew, 1973). Most of the pathological changes in paraquat poisoning involve the lung. There may be some associated renal tubular necrosis but this only occasionally contributes significantly to the death of the patient (Oreopoulos et al, 1968; Smith and Heath, 1974b). The most striking pulmonary lesion in paraquat poisoning both in man and animals has been described as an interstitial pulmonary fibrosis (Bullivant, 1966; Clark, McElligott and Hurst, 1966; Fennelly et al, 1968; Matthew et al, 1968; Vijeyaratnam and Corrin, 1971). There is often an associated acute inflammatory exudate, alveolar oedema, alveolar macrophages and a proliferation of the bronchiolar epithelium.

Only comparatively recently has the pathogenesis of the pulmonary lesions in paraquat poisoning been studied in experimental animals (Vijeyaratnam and Corrin, 1971; Smith, Heath and Kay, 1974; Smith and Heath, 1974a). These investigations have been greatly facilitated by the electron microscope and the application of this instrument to a study of the early stages of paraquat poisoning has already been discussed in relation to the membranous pneumocyte. In addition to this, the origin and nature of the pulmonary fibrosis in paraquat poisoning have been uncertain for several years. It was assumed that the fibrosis was interstitial and that paraquat lung was yet another example of diffuse fibrosing alveolitis. However, studies on rats revealed that there is an intra-alveolar infiltration of primitive mesenchymal cells or profibroblasts which then differentiate into mature fibroblasts (Smith et al, 1974; Smith and Heath, 1974a). The result is an intra-alveolar fibrosis consisting of cellular fibroblastic tissue and not a fibrosing alveolitis. The electron microscope showed that the ultrastructure of profibroblasts shared similarities with both fibroblasts and macrophages (Smith et al, 1974; Smith and Heath, 1974a). Toner et al (1970) described similar cells in a human lung biopsy specimen of paraquat poisoning but identified them as macrophages. The question as to whether the infiltrating cells are profibroblasts or macrophages is relatively unimportant since both cells may ultimately derive from the blood monocyte. The significant outcome of these investigations is that the intra-alveolar infiltrate of primitive cells differentiates into fibroblasts rather than becoming phagocytic. In the later stages of the pathogenesis of paraquat lung the damaged alveolar walls become engulfed by the intra-alveolar fibroblastic tissue so that the lung architecture is obliterated. At this stage the intra-alveolar nature of the fibrosis cannot be defined (Smith et al, 1974).

In many human cases of paraquat poisoning the pulmonary fibrosis is at an advanced stage of development by the time the patient dies and the pulmonary histopathology is examined. Consequently the nature of the pulmonary fibrosis is often unclear (Smith and Heath, 1974b). However, Toner et al (1970) described extensive intra-alveolar fibrosis in their human necropsy case, and in a study of four cases of paraquat poisoning one was at a sufficiently early stage to observe profibroblasts and fibroblasts exclusively within the alveolar spaces (Smith and Heath, 1974b). It appears, therefore, that in human paraquat poisoning the nature, and perhaps also the pathogenesis, of the pulmonary fibrosis is the same as that in the rat. It is thus not a fibrosing alveolitis but a type of pulmonary fibrosis which is so far unclassified. It is a fulminating, cellular, intra-alveolar fibrosis. The reason why paraquat should initiate the unusual cellular reaction remains to be elucidated.

Pyrrolizidine Alkaloids

It is now well established that the oral administration of a group of pyrrolizidine alkaloids derived from the seeds of various species of *Crotalaria* and *Senecio* will give rise to pulmonary arterial hypertension and associated hypertensive pulmonary vascular disease. Rats fed on a diet containing powdered *Crotalaria spectabilis* seeds at a concentration of 0.1 per cent for between 36 and 60 days show right ventricular hypertrophy and medial hypertrophy of their pulmonary arteries. A minority develop necrotising arteritis (Kay and Heath, 1966). Elevated pulmonary arterial pressure in rats so treated may be demonstrated directly by cardiac catheterisation (Kay, Harris and Heath, 1967). When the lungs are examined by electron microscopy one finds interstitial oedema with the formation of intraluminal endothelial vesicles, probably representing the early ultrastructural phase of pulmonary oedema, and more likely to be an effect of the pulmonary hypertension than its cause (Kay et al, 1969). There is also a proliferation of granular pneumocytes and excessive numbers of myelin figures and phospholipid lattices, no doubt from these cells, are seen within the alveolar spaces. Various histological changes occur in the lung tissues and pulmonary veins reminiscent of those found in man in mitral stenosis. These include osseous nodules, fibrous thickening of alveolar walls, intra-alveolar fibrosis, old haemorrhages and bronchiolar type epithelium lining of alveolar spaces (Smith, Kay and Heath, 1970). In rats there is cartilaginous metaplasia around pulmonary arteries. The similarity of these exudative lesions to those which occur in association with the pulmonary venous hypertension suggests that the primary action of monocrotaline may be on pulmonary veins. Certainly the intimal fibromuscular pads which characterise the pulmonary veins of the normal rat become accentuated in *Crotalaria spectabilis* toxicity. It may be that monocrotaline, the pyrrolizidine alkaloid contained in *Crotalaria spectabilis*, acts directly on the small pulmonary arteries causing them to constrict. Although there is a hyperplasia of mast cells under these conditions, there is no increase in plasma free or platelet bound serotonin to suggest that excessive secretion of this substance by mast cells underlies the elevation of pulmonary arterial pressure (Kay, Crawford and Heath, 1968).

It has now become clear that the production of pulmonary hypertension and hypertensive pulmonary vascular disease by pyrrolizidine alkaloids is not restricted to this one species but is characteristic of a group of plants. Fulvine is a closely related alkaloid that occurs in the plant *Crotalaria fulva* used in the preparation of bush-tea in Jamaica and now known to be the major aetiological agent in the production of veno-occlusive disease of the liver. When fulvine is administered to rats, it gives rise to the same form of hypertensive pulmonary vascular disease (HPVD) as that produced by monocrotaline (Kay et al, 1971). *Senecio jacobaea* is a plant sold in 'health stores' for a variety of ailments and when given to rats it leads to pulmonary hypertension,

HPVD and death from congestive cardiac failure (Burns, 1972). On a recent visit to Dar-es-Salaam the author was shown sections of lung from a case of primary pulmonary hypertension occurring in an African youth of 19 years. This boy came from the town of Kilwa in Southern Tanzania and is thought to have been given a herbal remedy for some illness by local witch doctors. There are no fewer than 170 species of *Crotalaria* growing in Tanzania and some are known to find their way into tribal potions. One of these species, *Crotalaria laburnoides*, is now under investigation as a possible producer of pulmonary hypertension.

The Aminorex Controversy

The above account of the effects of obscure plants on the pulmonary circulation of the rat might seem to be of interest only to academicians in white towers. This is far from the truth for these experiments introduce the new and exciting concept that dietary substances are capable of producing an elevated pulmonary arterial pressure. This concept assumed great practical importance in 1968 when a slimming tablet on the market was considered to be responsible for an epidemic of primary pulmonary hypertension in Western Europe. Aminorex (2-amino-5-phenyl-2 oxazoline) is an appetite-suppressing drug which was available in Switzerland from November 1965 to October 1968. In 1967 a sudden 20-fold increase in the incidence of primary pulmonary hypertension was observed in a Swiss medical clinic (Gurtner et al, 1968). It was noticed that a considerable number of these patients had taken aminorex to reduce weight. A similar increase in the incidence of primary pulmonary hypertension was encountered in other clinics in Switzerland, and also in Austria and Germany, where aminorex was available. The subjects who died showed pulmonary vascular disease characterised by plexiform lesions such as occurs in pre- or posttricuspid cardiac shunts, cirrhosis of the liver, or portal vein thrombosis (Fig. 18). An increased incidence of the disease has not been reported in countries where this drug was not available. A decline in the incidence of primary pulmonary hypertension has occurred in Switzerland since the withdrawal of aminorex. We administered a high oral dose of aminorex to rats for up to 43 weeks and to dogs for 20 weeks. A detailed quantitative pathological examination of the heart and pulmonary vasculature in these animals failed to reveal any evidence of hypertensive pulmonary vascular disease (Kay, Smith and Heath, 1971). Prolonged oral administration of aminorex to two adult Patas monkeys also failed to produce pulmonary hypertension or hypertensive pulmonary vascular disease (Smith et al, 1973). Hence the present position appears to be that it is not possible to induce pulmonary hypertension in animals using the drug. Although there is statistical evidence linking aminorex with pulmonary hypertension, there is no proof that aminorex causes HPVD in man. At the time of writing there is to be a Working Party of the World Health Organisation in Geneva in an attempt to resolve the controversy as to the cause of this epidemic of primary pulmonary hypertension in Europe. It seems important in the meanwhile to enquire into the diet and history of drug ingestion of any patient with unexplained pulmonary hypertension.

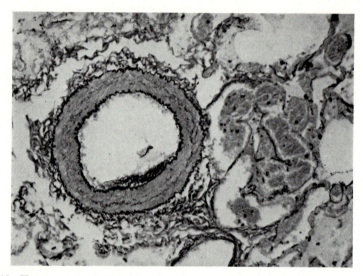

Figure 18   Transverse section of a muscular pulmonary artery from a German woman who had taken the anorexigen, aminorex fumarate. It shows medial hypertrophy and an eccentric crescent of intimal fibroelastosis. To the right is a dilatation lesion

Chlorphentermine

This is another drug used to depress appetite which brings about pathological changes in the lungs of experimental animals. When this sympathomimetic agent, which is available on the British market, is given intraperitoneally to rats it stimulates the appearance of numerous large cells with foamy cytoplasm in the alveolar spaces (Heath, Smith and Hasleton, 1973) (Fig. 19). Groups of them clump together and disintegrate to pack the alveoli with granular eosinophilic material (Fig. 20). As in the case of aminorex we have been unable to produce right ventricular hypertrophy or hypertensive pulmonary vascular disease with this drug in rats.

Electron microscopy of lung tissue from rats treated with chlorphentermine shows a hyperplasia in the alveolar walls of granular pneumocytes without desquamation of these cells. The alveolar spaces contain cellular debris, myelin figures and phospholipid lattices (Fig. 12) with large numbers of associated 'foam cells' which are macrophages that have ingested the intra-alveolar lamellar material (Smith, Heath and Hasleton, 1973). Similar lamellated inclusions are found in granular pneumocytes, membranous pneumocytes, bronchiolar Clara cells (Fig. 11) and endothelial cells of pulmonary capillaries. Similar changes have been described in rats following administration of the antidepressive drug Iprindole (Vijeyaratnam and Corrin, 1972). The appearances are those of a toxic alveolitis. Further studies of the chronic

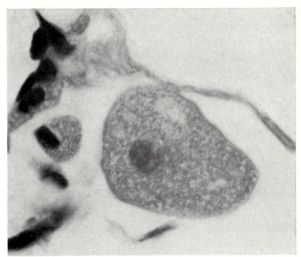

Figure 19 An intra-alveolar foam cell in a rat which had received an intraperitoneal injection of chlorphentermine. On electron microscopy such cells proved to be pulmonary macrophages which had ingested lamellar bodies derived from granular pneumocytes and possibly from Clara cells. Haematoxylin and eosin, × 1350

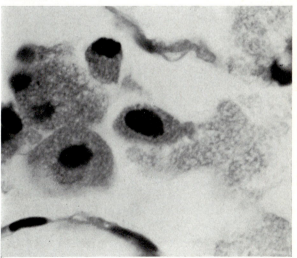

Figure 20 A group of intra-alveolar foam cells in a rat which had received an intraperitoneal injection of chlorphentermine. The cells have disintegrated in places to liberate their cytoplasmic contents. Haematoxylin and eosin, × 1350. (By permission of the Editor of *Thorax*)

toxicity of these drugs are indicated to ascertain whether this acute lesion progresses to fibrosing alveolitis or hypertensive pulmonary vascular disease.

Busulphan

An alveolitis may also be induced by busulphan (Myleran) which is used in the treatment of chronic myeloid leukaemia. The lungs show a pronounced proliferation of granular pneumocytes many of which disintegrate to produce intra-alveolar debris some of which shows fibrous organisation. There is associated interstitial pulmonary fibrosis. Electron microscopy confirms that the desquamated alveolar cells are granular pneumocytes containing characteristic lamellar bodies. Some of these bodies are liberated into the alveolar spaces with the formation of phospholipid myelin figures and lattices (Littler et al, 1969).

EXTRINSIC ALLERGIC ALVEOLITIS
(see also Chapter 7)

In recent years it has become clear that the parenchyma and blood vessels of the lung can also be damaged as the result of an antigen–antibody reaction provoked by inhalation of some form of organic dust. It would appear that such dusts can produce different allergic diseases of the lung depending upon whether the subject is atopic or not (Pepys, 1969). Inhalation of the dust in atopic patients leads to an acute reaginic type hypersensitivity reaction. In non-atopic persons inhalation of organic dusts can evoke precipitating antibodies against the dust or one of its components. Once these antibodies have been established in the circulation inhalation of the dust will cause a type III (Arthus-type) hypersensitivity reaction in the lungs (Van Toorn, 1970). The result of repeated reactions of this type can be severe damage to the lungs called 'extrinsic allergic alveolitis' (Riddle and Grant, 1967).

During the past decade a remarkable collection of dusts has been shown to cause extrinsic allergic alveolitis. Examples of the disease include farmer's lung (Pepys et al, 1962), pigeon breeder's (bird fancier's) lung (Reed, Sosman and Barbee, 1965), and bagassosis (Salvaggio et al, 1967). Other examples are pituitary snuff disease (Mahon et al, 1967), wheat weevil disease (Lunn and Hughes, 1967), malt worker's lung (Riddle et al, 1968), maple-bark stripper's disease (Emanuel, Wenzel and Lawton, 1966) and New Guinea lung disease (Blackburn and Green, 1966). Other probable examples are paprika splitter's lung (Hunter, 1969), vineyard sprayer's lung (Pimentel and Marques, 1969) and furrier's lung (Pimentel, 1970).

In the majority of these diseases precipitins have been demonstrated against a specific antigen. Exposure to the specific antigen in patients with extrinsic alveolitis sometimes causes an acute reaginic type I hypersensitivity reaction followed some hours later by a type III Arthus-type reaction. The first reaction is probably caused by IgE gamma globulin while the second is produced by IgG antibodies (Van Toorn, 1970).

The histopathological features of acute extrinsic allergic alveolitis are very characteristic but they become much less obvious as the disease becomes chronic so that the histological picture is non-specific and merely that of fibrosing alveolitis (Seal et al, 1968). Therefore, in cases of interstitial fibrosis of the lung an enquiry should be made into the exact occupations, past and present, of the patient (Van Toorn, 1970).

The earliest histopathological lesions to occur in extrinsic allergic alveolitis appear to have been described by Barrowcliff and Arblaster (1968) who reported the clinical and pathological findings in a fatal case of farmer's lung in a 17-year-old youth. His first exposure to mouldy hay occurred only weeks before his death. This case showed an acute nodular centrilobular bronchopneumonia with obstructve bronchiolitis. There was focal interstitial pneumonia with much proliferation of alveolar epithelium. A necrotic exudate was present containing neutrophils and eosinophils together with mononuclears, lymphocytes and plasma cells. Some alveoli contained much haemorrhagic fluid. Alveolar capillaries showed inflammatory changes with platelet and fibrin deposition and with neutrophil infiltration.

After farmer's lung has been established for three to four weeks sarcoid-like granulomas appear (Seal et al, 1968). These resolve slowly over a period of about a year. The acute stage of farmer's lung is also characterised by interstitial inflammatory changes. Early on the cellular infiltrate is composed predominantly of large mononuclear cells of histiocyte type. Later as interstitial fibrosis develops the cellular exudate comes to consist largely of lymphocytes and plasma cells. Obstructive bronchiolitis occurs in areas of lung with much confluent disease affecting the surrounding parenchyma. Seal and his associates did not find any acute inflammatory lesions in the walls of blood vessels. Instead they found merely proliferation of the intima and swelling of muscle fibres. Foreign body type giant cells were much in evidence and sometimes they contained clefts or birefringent material. Pimentel (1970) has also demonstrated follicles reminiscent of tuberculosis or sarcoidosis in furrier's lung. They included Langhans-type giant cells with a surrounding rim of lymphocytes. The follicles were frequently centrilobular near a respiratory bronchiole or in the mucosa and submucosa of segmental and subsegmental bronchi. Focal areas of necrosis with surrounding granulation tissue infiltrated with eosinophils were also present.

The chronic stage of farmer's lung is characterised by fibrosing alveolitis and focally the fibrous tissue may become confluent. The thickened alveolar septa become infiltrated by lymphocytes (Seal et al, 1968). Focal collections of lymphocytes are seen around bronchioles and pulmonary blood vessels. Scattered giant cells, often of foreign body type, are also seen. Eventually, as in all forms of interstitial pulmonary fibrosis, honeycomb change may supervene. The changes which occur in farmer's lung may be taken as characteristic of the whole group of extrinsic allergic alveolitis.

ACKNOWLEDGEMENTS

The author gratefully acknowledges the help given to him in the preparation of this chapter by Dr J. M. Kay, Dr P. H. Smith and Dr P. S. Hasleton. While working together with these colleagues on many research projects in the Department of Pathology at Liverpool he has greatly benefited from their stimulating discussions and constructive criticism. He also acknowledges with gratitude the permission of the Editors of *Thorax* to reproduce Figures

10, 11, 12 and 20; the Editor of *The Journal of Pathology* and Dr Kay to reproduce Figures 15 and 16; and the Editor of *The Journal of Physiology* to reproduce Figure 14. Professor Javier Arias-Stella kindly provided a slide from which Figure 8 was prepared.

REFERENCES

Alexander, I. G. S. (1968) Ultrastructure of the pulmonary alveolar vessels in Mendelson's (acid pulmonary aspiration) syndrome. *British Journal of Anaesthesia*, **40**, 408–414.

Almog, Ch. & Tal, E. (1967) Death from paraquat after subcutaneous injection. *British Medical Journal*, **3**, 721.

Arias-Stella, J. (1969) Human carotid body at high altitudes. Item 150 in the 69*th Programme and Abstracts of the American Association of Pathologists and Bacteriologists*, San Francisco, California.

Barrowcliff, D. F. & Arblaster, P. G. (1968) Farmer's lung: a study of an early acute fatal case. *Thorax*, **23**, 490–500.

Becker, A. E. (1966) The glomera in the region of the heart and great vessels. A microscopical-anatomical and histochemical study, p. 125 (MD thesis). Amsterdam: Drukkerij Aemstel-stad.

Bergofsky, E. H. (1969) Ions and membrane permeability in the regulation of the pulmonary circulation. In *The Pulmonary Circulation and Interstitial Space*, ed. Fishman, A. P. & Hecht, H. H., Ch. 18, p. 289. University of Chicago Press: Chicago.

Blackburn, C. R. B. & Green, W. (1966) Precipitins against extracts of thatched roofs in the sera of New Guinea natives with chronic lung disease. *Lancet*, **2**, 1396–1397.

Brewer, D. B., Heath, D. & Asquith, P. (1969) Electron microscopy of desquamative inter-stitial pneumonia. *Journal of Pathology*, **97**, 317–323.

British Medical Journal (1967) Leading article: Poisoning from paraquat, **3**, 690–691.

Bullivant, C. M. (1966) Accidental poisoning by paraquat: Report of two cases in man. *British Medical Journal*, **1**, 1271–1273.

Burns, J. (1972) The heart and pulmonary arteries in rats fed on *Senecio jacobaea*. *Journal of Pathology*, **106**, 187–194.

Campbell, S. (1968) Death from paraquat in a child. *Lancet*, **1**, 144.

Carson, E. D. (1972) Fatal paraquat poisoning in Northern Ireland. *Journal of the Forensic Science Society*, **12**, 437–443.

Clark, D. G., McElligott, T. F. & Hurst, E. W. (1966) The toxicity of paraquat. *British Journal of Industrial Medicine*, **23**, 126–132.

Cooke, N. J., Flenley, D. C. & Matthew, H. (1973) Paraquat poisoning. *Quarterly Journal of Medicine*, **168**, 683–692.

Cottrell, T. S., Levine, O. R., Senior, R. M., Wiener, J., Spiro, D. & Fishman, A. P. (1967) Electron microscopic alterations at the alveolar level in pulmonary oedema. *Circulation Research*, **21**, 783–797.

Cox, J. S. G. (1971) Disodium cromoglycate. *British Journal of Diseases of the Chest*, **65**, 189–204.

Dunnill, M. S. (1962) Quantitative methods in the study of pulmonary pathology. *Thorax*, **17**, 320–328.

Edwards, C. & Heath, D. (1969) Microanatomy of glomic tissue of the pulmonary trunk. *Thorax*, **24**, 209–217.

Edwards, C. & Heath, D. (1970) Site and blood supply of the intertruncal glomera. *Cardio-vascular Research*, **4**, 502–508.

Edwards, C. & Heath, D. (1972) Pulmonary venous chemoreceptor tissue. *British Journal of Diseases of the Chest*, **66**, 96–100.

Edwards, C., Heath, D. & Harris, P. (1971) The carotid body in emphysema and left ventri-cular hypertrophy. *Journal of Pathology*, **104**, 1–13.

Edwards, C., Heath, D., Harris, P., Castillo, Y., Krüger, H. & Arias-Stella, J. (1971) The carotid body in animals at high altitude. *Journal of Pathology*, **104**, 231–238.

Edwards, C., Heath, R. & Harris, P. (1972) Ultrastructure of the carotid body in high-altitude guinea-pigs. *Journal of Pathology*, **107**, 131–136.

Emanuel, D. A., Wenzel, F. J. & Lawton, B. R. (1966) Pneumonitis due to cryptostroma corticale (maple-bark disease). *New England Journal of Medicine*, **274**, 1413–1418.

Euler, U. S. von & Liljestrand, G. (1946) Observations on the pulmonary arterial blood pressure in the cat. *Acta Physiologica Scandinavica*, **12**, 301–320.

Fennelly, J. J., Gallagher, J. T. & Carroll, R. J. (1968) Paraquat poisoning in a pregnant woman. *British Medical Journal*, **3**, 722–723.

Finlay-Jones, J. M., Robertson, T. A. & Walters, M. N-l. (1971) The effect of anaesthetics on pulmonary ultrastructure. *Pathology*, **3**, 181–190.

Fulton, R. M., Hutchinson, E. C. & Jones, M. A. (1952) Ventricular weight in cardiac hypertrophy. *British Heart Journal*, **14**, 413–420.

Grover, R. F. & Kay, J. M. (1972) Personal communication.

Gurtner, H. P., Gertsch, M., Salzmann, C., Scherrer, M., Stucki, P. & Wyss, F. (1968) Häufen sich die primär vasculären Formen des Chronischen Cor pulmonale? *Schweizerische Medizinische Wochenschrift*, **98**, 1579–1589, 1695–1707.

Haas, F. & Bergofsky, E. H. (1972) Role of the mast cell in the pulmonary pressor response to hypoxia. *Journal of Clinical Investigation*, **51**, 3154–3162.

Hasleton, P. S. (1971) Clinico-pathological studies in emphysema. (MD thesis). University of Birmingham.

Hasleton, P. S. (1973) Right ventricular hypertrophy in emphysema. *Journal of Pathology*, **110**, 27–36.

Hauge, A. (1968) Role of histamine in hypoxic pulmonary hypertension in the rat. 1. Blockade or potentiation of endogenous amines, kinins, and ATP. *Circulation Research*, **22**, 371–383.

Hauge, A. & Melmon, K. L. (1968) Role of histamine in hypoxic pulmonary hypertension in the rat. II. Depletion of histamine, serotonin, and catecholamines. *Circulation Research*, **22**, 385–392.

Hayes, J. A. & Shiga, A. (1970) Ultrastructural changes in pulmonary oedema produced experimentally with ammonium sulphate. *Journal of Pathology*, **100**, 281–286.

Heath, D., Smith, P. & Hasleton, P. S. (1973) Effects of chlorphentermine on the rat lung. *Thorax*, **28**, 551–558.

Heath, D., Moosavi, H. & Smith, P. (1973) Ultrastructure of high altitude pulmonary oedema. *Thorax*, **28**, 694–700.

Hicken, P., Brewer, D. & Heath, D. (1966) The relation between the weight of the right ventricle of the heart and the internal surface area and number of alveoli in the human lung in emphysema. *Journal of Pathology and Bacteriology*, **92**, 529–546.

Hicken, P., Heath, D. & Brewer, D. (1966) The relation between the weight of the right ventricle and the percentage of abnormal air space in the lung in emphysema. *Journal of Pathology and Bacteriology*, **92**, 519–528.

Hunter, D. (1969) *The Diseases of Occupations*, 4th edn. London: English Universities Press.

Kapanci, Y., Weibel, E. R., Kaplan, H. P. & Robinson, F. R. (1969) Pathogenesis and reversibility of the pulmonary lesions of oxygen toxicity in monkeys. II. Ultrastructural and morphometric studies. *Laboratory Investigation*, **20**, 101–118.

Kay, J. M. & Edwards, F. R. (1973) Ultrastructure of the alveolar-capillary wall in mitral stenosis. *Journal of Pathology*, **111**, 239–245.

Kay, J. M. & Heath, D. (1966) Observations on the pulmonary arteries and heart weights of rats fed on *Crotalaria spectabilis* seeds. *Journal of Pathology and Bacteriology*, **92**, 385–394.

Kay, J. M., Harris, P. & Heath, D. (1967) Pulmonary hypertension produced in rats by ingestion of *Crotalaria spectabilis* seeds. *Thorax*, **22**, 176–179.

Kay, J. M., Crawford, N. & Heath, D. (1968) Blood-5-hydroxytryptamine in rats with pulmonary hypertension produced by ingestion of *Crotalaria spectabilis* seeds. *Experientia*, **24**, 1149–1150.

Kay, J. M., Smith, P. & Heath, D. (1969) Electron microscopy of *Crotalaria* pulmonary hypertension. *Thorax*, **24**, 511–526.

Kay, J. M., Heath, D., Smith, P., Bras, G. & Summerell, J. (1971) Fulvine and the pulmonary circulation. *Thorax*, **26**, 249–261.

Kay, J. M., Smith, P. & Heath, D. (1971) Aminorex and the pulmonary circulation. *Thorax*, **26**, 262–270.

Kay, J. M., Waymire, J. C. & Grover, R. F. (1974) Lung mast cell hyperplasia and pulmonary histamine-forming capacity in hypoxic rats. *American Journal of Physiology*, **226**, 178–184.

Korn, D., Bensch, K., Liebow, A. A. & Castleman, B. (1960) Multiple minute pulmonary tumors resembling chemodectomas. *American Journal of Pathology*, **37**, 641–672.

Krahl, V. E. (1960) The glomus pulmonale. *Bulletin of the School of Medicine, University of Maryland*, **45**, 36–38.

Lancet (1971) **2**, 1018–1019.

Lauweryns, J. M. & Peuskens, J. C. (1969) Argyrophil (kinin and amine producing?) cells in human infant airway epithelium. *Life Sciences*, **8**, 577–585.

Lauweryns, J. M., Peuskens, J. C. & Cokelaere, M. (1970) Argyrophil, fluorescent, and granulated (peptide and amine producing?) AFG cells in human infant bronchial epithelium. Light and electron microscopic studies. *Life Sciences*, **9**, 1417–1429.

Liebow, A. A., Steer, A. & Billingsley, J. G. (1965) Desquamative interstitial pneumonia. *American Journal of Medicine*, **39**, 369–404.

Littler, W. A., Kay, J. M., Hasleton, P. S. & Heath, D. (1969) Busulphan lung. *Thorax* **24**, 639–655.

Lunn, J. A. & Hughes, D. T. D. (1967) Pulmonary hypersensitivity to the grain weevil. *British Journal of Industrial Medicine*, **24**, 158–161.

McCann, B. G. & Brewer, D. B. (1974) A case of desquamative interstitial pneumonia progressing to honeycomb lung. *Journal of Pathology*, **112**, 199–202.

Mahon, W. E., Scott, D. J., Ansell, G., Manson, G. L. & Fraser, R. (1967) Hypersensitivity to pituitary snuff with miliary shadowing in the lungs. *Thorax*, **22**, 13–20.

Matthew, H., Logan, A., Woodruff, M. F. A. & Heard, B. (1968) Paraquat poisoning—lung transplantation. *British Medical Journal*, **3**, 759–763.

Meyrick, B. & Reid, L. (1968) The alveolar brush cell in rat lung—a third pneumocyte. *Journal of Ultrastructure Research*, **23**, 71–80.

Meyrick, B. & Reid, L. (1970) The alveolar wall. *British Journal of Diseases of the Chest*, **64**, 121–140.

Meyrick, B., Miller, J. & Reid, L. (1972) Pulmonary oedema induced by ANTU, or by high or low oxygen concentrations in rat—an electron microscope study. *British Journal of Experimental Pathology*, **53**, 347–358.

Moosavi, H., Smith, P. & Heath, D. (1973) The Feyrter cell in hypoxia. *Thorax*, **28**, 729–741.

Oreopoulos, D. G., Soyannwo, M. A. O., Sinniah, R., Fenton, S. S. A., McGeown, M. G. & Bruce, J. H. (1968) Acute renal failure in a case of paraquat poisoning. *British Medical Journal*, **1**, 749–750.

Patchefsky, A. S., Israel, H. L., Hoch, W. S. & Gordon, G. (1973) Desquamative interstitial pneumonia. Relationship to interstitial fibrosis. *Thorax*, **28**, 680–693.

Pearse, A. G. E. (1969) The cytochemistry and ultrastructure of polypeptide hormone-producing cells of the APUD series and the embryologic, physiologic and pathologic implications of the concept. *Journal of Histochemistry and Cytochemistry*, **17**, 303–313.

Pepys, J. (1969) Hypersensitivity diseases of the lungs due to fungi and organic dusts. *Monographs in Allergy*, Vol. 4. Basel: Karger.

Pepys, J., Riddell, R. W., Citron, K. M. & Clayton, Y. M. (1962) Precipitins against extracts of hay and moulds in the serum of patients with farmer's lung, aspergillosis, asthma and sarcoidosis. *Thorax*, **17**, 366–374.

Pimentel, J. C. (1970) Furrier's lung. *Thorax*, **25**, 387–398.

Pimentel, J. C. & Marques, F. (1969) 'Vineyard-sprayer's lung': a new occupational disease. *Thorax*, **24**, 678–688.

Reed, C. E., Sosman, A. & Barbee, R. A. (1965) Pigeon-breeder's lung. *Journal of the American Medical Association*, **193**, 261–265.

Reeves, J. T., Leathers, J. E., Eiseman, B. & Spencer, F. C. (1962) Alveolar hypoxia versus hypoxaemia in the development of pulmonary hypertension. *Medicina thoracalis*, **19**, 561–572.

Riddle, H. F. V. & Grant, I. W. B. (1967) Allergic alveolitis in a maltworker. *Thorax*, **22**, 478.

Riddle, H. F. V., Channell, S., Blyth, W., Weir, D. M., Lloyd, M., Amos, W. M. G. & Grant, I. W. B. (1968) Allergic alveolitis in a maltworker. *Thorax*, **23**, 271–280.

Salvaggio, J. E., Seabury, J. H., Buechner, H. A. & Kundur, V. G. (1967) Bagassosis: demonstration of precipitins against extracts of thermophilic actinomycetes in the sera of affected individuals. *Journal of Allergy and Clinical Immunology*, **39**, 106.

Scadding, J. G. & Hinson, K. F. W. (1967) Diffuse fibrosing alveolitis (diffuse interstitial fibrosis of the lungs). Correlation of histology at biopsy with prognosis. *Thorax*, **22**, 291–304.

Schneeberger-Keeley, E. E. & Karnovsky, M. J. (1968) The ultrastructural basis of alveolar–capillary membrane permeability to peroxidase used as a tracer. *Journal of Cell Biology*, **37**, 781–793.

Seal, R. M. E., Hapke, E. J., Thomas, G. O., Meek, J. C. & Hayes, M. (1968) The pathology of the acute and chronic stages of farmer's lung. *Thorax*, **23**, 469–489.

Shortland, J. R., Darke, C. S. & Crane, W. A. J. (1969) Electron microscopy of desquamative interstitial pneumonia. *Thorax*, **24**, 192–208.

Smith, P. & Heath, D. (1974a) The ultrastructure and time sequence of the early stages of paraquat lung in rats. *Journal of Pathology*, **114**, 177–184.

Smith, P. & Heath, D. (1974b) Paraquat lung—a reappraisal. *Thorax*, **29**, 643–653.

Smith, P., Kay, J. M. & Heath, D. (1970) Hypertensive pulmonary vascular disease in rats after prolonged feeding with *Crotalaria spectabilis* seeds. *Journal of Pathology*, **102**, 97–106.

Smith, P., Heath, D. & Hasleton, P. S. (1973) Electron microscopy of chlorphentermine lung. *Thorax*, **28**, 559–566.

Smith, P., Heath, D., Kay, J. M., Wright, J. S. & McKendrick, C. S. (1973) Pulmonary arterial pressure and structure in the Patas monkey after prolonged administration of aminorex fumarate. *Cardiovascular Research*, **7**, 30–38.

Smith, P., Heath, D. & Kay, J. M. (1974) The pathogenesis and structure of paraquat-induced pulmonary fibrosis in rats. *Journal of Pathology*, **114**, 57–67.

Smith, P., Heath, D. & Moosavi, H. (1974) The Clara cell. *Thorax*, **29**, 147–163.

Szidon, J. P., Pietra, G. G. & Fishman, A. P. (1972) The alveolar–capillary membrane and pulmonary oedema. *New England Journal of Medicine*, **286**, 1200–1204.

Toner, P. G., Vetters, J. M., Spilg, W. G. S. & Harland, W. A. (1970) Fine structure of the lung lesion in a case of paraquat poisoning. *Journal of Pathology*, **102**, 182–185.

Van Toorn, D. W. (1970) Coffee worker's lung: a new example of extrinsic allergic alveolitis. *Thorax*, **25**, 399–405.

Vijeyaratnam, G. S. & Corrin, B. (1971) Experimental paraquat poisoning. A histological and electron-optical study of the changes in the lung. *Journal of Pathology*, **103**, 123–129.

Vijeyaratnam, G. S. & Corrin, B. (1972) Pulmonary histiocytosis simulating desquamative interstitial pneumonia in rats receiving oral Iprindole. *Journal of Pathology*, **108**, 105–113.

Weibel, E. R. (1963) *Morphometry of the Human Lung*, p. 52. Berlin: Springer.

Weibel, E. R. (1973) Morphological basis of alveolar–capillary gas exchange. *Physiological Reviews*, **53**, 419–495.

Weibel, E. R. & Vidone, R. A. (1961) Fixation of the lung by formalin steam in a controlled state of air inflation. *American Review of Respiratory Disease*, **84**, 856–861.

White, R. J. (1973) Chronic cor pulmonale. *Medicine*, **18**, 1128–1130.

4

HYPOXIA IN LUNG DISEASE

D. C. Flenley

Possible definitions of the physiological function of the lungs must give high priority to the addition of oxygen to and the removal of carbon dioxide from the bloodstream. Equally, it is obvious that impairment of this gas exchanging function commonly arises in lung disease. This chapter first considers the biochemical usage of oxygen in man, then the possible abnormalities in mechanisms of oxygen transfer in the lungs, and of oxygen transport in the blood in disease. The role of hypoxia in controlling ventilation, and the clinical recognition and possible causes and consequences of hypoxaemia are then described, followed by consideration of the treatment of hypoxaemia, with a brief discussion of methods of oxygen therapy, including the problems and potential of long-term oxygen therapy in chronic cor pulmonale.

The Biochemical Uses of Oxygen

Molecular oxygen acts on the final acceptor of electrons for the electron transport chain of respiratory enzymes in the cellular mitochondria. These enzymes, including the cytochromes, flavine adenine dinucleotide and nicotine adenine dinucleotide (NAD), oscillate between the reduced and oxidised form as substrates are oxidised in the tricarboxylic acid cycle. A simplified scheme of mammalian biochemical energetics (Fig. 1) shows the intimate relationship between oxidative phosphorylation, with the production of high energy adenosine triphosphate (ATP), and the oxidation of NADH by the respiratory enzyme chain. In the absence of available oxygen, with resultant inactivity of the respiratory enzymes and oxidation of NADH by Krebs cycle, catabolism of acetyl coenzyme A (the common intermediate of catabolism of carbohydrate, fats and some proteins) cannot proceed. In this situation pyruvate molecules are reduced to lactate which thus accumulates as the hallmark of anaerobic glycolysis. This anaerobic pathway is very much less efficient in the production of ATP than is full aerobic oxidation, for the catabolism of one glucosyl unit of glycogen to two molecules of lactate only yields two ATP molecules, whereas complete oxidative catabolism to CO_2 and water via the Embden–Meyerhof glycolytic pathway and the tricarboxylic acid cycle produces 38 molecules of ATP. Unfortunately, tissue levels of lactate may be 10 times those of the blood draining that tissue so that quantification of oxygen lack from blood lactate levels is very imprecise.

The concentration of molecular oxygen which must be available to the mitochondria to allow active aerobic metabolism to proceed is not entirely certain. From studies on the cerebral cortex of the rat, it appears that a partial pressure of oxygen (Po_2) of probably 1 mmHg or less is adequate to maintain the components of the electron transfer respiratory enzymes in an oxidised state. If this figure can be extrapolated to other tissues (which is by no means certain), it would seem that maintenance of an oxygen tension of 1 mmHg or so at mitochondria will allow maximal catabolism of substrates by oxidative pathways (Lubbers, 1968).

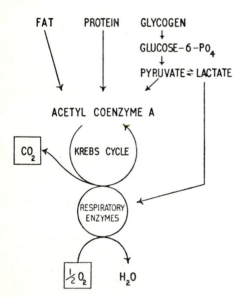

Figure 1   The biochemical use of oxygen in the mammalian cell, allowing the oxidative catabolism of foodstuffs to CO_2 and water, with the provision of high energy phosphate (ATP) via Krebs tri-carboxylic acid cycle

Delivery of Oxygen to Mitochondria

Molecular oxygen can only be delivered to mitochondria by diffusion from the red cells in the nearest capillary to the metabolizing cell. Oxygen molecules must therefore pass from haemoglobin across the red cell membrane, plasma layer, capillary walls, interstitial space, cellular membrane, cell sap and mitochondrial membrane to the respiratory enzymes, which are located in the internal cristae of the mitochondria, oxygen molecules passing down a concentration gradient determined by the differences in partial pressure of O_2 at these sites. Unfortunately, we have little quantitative knowledge in this area, for even attempts to measure 'tissue' oxygen tension directly by micro-oxygen electrodes must distort tissue locally. Such studies, however, emphasise the critical importance of the proximity of the capillary to the site of measurement for these determinations of 'tissue' oxygen tensions.

Oxygen released from haemoglobin in the capillary, which is the source of this diffusion gradient, must in turn come from the arterial blood, the 'mean capillary Po_2', lying somewhere between arterial and venous tensions. Indeed, by adaptation of the Bohr integration technique, originally proposed to quantitative oxygen transfer from alveolar gas in the lungs, an arithmetic estimate of the average capillary tension in a tissue can be calculated, if we know the arterial and venous tensions and oxygen uptake of that tissue (Flenley, 1967). However, it is to be emphasised that these ideas are only abstractions, for in actuality, structural and temporal variations in capillary blood flow will greatly influence the efficiency of oxygen delivery to an individual cell. In muscle, for example, where oxygen diffusion may be in part facilitated by the extravascular tissue pigment myoglobin, the capillary density can vary up to 25 times, depending upon the state of activity, and thus of demand for the provision of oxygen.

None the less, in clinical practice, these ideas do suggest that the Po_2 of the effluent venous blood, when related to the oxygen uptake of a tissue, may be a more adequate measure of the oxygenation status of that tissue than mere consideration of the oxygen input tension (the arterial Po_2), alone. Thus, consciousness is lost when the jugular venous Po_2 falls below 18 to 20 mmHg in man, yet the cerebral arterial Po_2 is much less clearly correlated with this event. It is essential in this context to consider the oxygen uptake as well as the tension, for a high effluent venous Po_2 could exist with relative or absolute deficiency of oxygen delivery to part of that tissue, as for example in a local infarction, but if we make the reasonable assumption that overall oxygen consumption cannot be increased beyond a maximal value by provision of more *oxygen* (although it can be increased by greater provision of oxidisable *substrate*, as in muscular contraction), it would then follow that a high venous Po_2 will be associated with a reduction in oxygen uptake of that organ or tissue, when compared to the preinfaction situation.

The input for this delivery of oxygen to the tissues is, of course, the arterial oxygen, which can be measured in terms of both partial pressure (Po_2) and oxygen content, these two being linked by the haemoglobin concentration and oxygen dissociation curve, which is in turn dependent upon the plasma and red cell pH (the Bohr effect), temperature, and red cell concentration of 2,3-diphosphoglycerate (see later).

The arterial oxygen tension in its turn depends upon gas transfer in the lungs, again by diffusion from alveoli, where the oxygen tension ($P_{A}o_2$) depends upon the adequacy of ventilation, to the red cell in the pulmonary capillary, across the diffusion pathway of surfactant layer, alveolar membrane, interstitial spaces, capillary membrane, plasma layer, and red cell membrane. Again, a most important determinant of the Po_2 in the alveolar capillary is the relationship of alveolar ventilation to perfusion, and of diffusion to perfusion.

Oxygen Transport in the Lungs

The basic ideas underlying oxygen transport in the lungs are simple: fresh air ventilates alveoli so admitting inspired gas to mix with evolving CO_2 in the alveolar gas; diffusion to the haemoglobin of the red cell; and onward movement of the red cell as the blood perfuses the alveolar capillary. The Riley three compartment model of gas exchange, consisting of dead space (ventilated but not perfused), ideal alveolus (where all gas exchange occurs) and shunt (perfused but not ventilated), remains a useful model, which can be used quantitatively. However, the fundamental importance to gas exchange in the 300 million individual alveoli of the adult lungs, lies in the balance of

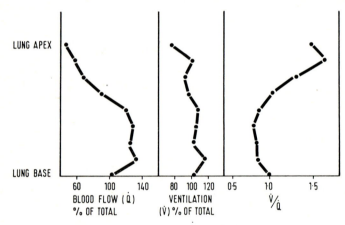

Figure 2   Regional distributions of ventilation (V), blood flow (Q), and ventilation to perfusion ratios ($\dot{V}/\dot{Q}$), from apex to base of the lungs of an upright normal man, as determined by radioactive xenon-133, either inspired (for measuring $\dot{V}$), or infused in solution intravenously (for measuring $\dot{Q}$), with external quantitative imaging of radioactivity by a gamma camera.

alveolar ventilation ($\dot{V}_A$) to capillary perfusion ($\dot{Q}_c$) which has recently been joined by the recognition that the diffusing capacity of the lung (D_L) is also a distributed function, so that the contribution of each individual alveolus to oxygen transfer will depend quantitatively upon both its $\dot{V}_A/\dot{Q}_c$ ratio, and $D_L/\dot{Q}_c$ ratio (McHardy, 1972).

Practical application of these physiological abstractions has depended largely upon study of gas exchange of inert gases, notably radioactive xenon-133, which is physiologically inert and relatively insoluble in plasma. Detection of regional radioactivity in the lungs following either inhalation of gaseous ^{133}Xe in solution in saline, with imaging by either fixed or scanning counters, or by gamma camera, has emphasised the importance of the gravitationally dependent variation in both perfusion and ventilation in the normal upright lung (Fig. 2). With normal pulmonary arterial pressure, it is probable that a significant proportion of the apices receive little blood flow in the upright posture in man, and are also less well ventilated than are the lung bases but that the regional $\dot{V}_A/\dot{Q}_c$ is biased towards a lower value at the bases, and higher value at the apices. These distributions depend in a complex fashion upon the gradient of pleural pressure from apex to base, which surrounds the lungs in situ.

Lung disease obviously disturbs these relationships, the consequences for gas exchange again largely depending upon the proportion of the total alveoli which are involved by the disease. Thus, in centrilobular emphysema, where the first and second order respiratory bronchioles may be largely destroyed, it seems apparent that transfer of gas molecules to and from the alveolar gas-exchanging perfused membrane will be seriously hindered. Again, loss of alveoli by fibrosis, or flooding by oedema or fibrinous exudate of pneumonia, will obviously impair ventilation, yet if the blood flow to that alveolus is equally impaired, overall gas exchange will not be grossly disturbed, unless the numbers of alveoli involved constitute an appreciable proportion of the lung volume, as both blood flow and ventilation may be diverted to other intact alveoli. However, if blood continues to flow through unventilated alveoli, the resultant addition of unoxygenated venous blood to the systemic arterial flow (venous admixture or shunt) will constitute a potent mechanism of arterial hypoxaemia, which in that instance is difficult to correct by increasing the inspired oxygen concentration, so that, for example, even with 100 per cent inspired oxygen, the arterial P_{O_2} cannot be kept over 50 mmHg when a 50 per cent shunt exists.

The old concept of 'alveolar–capillary block', where thickening of the alveolar membrane by diffuse pulmonary fibrosis (of whatever aetiology), was thought to present a barrier for diffusion of oxygen from alveolus to capillary, remains as a useful categorisation of a pattern of functional disturbance, with restriction of lung volumes, stiff lungs (decreased compliance), and hypoxaemia without CO_2 retention, particularly on exercise if not at rest. However, the exact physiological mechanism remains in dispute, the initial challenge to the 'diffusion block' concept from the more probable mismatching of ventilation to perfusion amongst alveoli, in turn giving way to the mismatching of $D_L/\dot{Q}_c$ ratios amongst alveoli.

In this, as in other more common lung diseases (bronchial asthma, pneumonia, pulmonary oedema, pulmonary thromboembolism), hypoxaemia is often combined with a low or normal P_{CO_2} (type I respiratory failure, see later). This apparent paradox, that oxygenation is impaired despite supranormal CO_2 removal, arises in large part from the differences in slope of the oxygen and CO_2 dissociation curves of blood, for underventilation of some of alveoli cannot be compensated for by overventilation of another group of alveoli, at least in the case of oxygen (West, 1969).

As the volume of gas in the lungs falls towards residual volume during expiration, the pleural pressure in the lower lung zones exceeds the pressure within the lower zone airways, so that these airways close, thereby preventing ventilation of the alveoli in these dependent regions of the lungs. The lung volume at which this airway closure occurs is known as the 'closing volume', and may be detected by an abrupt change in the concentration of an inert marker gas, as detected at the lips during a slow expiration (Fig. 3) (Holland et al, 1968). This closing volume rises with age, due to loss of lung elastic recoil, and is raised even more in the supine position, so that in normal sub-

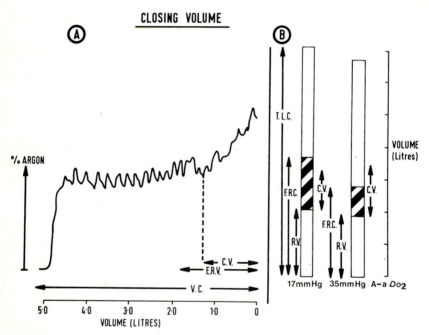

Figure 3 (A) The measurement of 'closing volume' (CV) by recording the concentration of argon of the lips following a slow inspirate of an argon bolus, followed by a slow expiration of the full vital capacity (VC), in a normal subject, whose CV is less than expiratory reserve volume (ERV). (B) In this normal subject, the CV + residual volume (RV) does not exceed the functional residual capacity (FRC), so that the alveolar to arterial oxygen tension gradient $(A - a\ Do_2)$ is normal at 17 mmHg (left hand column). In another subject where CV + RV does exceed the FRC (right hand column), the $A - a\ Do_2$ is abnormally raised at 35 mmHg. (Data from Craig et al, 1971)

jects over 44 years, it exceeded the expiratory reserve volume when lying down, so that during normal tidal breathing, some alveoli in dependent lung zones were then unventilated (McCarthy et al, 1972).

Blood Oxygen Transport

The amount of oxygen carried by the arterial blood depends upon the Po_2, pH and haemoglobin concentration. The relationship between Po_2 and the oxygen saturation (So_2), the oxygen dissociation curve, has long been known to depend upon the pH (Bohr effect), and P_{CO_2}, but in recent years another important ligand affecting this relationship has been discovered: 2,3-diphosphoglycerate (Benesch and Benesch, 1967; Kilmartin and Rossi-Bernardi, 1973). This intermediate of red cell carbohydrate metabolism can combine reversibly with reduced haemoglobin, with which it is in equivalent concentrations in the red cell, and so affects the affinity of haemoglobin for oxygen. The effect can be described by changes in P_{50}, or the oxygen tension for one half full saturation, which is conventionally described at pH 7.4,

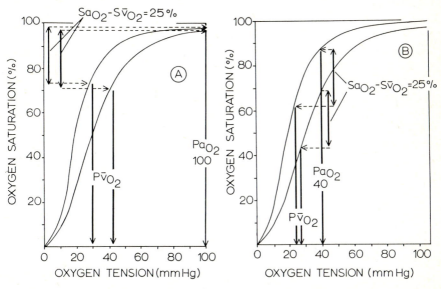

Figure 4 (A) The oxygen dissociation curve with a P_{50} (see text) of 20 mmHg (left hand curve), or 30 mmHg (right hand curve). In (A) the arterial oxygen tension (P_aO_2) is 100 mg, and the arteriovenous oxygen difference ($S_aO_2 - S_{\bar{v}}O_2$) 25 per cent so that the mixed venous oxygen tensions ($P_{\bar{v}}O_2$) is either 30 mmHg (when the P_{50} is 20 mmHg) or 42 mmHg (when the P_{50} is 30 mmHg). (B) The P_aO_2 is 40 mmHg, but the $S_aO_2 - S_{\bar{v}}O_2$ remains at 25 per cent, yet now the change in P_{50} has very little effect on the resultant mixed venous oxygen tension ($P_{\bar{v}}O_2$)

$P_{50(7.4)}$ to correct for the Bohr effect (Fig. 4). Recently, the levels of 2,3-DPG in the red cell have themselves been shown to depend upon red cell pH (which is in a linear relationship to the pH of plasma as measured by the glass electrode in whole blood). In health, when plasma pH is 7.40, red cell pH lies between 7.14 and 7.18. The 2,3-DPG is synthesised and hydrolysed by separate enzymes which are both pH dependent, so that DPG levels in the red cell depend upon pH. These complex interactions between 2,3-DPG, pH and P_{50} are of considerable importance in metabolic disturbances of acid base balance (as in diabetic ketoacidosis) and following transfusion with stored blood (which is low in 2,3-DPG) but seem to have much less significance in hypoxic respiratory acidosis, for a shift in P_{50} affects both arterial and venous ends of the dissociation curve in this situation (Fig. 4). Furthermore, in chronic hypercapnia, 2,3-DPG and P_{50} both vary spontaneously above and below the normal range (Fairweather, Walker and Flenley, 1974).

A low cardiac output, as in shock, will compound the effect of any deficiency of arterial oxygenation, in so far as delivery of oxygen to cellular mitochondria is concerned. In cardiogenic shock, arterial hypoxaemia is frequent, and may be relatively resistant to even high concentrations of inspired oxygen (MacKenzie et al, 1964). In this situation, a raised arterial lactate often heralds a fatal outcome which still results in over 80 per cent of such cases. The mechanism of arterial hypoxaemia in this condition is not clear, but is probably multifactorial, with interstitial pulmonary oedema contributing to small airway closure, microthrombi formation in lung capillaries, and overall reduction of the number of effectively ventilated and perfused alveoli from the severe reduction in cardiac output. A similarly grave prognosis is seen in other conditions where the lethal combination of a fall in cardiac output is combined with arterial hypoxaemia, as in cardiac tamponade, crushed chest injury, tension pneumothorax and intractable pulmonary oedema. Conversely, in many cases of bacteraemic shock, although the systemic blood pressure can be low with a reduced cardiac output, enzymatic inactivation, as in dinitrophenol or salicylate poisoning, causes oxygen utilisation to be partially uncoupled from production of energy rich ATP in the mitochondria.

The Hypoxic Drive to Breathing

The hypoxic drive to breathing arises principally from the peripheral arterial chemoreceptors of which the carotid bodies are most important in man, for the drive is eliminated following their surgical removal (Lugliani et al, 1971). (Fig. 5). The intensity of this ventilatory drive can vary between different individuals; for example, high altitude residents who suffer from chronic mountain polycythaemia may have no demonstrable drive from hypoxia (Severinghaus, Bainton and Carcelen, 1966b). This phenomenon has also been confirmed in subjects in the high Andes, the Himalayas (Milledge and Lahiri, 1967) and also in Leadville, Colorado, at a height of around 10 000 ft (Weil et al, 1971). However, the phenomenon does not appear to represent a genetic variation, for children native to Leadville have been found to have a normal hypoxic drive, whereas it may be deficient in their parents who have been exposed to altitude hypoxia for longer (Byrne-Quinn, Sodal and Weil, 1972). Consistent absence of hypoxic drive has been described in children following total correction of Fallot's tetralogy, leading to the suggestion that exposure to chronic hypoxaemia in early postnatal life might have resulted in loss of the hypoxic ventilatory drive (Sørensen and Severinghaus, 1968).

Flenley, Franklin and Millar (1970) described 2 out of 12 patients with chronic bronchitis and emphysema in whom the ventilatory response to CO_2 was unchanged when the arterial Po_2 was varied from 40–60 mmHg to 100–200 mmHg, implying an absence of hypoxic drive to breathing in these two patients (Fig. 6), who both suffered from severe cor pulmonale, marked secondary polycyaemia, severe persistent airways obstruction, and CO_2 retention. This observation, which has been confirmed in studies of similar patients by Kepron and Cherniack (1973), led to the suggestion that pre-morbid variations in the intensity of the hypoxic drive might underlie some of the variations in clinical presentation of patients suffering from chronic bronchitis and emphysema. The contrast between the 'blue and bloated' patient, in whom the hypoxic drive to breathing might be depressed and the

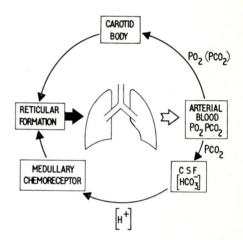

Figure 5 A simplified scheme of the chemical control of breathing, showing the carotid body as stimulated by a fall in arterial Po_2 (with some stimulation from a rise in Pco_2), and the medullary chemoreceptor stimulated by changes in the acidity (H^+) of the cerebrospinal (CSF), to a degree dependent on the arterial Pco_2 and the CSF bicarbonate concentration

'pink and puffing' in whom the hypoxic drive might be normal, might thereby be explained. This hypothesis awaits confirmation, but variations in intensity of the hypoxic drive have already been described in apparently normal healthy men studied during exercise at sea level (Flenley et al, 1973b). In 4 out of 37 normal subjects the drive appeared to be absent, and this lack of response was found to persist when two of these four subjects were studied one year later. Further work is needed to establish the prevalence in variation in the hypoxic drive to breathing in the normal population. In this context, it has recently become apparent that the ventilatory response to CO_2 stimulation, in the absence of hypoxia, can vary some 10-fold in apparently normal subjects, with a level of 0.8 to 8.0 litres/min/mmHg (Lyall and Cameron, 1974). If such an impaired ventilatory drive from hypoxia does exist in patients with chronic bronchitis, they would be expected to be less sensitive to ventilatory depression following oxygen therapy. However, many factors contribute to the control of breathing in these patients during an acute

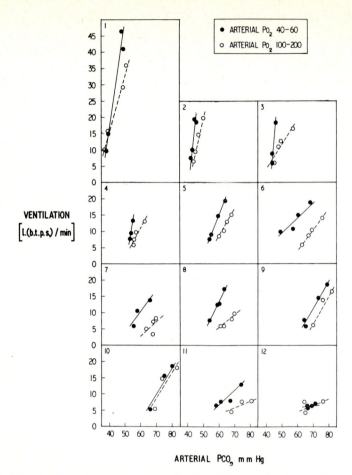

Figure 6 The ventilatory response to rises in arterial Pco_2 at two levels of arterial Po_2 in 12 patients with chronic bronchitis and emphysema, with various degrees of CO_2 retention when breathing air. In two cases (10 and 12), with severe CO_2 retention and hypoxia when breathing air, there was no further increase in ventilation when hypoxia was combined with a rise in Pco_2, indicating that the ventilatory response to hypoxia was blunted in these two patients. (From Flenley, Franklin and Millar (1970) by permission of the Editor of *Clinical Science*)

exacerbation of chest infection. Thus, the removal of peripheral chemo-receptor stimulation might play a lesser role than does the relief of locally intense hypoxia in the brain stem leading to a reduction in local production of lactic acid which may in turn reduce the central ventilatory drive from acidic stimulation of the medullary chemoreceptor (Fig. 5). However, at least in the lumbar cerebrospinal fluid, we did not find raised levels of lactate in such patients during an acute exacerbation of their chest infection (Alroy and Flenley, 1967).

Recognition of Hypoxaemia

The clinical recognition of hypoxaemia depends upon central cyanosis, seen in the warm mucous membranes of the tongue, cheeks and conjunctivae. This sign can be difficult to detect, particularly in tungsten or some fluorescent lighting. Recognition can vary from detection by only 50 per cent of observers unless the patient's arterial oxygen saturation was below 85 per cent (Po_2 probably between 47 and 55 mmHg, depending on the arterial pH) (Comroe

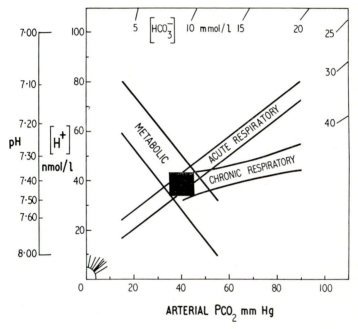

Figure 7 Non-logarithmic acid–base diagram relating arterial acidity (H+), (or pH), to arterial Pco_2, with isopleths of (HCO$_3^-$) radiating from the origin. The black rectangle signifies the normal range, the acute respiratory, chronic respiratory and metabolic confidence bands identifying the values observed in these single disturbances of acid–base balance in the blood of man in vivo. (From Flenley (1971) by permission of the Editor of the *Lancet*)

and Botelho, 1947), to recognition on 98 per cent of occasions by two skilled anaesthetists when their patients' arterial oxygen saturation was below 91 per cent (Po_2 57–64 mmHg, again if pH varied from 7.35 to 7.45) (Kelman and Nunn, 1966). This latter detection was attained when the patients were examined in 'daylight' fluorescent lighting. Other indices of hypoxia, including tachycardia, hyperventilation and anxiety, are notoriously variable and the aviation literature particularly emphasises the insidious changes of progressive hypoxia without awareness by either the subject or his colleagues, until unconsciousness suddenly supervenes.

In clinical practice, of course, the suspicion of central cyanosis can readily be confirmed by arterial blood analysis, which should be available in any district general hospital, for today few would doubt that the proper management of respiratory failure demands this facility on a 24 h service basis. Brachial or radial arterial puncture, under local anaesthesia, with anaerobic withdrawal of blood into an all-glass syringe, is a simple and safe procedure in the adult. The old suspicion that the pain of arterial puncture causes transient hyperventilation, so invalidating the results, has not been confirmed by direct investigation (Glauser and Morris, 1972). Femoral arterial puncture not infrequently leads to serious errors from analysis of blood from the femoral vein, despite warnings that the only proof of arterial origin of the blood is a visual demonstration of pulsatile movement of the barrel of the syringe. In addition to Po_2, pH and Pco_2 measurements on the arterial blood sample allow precise evaluation of the acid base status of the patient, which can aid both diagnosis and therapeutic management (Fig. 7).

The Consequences of Hypoxaemia

The consequences of acute exposure to prolonged hypoxaemia are seen in a pure form, uncomplicated by other disease, when healthy subjects are suddenly exposed to altitude. The Indo-Chinese War, fought at an altitude of over 10 000 ft in the Himalayas provided the opportunity to study this problem in large groups of subjects (Singh et al, 1969). Acute altitude sickness, characterised by breathlessness, headache, nausea, anorexia, and muscular weakness, which rarely proceeded to blurred vision, collapse, coma and paralysis, was seen in between 1 and 80 cases per 1000 subjects at risk. Symptoms developed from 6 to 96 h following the sudden exposure to 11 000 ft, when the arterial oxygen tension would be about 40 to 50 mmHg. Oliguria frequently preceded the development of symptoms, in contrast to the diuresis which is more usual in subjects who do not develop high altitude sickness. The exact role of hypoxaemia in causation of acute altitude sickness is uncertain, for the hyperventilatory adaptation to altitude, which arises initially from hypoxic stimulus through the carotid chemoreceptors, results in a lowering of the arterial Pco_2 with a respiratory alkalosis, so that typical blood gas figures at these altitudes would be Po_2 42 mmHg, Pco_2 34 mmHg, pH 7.47 (Severinghaus et al, 1966a). Oxygen administration does not relieve the symptoms at once, but they can be prevented by frusemide, or acetazolamide, given prophylactically. These drugs both affect acid base balance, so that the combination of hypoxaemia with respiratory alkalosis may be important in the development of high altitude sickness.

High altitude pulmonary oedema is less frequent than acute altitude sickness, and it can be fatal. Subjects who are susceptible to this condition, which usually develops after two or three days at altitude often following a hard day's exertion, appear to have an excessive rise in pulmonary arterial pressure on exposure to hypoxia, and this pressure can rise to a mean level of over 50 mmHg on exercise at altitude (Hultgren, Grover and Hartley, 1971). Frusemide is again effective in both treatment and prevention, and although the exact mechanism remains unknown, pulmonary hypertension would seem to be important. Hypoxic damage to the pulmonary capillary membrane, with resultant increase in permeability, might allow this increased pressure to drive fluid into the interstitial and alveolar spaces (Whayne and Severinghaus, 1968).

Pulmonary hypertension

Chronic hypoxaemia can be studied in both sojourners and natives at high altitude, and is characterised by pulmonary hypertension with right ventricular hypertrophy, and secondary polycythaemia. It has long been known that pulmonary vasoconstriction is induced by acute exposure to hypoxia, for example, a reduction in arterial Po_2 to about 50 mmHg, by breathing a 13 per cent oxygen mixture, will cause a rise in mean pulmonary arterial pressure $(P\overline{PA})$ from 12 mmHg at rest when breathing air, to around 20 to 22 mmHg when breathing the hypoxic mixture. This vasoconstriction probably arises in both pre- and postcapillary segments of the pulmonary vascular tree (Lee, 1971). In chronic mountain sickness (Monge's disease), the rise in pulmonary arterial pressure is excessive. Thus in 12 healthy adult residents at 14 000 ft, Peñaloza, Sime and Ruiz (1971) found the average arterial oxygen saturation to be 81 per cent (probably equivalent to an arterial Po_2 of about 46 mmHg), with the average $P\overline{PA}$ being 23 ± 5.1 mmHg, as compared to a $P\overline{PA}$ of 13.0 ± 3.5 mmHg in sea level residents with a similar cardiac output at rest. In contrast, 10 patients with chronic mountain sickness were found by these investigators to have a much lower arterial Po_2 (probably about 37 mmHg), although living at the same altitude, yet to have a $P\overline{PA}$ of 47 ± 17.7 mmHg. These latter patients had the characteristic features of this disease, consisting of extreme polycythaemia, cor pulmonale with right ventricular hypertrophy, and peripheral oedema. It is in this type of patient that Severinghaus et al (1966b) found the hypoxic ventilatory drive to be blunted.

Pathological examination of the pulmonary circulation in residents at high altitude often shows duplication of the internal elastic laminae of pulmonary arterioles, with hypertrophy of the muscular layers of these vessels, and right ventricular hypertrophy, as shown by a right ventricular weight of over 65 g. Hypoxic conditions of whatever aetiology produce similar results. In a postmortem study, Heath, Edwards and Harris (1970) found the weight of the right ventricle to correlate well with the weights of the carotid bodies in patients with emphysema, and they presumed that the right ventricular hypertrophy was evidence of hypoxaemia during life. Similar hypertrophy of carotid bodies (see also Chapter 3) has been noted in man resident in high altitudes and also in animals native to high altitude (Edwards et al, 1971).

Hunter et al (1974) have recently shown that the right ventricle grew abnormally rapidly in rats and mice exposed to experimental hypoxia in a decompression chamber, and that this hypertrophy could be reversed by subsequent return of the animals to normal oxygen tensions. Pulmonary vascular resistance increased during hypoxaemia of these animals with development of the characteristic pathological changes described above.

Secondary polycythaemia in adults

In normal healthy subjects native to different altitudes, Weil et al (1968) have established that there is a linear relationship between the degree of secondary polycythaemia, as measured by the circulating red cell mass, and the arterial oxygen saturation. However, in chronic hypoxaemia resulting from lung disease, some observers have observed a similar relationship between red cell mass and arterial oxygen saturation (Chan, 1969), whilst others have found the response to hypoxaemia to be less than in normal subjects (Cocking and Darke, 1972). Recently, Harrison (1973) has described 19 patients with cor pulmonale and a raised peripheral venous haematocrit in whom the red cell mass is greater than expected when compared to their arterial oxygen saturation. It seems unlikely that these differences in response will be explained until accurate chemical or immune assays of human erythropoeitin become available.

Controversy also surrounds the effects of secondary polycythaemia on the pulmonary circulation. Segel and Bishop (1966) found that venesection, which restored the red cell mass of a group of severely polycythaemic bronchitics to normal, had little effect in reducing their pulmonary arterial pressure. This surprising result, which was confirmed in patients with primary polycythaemia (Segel and Bishop, 1967) has now been challenged by Duroux et al (1974), who have found that rapid replacement of whole blood by dextran of 40 000 molecular weight left the arterial blood gas tensions of 17 patients with severe obstructive lung disease unchanged (P_{O_2} 44 ± 9, P_{CO_2} 60 ± 12 mmHg), but reduced the mean pulmonary artery pressure, despite an increase in cardiac output. They concluded that the acute reduction of haematocrit from 65 to 47 per cent following the dextran infusion contributed substantially to the reduction in pulmonary hypertension, suggesting that the viscosity of polycythaemic blood is an important cause of pulmonary hypertension, and thus cor pulmonale, in patients with chronic hypoxic lung disease.

Respiratory Failure

Respiratory failure can be defined as existing in a patient, who when breathing air at sea level, has an arterial oxygen tension below 60 mmHg, as a result of lung disease. If the arterial P_{CO_2} is at or below normal (35–45 mmHg), this is *type I respiratory failure*, whereas if the arterial P_{CO_2} is above 49 mmHg, this is *type II respiratory failure* (Campbell, 1965). This distinction of the two types of respiratory failure carries important therapeutic implications.

Causes of *type I respiratory failure* (low Po_2, low or normal Pco_2) are listed in Table 1.

Type I respiratory failure is common in any condition which obstructs or destroys a significant number of alveoli or their airways. It is often assumed that the low Pco_2 so often accompanying hypoxaemia is due to ventilatory stimulation from the peripheral chemoreceptors. However, in normal man, the arterial Po_2 must be lowered to around 40 to 50 mmHg before significant hyperventilation develops, particularly if the physiological feedback is closed so that the Pco_2 does fall with the increase in ventilation so in turn reducing

Table 1 Causes of respiratory failure type I
(hypoxaemia without CO_2 retention)

Chronic bronchitis and emphysema
Pneumonia
Pulmonary oedema
Atelectasis
Pulmonary fibrosis
Bronchial asthma
Spontaneous pneumothorax
Pulmonary embolism
Thromboembolic pulmonary hypertension
Bronchiectasis
Cardiogenic shock
Traumatic and septic shock
Fat embolism
Crushed chest injury
Kyphoscoliosis
Barbiturate poisoning
Postoperation
Obesity
Pulmonary arteriovenous fistulae

the ventilatory drive. Again, correction of hypoxaemia in these conditions rarely restores the Pco_2 to normal, suggesting that the hyperventilation arises from other causes, probably through vagal afferent fibres from irritant receptors or juxtapulmonary capillary (J) receptors (Paintal, 1963), since in experimental sterile pneumonia in the rabbit, hyperventilation can be reduced by blocking the vagus from the pneumonic lung (Trenchard, Gardner and Guz, 1972). The low Pco_2 in type I respiratory failure carries implications for oxygen transport, because hypocapnia interacts with hypoxia in modifying circulatory control. This is particularly apparent in the cerebral circulation. Diminution of oxygen supply, due to arterial hypoxaemia, leads of course, to the further impairment of O_2 delivery to cells if regional blood flow is reduced. It seems possible that some of the anxiety and distress of both pulmonary oedema and bronchial asthma may be contributed to by the hazardous state of cerebral oxygenation which results from the combination of low Po_2 and low Pco_2.

Hypoxaemia arises very often in *chronic bronchitis and emphysema* and indeed, from the known relationships between FEV_1 and arterial blood gas tensions in these patients, and the prevalence of chronic bronchitis causing airways obstruction in Britain, it seems probable that about 500 000 patients in Britain may have an arterial Po_2 below 60 mmHg. However, hypoxaemia in chronic bronchitis, unlike bronchial asthma, is very frequently associated with CO_2 retention. Such a complication increases the gravity of prognosis (Renzetti, McClement and Litt, 1966). It is important to appreciate that the combination of hypoxaemia and CO_2 retention in a conscious patient must imply that ventilatory control is severely deranged, for this combination of two uniquely powerful chemical ventilatory stimuli would normally lead to such powerful ventilatory change as to restore normal Po_2 and Pco_2, if the lungs were normal.

Carbon dioxide retention in chronic bronchitis is frequently chronic, a problem which is readily recognised if use is made of new information on 95 per cent confidence limits of the hydrogen ion (or pH)/Pco_2 relationships in arterial blood in vivo (Flenley, 1971) (Fig. 7).

Hypoxaemia in *bronchial asthma*, was first clearly documented in a large series of cases in 1967 (Tai and Read, 1967) but has since been amply confirmed. Hypoxaemia occurs most frequently in severe asthma where it is usually associated with low Pco_2 indicating hyperventilation despite the increased airways obstruction and lung hyperinflation, which greatly increase the work of breathing (Fig. 8). The hypoxaemia almost certainly results from gross mismatching of ventilation to perfusion, for perfusion can be severely impaired in some regions, as shown by lung scan, as can regional ventilation. In addition to hypoxaemia in severe asthma, mild hypoxaemia, with widening of the alveolar to arterial oxygen tension gradient, has recently been documented in asymptomatic asthma between attacks, when the airways resistance is relatively normal. In this situation hypoxaemia can be attributed to patchy occlusion of small airways, particularly in the lower zones of the lungs, as shown by an abnormally high 'closing volume' (McCarthy and Milic-Emili, 1973). It is also important to recognise that bronchodilators may potentiate hypoxaemia in severe asthma, presumably by increasing the mismatch of alveolar ventilation to perfusion. This action appears particularly probable with adrenaline, or isoprenaline, but this is less of a problem with the $beta_2$ sympathetic stimulants, salbutamol and terbutaline. In clinical practice, of course, such dangers can be avoided by using bronchodilators in the severe asthmatic only when he is receiving oxygen.

In *fibrosing alveolitis* hypoxaemia may not be apparent at rest, until the final stages of the disease, but the alveolar to arterial oxygen tension gradient $(A-a\, Do_2)$ is increased earlier, and hypoxaemia on exercise is a well-recognised part of the pattern of functional disturbance, with restriction of lung

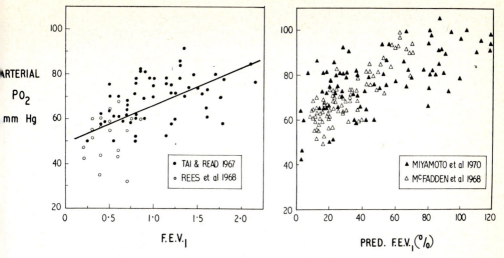

Figure 8 The relationship between the arterial Po_2 and FEV_1 (or percentage of predicted normal FEV_1) in severe asthma, as described in four series in the literature. Hypoxaemia is usual as the FEV_1 falls below 0.5 litre (or 20 per cent of predicted). (From *Bronchial Asthma: Mechanisms and Therapeutics*, by permission of Little, Brown & Co and *New Directions in Asthma*, by permission of the American College of Chest Physicians)

Table 2 Causes of respiratory failure type II (ventilatory failure—hypoxaemia with a raised arterial Pco_2)

Chronic bronchitis and emphysema
Bronchial asthma
Crushed chest injury
Following resuscitation from cardiac arrest
Drug overdosage
Myasthenia gravis
Polyneuropathy, myopathies, porphyria
Cervical cord injuries
Head injuries
Primary alveolar hypoventilation
Poliomyelitis
Pulmonary oedema
Hypothermia
Hypertrophy of tonsils and adenoids
Near-drowning
Complicating peritonitis
Suxamethonium apnoea

volumes, stiff lungs, and low transfer factor. Recently the widened $A-a\ Do_2$ has been related to gross maldistribution of regional ventilation/perfusion ratios in this condition, an assessment using ^{133}Xe (McCarthy and Cherniack, 1973), which, of course, only detects perfusion to lung regions which receive some ventilation.

Hypoxaemia *in obesity* is relatively common, and is now recognised to result in large part from the shunting of blood past unventilated alveoli in the lower lung zones (Holley et al, 1967). This arises from reduction in expiratory reserve volume, as the patient tends to breathe at a lower lung volume due to compression of the thorax by fat. As a result, the transmural pressure across some small airways at the base of the lung is such that they remain closed throughout the normal tidal breath; this 'closing volume' impinging then on the tidal volume range. Primary alveolar hypoventilation can occur in the obese patient, but if rigid criteria for definition of this syndrome are applied (Bates, Macklem and Christie, 1971) this will be recognised to be a rare disease, whereas hypoxaemia is common in the obese.

Causes of *type II respiratory failure* are given in Table 2.

Treatment of Hypoxaemia

The *treatment of type I respiratory failure* depends upon restoration of a normal arterial oxygen tension by administration of oxygen. As the P_{CO_2} is low or normal by definition, ventilatory control is normal, and there is no risk of provoking CO_2 retention by a device delivering high concentrations of oxygen. Six litres of oxygen/min by either a Polymask (BOC) or MC mask (BXL Limited) provides around 60 per cent oxygen at the lips. Both masks allow some rebreathing, thereby humidifying the inspired gas, and also raising the inspired CO_2 to between 0.5 to 2 per cent, which could be helpful in counteracting the respiratory alkalosis so typical of type I respiratory failure. Unfortunately, patients with this type of respiratory failure are nearly always breathless and therefore tolerate any mask poorly. The only alternative is the oxygen tent, which is both inefficient, costly in use of oxygen and claustrophobic. Temperature and humidity must be controlled in the tent, and the fire risk is greater than with masks or nasal catheters. The 'Mark V Refrigeration Oxygen Tent' (Oxygenaire) provides both refrigeration and circulation of the air by a fan, and also has a facility for CO_2 wash-out. This tent can produce oxygen concentrations between 50 and 57 per cent with a CO_2 concentration of less than 1 per cent, with the carbon dioxide wash-out off, but when this wash-out is on, the oxygen concentration can vary between 26 and 31 per cent at a flow rate of 4 to 10 litres of oxygen/min and the CO_2 concentration will then be below 0.4 per cent (Report, 1969).

Sixty per cent oxygen, giving an inspired tension of around 400 mmHg, is adequate for most cases of type I respiratory failure, and will produce an arterial oxygen tension of over 100 mmHg. However, if the volume of blood shunted through non-ventilated alveoli of the lungs rises much above 20 per cent of the cardiac output, this arterial P_{O_2} will no longer be obtained. Addition of oxygen by nasal prongs flowing at 2 to 4 litres/min along with a Polymask or MC mask receiving 6 litres/min will raise the inspired oxygen tension towards 80 to 90 per cent (550–600 mmHg), which will then give an arterial P_{O_2} of about 100 mmHg, even if the shunt rises as high as 25 per cent.

Maintenance of adequate oxygenation with higher shunt percentages may require mechanical ventilation with positive end expiratory pressure (PEEP), which may reduce the shunt by reopening some alveoli.

In *type II respiratory failure*, where hypoxaemia is combined with CO_2 retention, treatment must steer between the two dangers of death from hypoxaemia and death from respiratory acidosis, resulting from the removal of the hypoxic drive to breathing which follows the raising of the arterial Po_2. In most cases of type II respiratory failure, other than those due to chronic bronchitis and emphysema, this dilemma is solved by mechanical ventilation. The relative frequency of conditions needing ventilation will depend upon the hospital and population served. Thus, Pontoppidan, Geffin and Lowenstein (1972), found that of 1400 cases treated in the Respiratory Care Unit of the Massachusetts General Hospital in 1971, only 10 per cent suffered from chronic pulmonary disease, whereas surgical cases (following open heart surgery, thoracic, neurological or abdominal surgery), were most frequent, followed by drug overdoses, crushed chest injury and neuro-muscular disorders. The overall mortality of ventilator treatment was between 10 and 20 per cent, but many of these patients died from causes unrelated to their lung condition. The criteria for institution of ventilator support employed by these authors include vital capacity below 15 ml/kg body weight (i.e. below 1200 ml in most adults); FEV_1 below 10 ml/kg (around 700 ml), arterial Po_2 persistently below 70 mmHg when receiving oxygen by mask, Pco_2 over 55 mmHg, and dead space to tidal volume ratio over 60 per cent. They note, of course, that these criteria do not necessarily apply in patients with chronic bronchitis and emphysema.

Major remaining problems with mechanical ventilation include impairment of venous return (particularly when PEEP is used) with a resultant fall in cardiac output; increase of lung water with interstitial oedema; ulceration of the larynx following prolonged intubation; and pulmonary oxygen toxicity. A rise in pressure is transmitted to the intrathoracic veins, particularly if the chest wall is stiff, the lungs are compliant and the tidal volume of ventilation is large, with a long duration of high inflation pressures during the breathing cycle. In most patients an increase in venomotor tone allows venous return to be maintained during ventilation, but when the sympathetic nervous system is defective as in polyneuritis, cervical cord transection and in patients being treated with certain antihypertensive drugs, this no longer applies. Persistent hypoxaemia (arterial Po_2 below 70 mmHg) which cannot be corrected without raising the inspired oxygen tension over 50 per cent on the ventilator, thereby running the risk of pulmonary oxygen toxicity (see later), is regarded by Pontoppidan et al as an indication for PEEP. The response to PEEP is not predictable for although the cardiac output will fall in most patients, this does not necessarily hinder the transport of oxygen for this fall in output may be overcome by the gain in arterial Po_2. Thus in 19 subjects Lutch and Murray (1972) found that PEEP decreased the alveolar to arterial oxygen tension gradient, reduced the cardiac output in all patients, but did not change either oxygen uptake or the calculated mixed venous oxygen tension.

Most authorities now agree that a cuffed endotracheal tube can only be used for up to eight days in the adult without running a serious risk of permanent laryngeal or tracheal damage, though this risk can be minimised by using a low pressure prestretched cuff (Grillo, Cooper and Geffin, 1971).

Pulmonary oxygen toxicity has been known since Lorrain-Smith's work in 1898. The syndrome developed relevance for clinical practice when it became possible to continuously ventilate patients with high concentrations of oxygen. An extensive review by Clark and Lambertsen (1971) emphasises that the pathological lesion falls into an acute exudative phase, with interstitial and alveolar oedema, swelling of capillary endothelial cells and destruction of alveolar type I cells followed by a subacute proliferative phase, characterised by interstitial fibrosis, fibroblastic proliferation and hyperplasia of alveolar type II cells. The early exudative phase can be completely resolved if the damaging oxygen is removed. Clinical symptoms are variable, consisting of pain in the chest, tenacious tracheal secretions, with coarse crepitations, and eventual development of diffuse bilateral pulmonary opacities on x-ray. Changes in pulmonary function occur early, particularly a fall in dynamic compliance with progressive reduction in vital capacity, widening of the alveolar to arterial oxygen tension gradient being a later development. There is a wide variability in the tolerance of human lungs to oxygen damage, but in the most susceptible subjects the vital capacity shows a perceptible fall after 10 h of continuous exposure to 100 per cent oxygen at atmospheric pressure. Most normal subjects will show a 15 per cent fall in vital capacity after 30 h of such exposure. The mechanism of the damage is not certain, but it seems probable that oxygen can directly damage the alveolar cells, causing decrease in their protein synthesis (Gacad and Massaro, 1973). Although surfactant activity is decreased following oxygen damage, it seems that this effect is secondary. The condition can probably be prevented by intermittent reduction of the inspired oxygen, but in clinical practice the most important principle is to ensure that the inspired oxygen concentration never exceeds 50 per cent for prolonged periods of time. Widespread recognition that pressure cycled ventilators can give inspired oxygen concentrations of up to 90 per cent, despite using the 'airmix' control, has probably reduced the prevalence of the condition. The lethal lung damage following the poison paraquat may result from sensitisation of alveolar cells to damage by even normal levels of oxygen (Fisher, Clements and Wright, 1973).

Type II respiratory failure in chronic bronchitis and emphysema is most frequently encountered by physicians. Controlled oxygen therapy is the mainstay of treatment in this condition, with ventilator treatment only being necessary when this treatment fails. Oxygen is administered by a low concentration device, such as the Edinburgh Mask, giving approximately 30 per cent at 2 litres/min; the 28 per cent Ventimask, using 4 litres oxygen/min; or simply by nasal prongs which at 2 litres oxygen/min give about 30 per cent inspired concentration. Most of these patients will have acute or chronic CO_2 retention, and it is probably wiser to guide treatment by the arterial pH than by the P_{CO_2} alone (Flenley, 1971). In 1964 we proposed that aims of treatment in these patients when using controlled oxygen therapy were an arterial P_{O_2} above 50 mmHg and an arterial pH above 7.25 (Hutchison, Flenley and Donald, 1964). Experience in the past decade with over 200 further cases has confirmed that these are reasonable criteria for treatment. However, a desultory debate continues as to the lower level of arterial P_{O_2} than can be tolerated in these patients. This is undoubtedly less than in patients with hypoxaemia due to acute pulmonary oedema (Flenley et al, 1973a), because of the higher cardiac output in the chronic bronchitic, but accurate determination of the lowest level of arterial P_{O_2} that is compatible with survival would require unethical studies, and this debate will therefore not be resolved by experiment in man.

If these criteria cannot be attained by controlled oxygen therapy, it is our practice then to consider mechanical ventilation for these patients. The place of respiratory stimulants remains controversial (*Lancet*, 1973). Doxapram hydrochloride may be the most effective stimulant when given by continuous infusion; this drug prevented significant rises in arterial P_{CO_2} in 38 cases out of 40 when controlled oxygen therapy was used to raise the arterial P_{O_2} to 60–70 mmHg in bronchitis patients with acute CO_2 retention (Moser et al, 1973). The side effects of Doxapram include hypertension, agitation and tremor, and probably increases in cardiac output and pulmonary arterial mean pressure ($P_{\overline{PA}}$).

Long-term oxygen therapy in chronic cor pulmonale

Once type II respiratory failure and cor pulmonale have developed, the prognosis in chronic obstructive bronchitis is appalling. Of 92 patients with cor pulmonale (average arterial P_{O_2} 56 mmHg, P_{CO_2} 53 mmHg) only one quarter were alive after four years (Renzetti et al, 1966). Improvement of this dismal outlook by correction of hypoxaemia still remains to be proved, and is currently the subject of a controlled multicentre trial in Britain. Continuous low-dosage oxygen therapy can reverse secondary polycythaemia in these patients and also reduce pulmonary arterial mean pressure even three weeks after completion of four to eight weeks of continuous oxygen treatment (Abraham, Cole and Bishop, 1968). In stable chronically hypoxic bronchitics acute alleviation of hypoxaemia does *not* lower the $P_{\overline{PA}}$ (Abraham et al, 1969), whereas in an acute exacerbation of chronic bronchitis, controlled oxygen therapy can significantly lower $P_{\overline{PA}}$.

The potential value of continued correction of oxygen lack was first directly tested in the mile high city of Denver, Colorado, where the altitude is not only sufficient to reduce 'normal' arterial P_{O_2} to around 70 mmHg, but also to shorten the lives of hypoxic bronchitics when compared with those living at sea level. Neff and Petty (1970) described 33 patients with severe irreversible airways obstruction, aged between 50 and 70 years, who were continuously given 2 to 4 litres of oxygen/min by nasal catheters, from a liquid oxygen source, for between 7 and 41 months. Before oxygen therapy they had an arterial Po_2 between 35 and 55 mmHg, and this was below 45 mmHg in 17 of the patients with cor pulmonale. The oxygen treatment raised the Po_2 to around 60 mmHg. Two-thirds of the patients with cor pulmonale were alive two years later, which compares with only one-third of 13 patients with a comparable degree of hypoxia who were treated without oxygen, though the latter patients lived at sea level (Boushy and Coates, 1964). The Denver studies were not formally controlled, for there was no comparison with similar patients treated concurrently without oxygen. However, there was no improvement in survival in the 16 patients treated with oxygen in whom the arterial Po_2 was above 45 mmHg when they were breathing air at the start of the study, so that long-term oxygen only appeared to prolong life in patients with moderate to severe hypoxaemia. These studies have been criticised (Stevens, 1970), particularly on the point of comparison with patients living at sea level but, in answer, Neff and Petty (1970) pointed out that only 26 per cent of patients with cor pulmonale who lived at altitude survived for $2\frac{1}{2}$ years, when treated without oxygen, compared with 72 per cent survival at this time in their patients with cor pulmonale who did have oxygen.

In Britain, Stark, Finnegan and Bishop (1972) described 11 men with cor pulmonale due to chronic bronchitis and hypoxia (average Po_2 49 mmHg) who were treated with 2 litres/min of oxygen for eight weeks. During treatment the Po_2 was raised to about 70 mmHg. The patients were divided into three groups: some received oxygen for 18 h/day, whilst others received it for 15 or 12 to 13 h daily. The $P\overline{PA}$ was raised in all patients when breathing air at the start of the study, and significant falls in both $P\overline{PA}$ and pulmonary vascular resistance occurred in patients receiving oxygen for 18 or 15 h/day, but not in those receiving 12 to 13 h daily. Anderson et al (1973) treated 14 similarly hypoxic bronchitic patients with long-term oxygen for 12 h in the day, but only three patients derived benefit, as judged by a reduction in the expected number of acute exacerbations of cor pulmonale, and most cases continued to deteriorate. It therefore appears that long-term oxygen is only likely to be valuable if administered for at least 15 h of the day. Stark, Finnegan and Bishop (1973), described five patients treated with long-term oxygen for between 6 and 24 months, for a period of 15 h in a day. After 23 to 59 weeks' treatment they found $P\overline{PA}$ and pulmonary vascular resistance to be reduced, and all five patients no longer had pulmonary hypertension at rest. Two of the patients were able to return to work.

These studies have shown that long-term oxygen is possible in a domiciliary setting, but there is no doubt that the treatment is expensive and does involve the patient in a degree of inconvenience. Oxygen can be supplied in cylinders though even without any wastage of gas this will require at least 10 standard size (1360 litres; 48 cu. ft) cylinders each week, at a consumption of 2 litres of oxygen a minute for 15 h treatment each day. Large cylinders, containing either 3400 litres (120 cu. ft) or 6800 litres (240 cu. ft) of oxygen, are extremely heavy, and at the moment special arrangements have to be made for their delivery to domiciliary patients in Britain. There are two alternative systems to cylinders. The first, the oxygen concentrator (Cotes, Douglas-Jones and Saunders, 1969; Stark and Bishop, 1973), differentially absorbs nitrogen from air on to molecular sieves, thereby producing up to 60 per cent oxygen. Current models of this equipment are the size of a small refrigerator, and run on domestic electricity. The second alternative is the liquid oxygen Walker system (Union Carbide Limited). This equipment, which has been extensively used in N. America, consists of two units: the Mark II oxygen reservoir and the Walker Unit. The former contains 18.1 kg (40 lb) of liquid oxygen and can be carried into the patient's home by one delivery man. This reservoir unit supplies oxygen for use in the home and will require to be exchanged for a full unit twice a week. The Walker Unit, the second component of the system, is a compact portable oxygen supply that can be carried by the patient on a shoulder strap. The Walker weighs about 5 kg (11 lb) when full, and holds the equivalent of about 1000 litres of oxygen, sufficient to provide for 8 h treatment at 2 litres/min. The patient can fill the Walker Unit in his own home from his reservoir. This is the only effective system that allows oxygen therapy for the hypoxic bronchitic during exercise, when the arterial Po_2 of these patients usually falls even lower. Correction of hypoxaemia also reduces the exercise ventilation of these patients, thus making them less breathless on exertion (King et al, 1974).

The cost of providing oxygen on a continuous basis is considerable. Oxygen supplied in 1360 litre cylinders costs around £1500 per year at current rates in Britain for a continuous supply of 2 litres/min of oxygen for 15 h in the day. The cost is reduced by the larger cylinders, but these are very inconvenient to handle. The oxygen concentrator currently costs around £900, with considerable expenditure on running costs and maintenance in the year. The liquid system is not yet commercially available in Britain, but the cost would probably be comparable. Against these expenses should be set the economic benefit of reduction of time in hospital, which seems to be a likely outcome of long-term treatment with oxygen in these patients, and also the possibility that some will be able to return to work.

REFERENCES

Abraham, A. S., Cole, R. B., Green, I. D., Hedworth-Whitty, R. B., Clarke, S. W. & Bishop, J. M. (1969) Factors contributing to the reversible pulmonary hypertension of patients with acute respiratory failure studied by serial observations during recovery. *Circulation Research*, **24**, 51–60.

Abraham, A. S., Cole, R. B. & Bishop, J. M. (1968) Reversal of pulmonary hypertension by prolonged oxygen administration to patients with chronic bronchitis. *Circulation Research*, **23**, 147–157.

Alroy, G. G. & Flenley, D. C. (1967) The acidity of the cerebrospinal fluid in man with particular reference to chronic ventilatory failure. *Clinical Science*, **33**, 335–343.

Anderson, P. B., Cayton, R. M., Holt, P. J. & Howard, P. (1973) Long-term oxygen therapy in cor pulmonale. *Quarterly Journal of Medicine*, **42**, 563–573.

Bates, D. V., Macklem, P. T. & Christie, R. V. (1971) *Respiratory Function in Disease*, 2nd edn. Philadelphia: Saunders.

Benesch, R. & Benesh, R. E. (1967) Effect of organic phosphates from human erythrocytes on allosteric properties of haemoglobin. *Biochemical and Biophysical Research Communications*, **26**, 162–167.

Boushy, S. F. & Coates, E. D. Jr (1964) The prognostic value of pulmonary function tests in emphysema with special reference to arterial blood studies. *American Review of Respiratory Disease*, **90**, 553–563.

Byrne-Quinn, E., Sodal, I. E. & Weil, J. V. (1972) Hypoxic and hypercapnic ventilatory drives in children native to high altitude. *Journal of Applied Physiology*, **32**, 44–46.

Campbell, E. J. M. (1965) Respiratory failure. *British Medical Journal*, **1**, 1451–1460.

Chan, B. W. B. (1969) Polycythaemia in coal miners with chronic lung disease. *British Medical Journal*, **2**, 349–350.

Clark, J. M. & Lambertsen, C. J. (1971) Pulmonary oxygen toxicity: a review. *Pharmacological Reviews*, **23**, 37–133.

Cocking, J. B. & Darke, C. S. (1972) Blood volume studies in chronic obstructive non-specific lung disease. *Thorax*, **27**, 44–51.

Comroe, J. H. & Botelho, S. (1947) The unreliability of cyanosis in the recognition of arterial anoxemia. *American Journal of Medical Sciences*, **214**, 1–6.

Cotes, J. E., Douglas-Jones, A. G. & Saunders, M. J. (1969) A 60 per cent oxygen supply for medical use. *British Medical Journal*, **4**, 143–146.

Craig, D. B., Wahba, W. M., Don, H. F., Couture, J. G. & Becklake, M. R. (1971) 'Closing volume' and its relationship to gas exchange in seated and supine positions. *Journal of Applied Physiology*, **31**, 717–721.

Duroux, P., Caubarrere, I., Gonzalea, C., Fernandez, F., Ruff, F. & Even, P. (1974) Effects of blood viscosity upon the pulmonary circulation in chronic lung disease with polycythaemia. *European Journal of Clinical Investigation*, **4**, 360.

Edwards, C., Heath, D., Harris, P., Castillo, Y., Krüger, H. & Arias-Stella, J. (1971) The carotid body in animals at high altitude. *Journal of Pathology*, **104**, 231–238.

Fairweather, L., Walker, J. & Flenley, D. C. (1974) 2,3-Diphosphoglycerate concentration and the dissociation of oxyhaemoglobin in ventilatory failure. *Clinical Science and Molecular Medicine*, **47**, 577–588.

Fisher, H. K., Clements, J. A. & Wright, R. R. (1973) Enhancement of oxygen toxicity by the herbicide paraquat. *American Review of Respiratory Disease*, **107**, 246–252.

Flenley, D. C. (1967) The rationale of oxygen therapy. *Lancet*, **1**, 270–273.

Flenley, D. C. (1971) Another non-logarithmic acid-base diagram? *Lancet*, **1**, 961–965.

Flenley, D. C., Fanklin, D. H. & Millar, J. S. (1970) The hypoxic drive to breathing in chronic bronchitis and emphysema. *Clinical Science*, **38**, 503–518.

Flenley, D. C., Miller, H. C., King, A. J., Kirby, B. J. & Muir, A. L. (1973a) Oxygen transport in acute pulmonary oedema and in acute exacerbations of chronic bronchitis. *British Medical Journal*, **1**, 78–81.

Flenley, D. C., Cooke, N. J., King, A. J., Leitch, A. G. & Brash, H. M. (1973b) The hypoxic drive to breathing studied during exercise in normal man and in hypoxic patients with chronic bronchitis and emphysema. *Bulletin de Physio-Pathologie Respiratoire*, **9**, 689–693.

Gacad, G. & Massaro, D. (1973) Hyperoxia: influence on lung mechanics and protein synthesis. *Journal of Clinical Investigation*, **52**, 559–565.

Glauser, F. L. & Morris, J. F. (1972) Accuracy of routine arterial puncture for determination of oxygen and CO_2 tensions. *American Review of Respiratory Disease*, **106**, 776–779.

Grillo, H. C., Cooper, J. D. & Geffin, B. (1971) A low pressure cuff for tracheostomy tubes to minimise tracheal injury: a comparative clinical trial. *Journal of Thoracic and Cardiovascular Surgery*, **62**, 898–907.

Harrison, B. D. W. (1973) Polycythaemia in a selected group of patients with chronic airways obstruction. *Clinical Science*, **44**, 563–570.

Heath, D., Edwards, C. & Harris, P. (1970) Post-mortem size and structure of the human carotid body. Its relation to pulmonary disease and cardiac hypertrophy. *Thorax*, **25**, 129–140.

Holley, H. S., Milic-Emili, J., Becklake, M. R. & Bates, D. V. (1967) Regional distribution of pulmonary ventilation and perfusion in obesity. *Journal of Clinical Investigation*, **46**, 475–481.

Holland, J., Milic-Emili, J., Macklem, P. T. & Bates, D. V. (1968) Regional distribution of pulmonary ventilation and perfusion in elderly subjects. *Journal of Clinical Investigation*, **47**, 81–92.

Hultgren, H. N., Grover, R. F. & Hartley, L. H. (1971) Abnormal circulatory responses to high altitude in subjects with a previous history of high-altitude pulmonary oedema. *Circulation*, **44**, 759–770.

Hunter, C., Barer, G. R., Shaw, J. W. & Clegg, E. J. (1974) Growth of the heart and lungs in hypoxic rodents—a model of human hypoxic disease. *Clinical Science and Molecular Medicine*, **46**, 375–391.

Hutchison, D. C. S., Flenley, D. C. & Donald, K. W. (1964) Controlled oxygen therapy in respiratory failure. *British Medical Journal*, **2**, 1159–1166.

Kelman, G. R. & Nunn, J. F. (1966) Clinical recognition of hypoxaemia under fluorescent lamps. *Lancet*, **1**, 1400–1403.

Kepron, W. & Cherniack, R. M. (1973) The ventilatory response to hypercapnia and to hypoxaemia in chronic obstructive lung disease. *American Review of Respiratory Disease*, **108**, 843–850.

Kilmartin, J. V. & Rossi-Bernardi, L. (1973) Interaction of haemoglobin with hydrogen ions, carbon dioxide and organic phosphates. *Physiological Reviews*, **53**, 836–890.

King, A. J., Cooke, N. J., Leitch, A. G. & Flenley, D. C. (1973) The effects of 30 per cent oxygen on the respiratory response to treadmill exercise in chronic respiratory failure. *Clinical Science*, **44**, 151–162.

Lancet (1973) A new stimulant for ventilatory failure? **1**, 753–754.

Lee, G. de J. (1971) Regulation of the pulmonary circulation. *British Heart Journal*, **33**, Suppl. 15–26.

Lubbers, D. W. (1968) *Oxygen Transport in Blood and Tissue*, ed. Lubbers, D. W. et al. Stuttgart: Thieme.

Lugliani, R., Whipp, B. J., Seard, C. & Wasserman, K. (1971) Effect of bilateral carotid body resection on ventilatory control at rest and during exercise in man. *New England Journal of Medicine*, **285**, 1105–1111.

Lutch, J. S. & Murray, J. F. (1972) Continuous positive-pressure ventilation: effects on systemic oxygen transport and tissue oxygenation. *Annals of Internal Medicine*, **76**, 193–202.

Lyall, J. R. W. & Cameron, I. R. (1974) The relation between vital capacity and the respiratory response to inhaled carbon dioxide. *European Journal of Clinical Investigation*, **4**, 338.

McCarthy, D. & Cherniack, R. M. (1973) Regional ventilation–perfusion and hypoxia in cryptogenic fibrosing alveolitis. *American Review of Respiratory Disease*, **107**, 200–208.

McCarthy, D. & Milic-Emili, J. (1973) Closing volume in asymptomatic asthma. *American Review of Respiratory Disease*, **107**, 559–570.

McCarthy, D. S., Spencer, R., Greene, R. & Milic-Emili, J. (1972) Measurement of 'closing volume' as a simple and sensitive test for early detection of small airway disease. *American Journal of Medicine*, **52**, 747–753.

McFadden, E. R. J. & Lyons, H. A. (1968) Arterial-blood gas tension in asthma. *New England Journal of Medicine*, **278**, 1027–1032.

McHardy, G. J. R. (1972) Diffusing capacity and pulmonary gas exchange. *British Journal of Diseases of the Chest*, **66**, 1–19.

MacKenzie, G. J., Taylor, S. H., Flenley, D. C., McDonald, A. H., Staunton, H. P. & Donald, K. W. (1964) Circulatory and respiratory studies in myocardial infarction and cardiogenic shock. *Lancet*, **2**, 825–832.

Milledge, J. S. & Lahiri, S. (1967) Respiratory control in Lowlanders and Sherpa Highlanders at altitude. *Respiration Physiology*, **2**, 310–322.

Miyamoto, T., Mizuno, K. & Furuya, K. (1970) Arterial blood gases in bronchial asthma. *Journal of Allergy*, **45**, 248.

Moser, K. M., Luchsinger, P. C., Adamson, J. S., McMahon, S. M., Schlueter, D. P., Spivack, M. & Weg, J. G. (1973) Respiratory stimulation with intravenous doxapram in respiratory failure. A double-blind co-operative study. *New England Journal of Medicine*, **288**, 427–431.

Neff, T. A. & Petty, T. L. (1970) Long-term continuous oxygen therapy in chronic airway obstruction. *Annals Internal Medicine*, **72**, 621–626.

Paintal, A. S. (1973) Vagal sensory receptors and their reflex effects. *Physiological Reviews*, **53**, 159–227.

Peñaloza, D., Sime, F. & Ruiz, L. (1971) Cor pulmonale in chronic mountain sickness: present concept of Monge's Disease. In *High Altitude Physiology. Ciba Foundation Symposium*, ed. Porter, R. & Knight, J., pp. 41–60. Edinburgh and London: Churchill Livingstone.

Pontoppidan, H., Geffin, B. & Lowenstein, E. (1972) Acute respiratory failure in the adult. *New England Journal of Medicine*, **287**, 690, 743, 799.

Rees, H. A., Millar, J. S. & Donald, K. W. (1968) A study of the clinical course and arterial blood–gas tensions of patients in status asthmaticus. *Quarterly Journal of Medicine*, **37**, 541–561.

Renzetti, A. D., McClement, J. H. & Litt, B. D. (1966) The Veterans Administration Co-operative Study of Pulmonary Function. III. Mortality in relation to respiratory function in chronic obstructive pulmonary disease. *American Journal of Medicine*, **41**, 115–129.

Report (1969) *Uses and Dangers of Oxygen Therapy*. Report of a sub-committee of the Standing Medical Advisory Committee. Scottish Home and Health Dept, HMSO.

Segel, N. & Bishop, J. M. (1966) The circulation in patients with chronic bronchitis and emphysema at rest and during exercise, with special reference to the influence of changes in blood viscosity and blood volume on the pulmonary circulation. *Journal of Clinical Investigation*, **45**, 1555–1568.

Segel, N. & Bishop, J. M. (1967) Circulatory studies in polycythaemia vera at rest and during exercise. *Clinical Science*, **32**, 527–549.

Severinghaus, J. W., Chiodi, H., Eger, E. I., Brandstater, B. & Hornbein, T. F. (1966a) Cerebral blood flow in man at high altitude. *Circulation Research*, **19**, 274–282.

Severinghaus, J. W., Bainton, C. R. & Carcelen, A. (1966b) Respiratory insensitivity to hypoxia in chronically hypoxic man. *Respiratory Physiology*, **1**, 308–334.

Singh, I., Khanna, P. K., Srivastava, M. C., Lal, M., Roy, S. B. & Subramanyam, C. S. V. (1969) Acute mountain sickness. *New England Journal of Medicine*, **280**, 175–184.

Sørensen, S. C. & Severinghaus, J. W. (1968) Respiratory insensitivity to acute hypoxia persisting after correction of tetralogy of Fallot. *Journal of Applied Physiology*, **25**, 221–223.

Stark, R. D., Finnegan, P. & Bishop, J. M. (1972) Daily requirements of oxygen to reverse pulmonary hypertension in patients with chronic bronchitis. *British Medical Journal*, **3**, 724–728.

Stark, R. D., Finnegan, P. & Bishop, J. M. (1973) Long-term domiciliary oxygen in chronic bronchitis with pulmonary hypertension. *British Medical Journal*, **3**, 467–470.

Stark, R. D. & Bishop, J. M. (1973) New method for oxygen therapy in the home using an oxygen concentrator. *British Medical Journal*, **2**, 105–106.

Stevens, P. M. (1970) Altitude and O_2 therapy in chronic lung disease. *Annals of Internal Medicine*, **73**, 659–660.

Tai, E. & Read, J. (1967) Blood–gas tensions in bronchial asthma. *Lancet*, **1**, 644–646.

Trenchard, D., Gardner, D. & Guz, A. (1972) Role of pulmonary vagal afferent nerve fibres in the development of rapid shallow breathing in lung inflammation. *Clinical Science*, **42**, 251–263.

Weil, J. V., Byrne-Quinn, E., Sodal, I. E., Filley, G. F. & Grover, R. F. (1971) Acquired attenuation of chemoreceptor function in chronically hypoxic man at high altitude. *Journal of Clinical Investigation*, **50**, 186–195.

Weil, J. V., Jamieson, G., Brown, D. W. & Grover, R. F. (1968) The red cell mass: arterial oxygen relationship in normal man. *Journal of Clinical Investigation*, **47**, 1627–1639.

West, J. B. (1969) Ventilation–perfusion inequality and overall gas exchange in computer models of the lung. *Respiratory Physiology*, **7**, 88–110.

Whayne, T. F. & Severinghaus, J. W. (1968) Experimental hypoxic pulmonary oedema in the rat. *Journal of Applied Physiology*, **25**, 729–732.

5
LUNG MORPHOLOGY

K. Horsfield

Morphology is the study of the shape of things. In the lung this science has progressed from the older, purely descriptive anatomy to the present day situation in which all aspects of lung structure are being closely related to their function. Modern morphology and physiology are thus inseparable, and knowledge of the one is required in order to understand the other. Perhaps the most important change in our approach to the study of anatomy was brought about by the work of Weibel (1963). He showed how mathematical principles could be applied to the sampling, measuring and counting of anatomical structures so as to make it possible to give a statement of the whole from a study of part of a complex structure.

The basic function of the lung is to bring gas and blood into close proximity over a large enough surface area to permit oxygen and carbon dioxide to exchange at a rate equal to their metabolic utilisation and production. This exchange occurs at the alveolar capillary membrane, which has a surface area of about 80 m², and both gas and blood are transported to it by branching systems of tubes. Air returns by the same system which brings it and thus flow is reciprocating, whilst blood is carried to the membrane and away from it by two separate systems, the arteries and the veins, in which flow is uni-directional. This arrangement explains why there is a 'dead space' in the airways but not in the vasculature.

THE DESCRIPTION OF BRANCHING SYSTEMS IN THE LUNG

These three branching structures are very complex, the airways consisting of approximately fifteen million branches, and the two vascular trees each of hundreds of millions. In order to describe and analyse such complex structures some orderly and systematic method must be employed. Before doing this it is convenient first to give a general description of the airways.

The trachea divides into the right and left main bronchi, and these together with both lower lobe bronchi constitute the large bronchi which are situated outside the lung substance. All other bronchi including the upper lobe bronchi are situated within the lung, and as they enter it they take with them an invagination of the visceral pleura. This forms a peribronchial sheath, separated from the bronchi by a potential space. How far into the lung this sheath extends has not been clearly worked out, but it may extend as far as the small bronchi. The intrapulmonary airways as far as the broncho-pulmonary segment bronchi constitute the medium bronchi, and distal to these are found the small bronchi. Large, medium and small bronchi all contain cartilage within their walls, distal airways without cartilage in their walls being termed bronchioles. The most distal bronchiole on which no alveoli are found is the terminal bronchiole, and the segment of lung supplied by this is an acinus. Beyond the terminal bronchiole alveoli are found on the walls of the airways; these are the respiratory bronchioles. Finally, alveoli

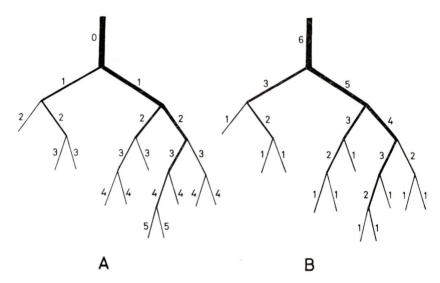

A   **B**

Figure 1   (A) Generations numbered downwards from the mainstem. (B) Orders numbered upwards to the main stem by Horsfield's method, in which order increases at each branching point. Generation 2 contains branches which are all of different diameters, while order 2 or order 3 contain branches of similar diameter

completely surround the airways which are termed alveolar ducts. The most distal of these end blindly in alveoli and constitute the alveolar sacs.

The above descriptive terms do not meet the needs of modern morphologists, who have developed their own methods to facilitate the mathematical analysis of branching structures. Several such methods exist, and these have been developed independently by the geomorphologists and the anatomical morphologists. They will be described using the bronchial tree as an example. The simplest method is to count down the tree from the trachea, each bifurcation giving rise to a new 'generation' (Weibel, 1963) or a 'division down' (Horsfield and Cumming, 1968). In this method the trachea is generation 0, its two daughter branches, the right and left main bronchi, generation 1, and so on, the generation increasing by one at each bifurcation (Fig. 1A).

A more complex method, of which there are several variations (Haggett and Chorley, 1969), is to start counting at the smallest, most peripheral, branches. These are called order 1 and from them counting is continued upwards to the trachea, which constitutes the highest ordered branch. Two such methods will be described, that of Horsfield and Cumming (1968) and that of Strahler (1953, 1957).

In the method described by Horsfield two order 1 branches meet to form an order 2 branch, two order 2 branches form an order 3 branch, and so on up the system. If two daughter branches of dissimilar order meet, the

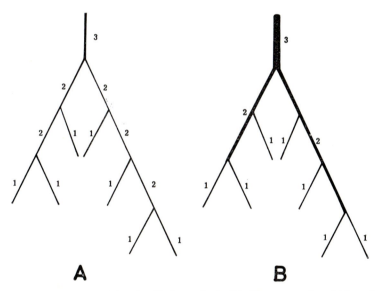

Figure 2 Orders numbered by Strahler's method. (A) First stage, in which order only increases when two similarly ordered branches meet. (B) Second stage, in which contiguous branches of the same order are considered to constitute one branch

parent branch is one order higher than the greater of the two daughter branches (Fig. 1B). Thus there is an increase in order at every branching point in the system.

Strahler (1953, 1957) described a method of counting rivers and their tributaries. It differs from that of Horsfield in that when two branches of differing order meet, the parent branch continues with the same order as the higher ordered daughter branch. Thus, order can only increase when two meeting daughter branches have the same order (Fig. 2A). When the total system has been ordered in this way contiguous branches of the same order, which may number two or more, are considered to constitute one branch (Fig. 2B). Such a compound branch will have more than two daughter branches.

These three methods of describing branching structures have different uses, and these will now be discussed.

The use of the term 'generation' comes most naturally to clinicians. When a chest x-ray or bronchogram is being examined, or a bronchoscopy performed, it is natural to count downwards starting at the trachea. The term is therefore useful in describing a positional relationship between the trachea and a given branch in the proximal airways. When the objective is to group together for descriptive or analytical purposes a number of bronchi of similar chracteristics the use of 'generation' is open to objection and may be misleading. This is because the bronchial tree is a relatively asymmetrical structure and branches of a given generation may vary widely in diameter, structure and function (Fig. 1A). An example of the degree of asymmetry of the bronchial tree is given by the structures which constitute generation 11. Depending on whether the pathway is short or long, generation 11 may be an alveolar duct, respiratory bronchiole, bronchiole or bronchus up to 2.5 mm in diameter.

The use of the term 'order' on the other hand, is almost impossible in the clinical situation. Even with a high quality bronchogram it is impossible to show all the peripheral bronchioles, so that orders cannot be counted. For the purpose of morphological analysis, however, orders are to be preferred, because branches of similar diameter, structure and function are grouped together (Fig. 1B). Furthermore, this method reveals some interesting mathematical relationships (Horsfield and Cumming, 1968).

The Bronchial Tree

Analysis of bronchial tree morphology is an important aid to the understanding of many physiological problems. A simple example is provided by the question how far down, on average, would the square wave front of a 500 ml inspirate penetrate into the airways? The answer is as far as the first generation of alveolar ducts. From this simple statement stem other important problems, such as what is the diffusing distance of the alveoli and how rapidly does this process occur? Detailed morphological knowledge is required to provide answers to such basic questions.

Weibel (1963) obtained morphometric data by measuring the diameter and length of branches of a resin cast of the bronchial tree, grouping the branches by generation. The measurements, which were complete for the first four generations, became increasingly incomplete down to the tenth generation in which only 21 per cent of branches were measured. Nevertheless, he was able to demonstrate linear relationships for log diameter and log length versus generation over this range.

A more detailed analysis was made by Horsfield and Cumming (1968) who also measured a resin cast. Their measurements were almost complete down to bronchi of 0.7 mm diameter, and samples of cast from 0.7 mm diameter down to the distal respiratory bronchioles were also measured. The

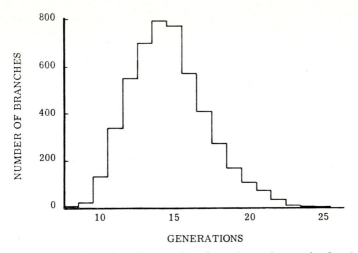

Figure 3 Distribution of number of generations from the trachea to the first branch of 0.7 mm diameter or less along every pathway. (From Horsfield (1974) by permission of the Editor of *British Journal of Diseases of the Chest*)

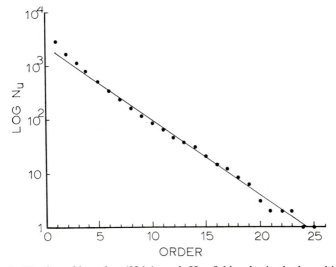

Figure 4 Number of branches (N_u) in each Horsfield order in the bronchial tree

distribution of divisions down (generations) from the trachea to branches of 0.7 mm diameter or less is shown in Figure 3, and ranges from 8 to 25, with a mode of 14. By combining this distribution with that obtained from the peripheral samples the range of divisions down from trachea to distal respiratory bronchioles was estimated to be from 10 to 32 with a mean of 18. This is a good measure of the asymmetry of the bronchial tree.

The data of Horsfield and Cumming have also been analysed using orders. With Horsfield's method there were 25 orders from branches of 0.7 mm diameter up to the trachea. When the number of branches in each order, and the mean number of distal respiratory bronchioles supplied by branches of each order, are plotted logarithmically against order, linear plots are obtained

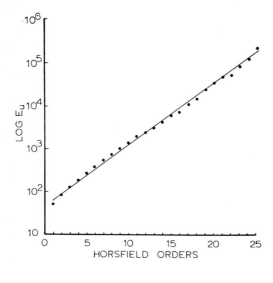

Figure 5   Mean number of distal respiratory bronchioles (E_u) supplied by branches of each Horsfield order in the bronchial tree

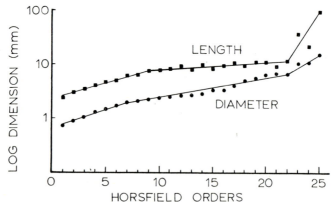

Figure 6   Mean diameter and length of branches of each Horsfield order in the bronchial tree

(Figs. 4, 5). Similar plots of log mean diameter and log mean length against order each show three linear sections (Fig. 6). These data are shown in Table 1.

The same data have been analysed by Strahler's method. It will be appreciated that since two or more contiguous bronchi may be labelled as one branch, the total number of branches and the total number of orders will be less than for the same system analysed by Horsfield's method. The data are given in Table 2, and log number of branches, log diameter and log length are plotted against order in Figures 7 and 8. It can be seen that the plots are more nearly linear than are the corresponding plots using Horsfield orders. Considering the plot of the number of branches in each order, the absolute value of the slop obtained from the regression equation is log 2.81. The value

Table 1   Model of the bronchial tree

Order	No. of branches	Diam. (mm)	Length (mm)	Distal RBs
31	1	16.00	100.00	233 920
30	1	11.10	22.00	128 576
29	2	9.70	32.80	94 836
28	2	7.20	9.50	61 088
27	2	7.20	12.75	44 256
26	4	6.67	11.27	32 064
25	6	5.74	12.88	23 232
24	7	5.35	9.70	16 832
23	11	4.27	10.81	12 192
22	15	3.49	9.53	8 832
21	20	3.47	8.57	6 400
20	27	3.09	9.88	4 640
19	38	2.88	7.96	3 360
18	53	2.77	9.18	2 432
17	73	2.67	8.18	1 760
16	99	2.51	8.08	1 280
15	138	2.35	7.74	928
14	191	2.18	6.40	672
13	262	2.00	6.27	480
12	364	1.77	5.17	352
11	501	1.56	4.77	256
10	693	1.35	4.22	192
9	957	1.13	3.56	128
8	1 321	0.95	3.12	96
7	2 516	0.76	2.54	64
6	7 310	0.63	1.10	32
5	14 620	0.53	1.31	16
4	29 240	0.48	1.05	8
3	58 480	0.43	0.75	4
2	116 960	0.40	0.59	2
1	233 920	0.40	0.48	1

Distal RBs = distal respiratory bronchioles (order 1 branches) supplied by a branch.

2.81 is called the 'branching ratio' which means that the number of branches in successive orders down the tree increases by a factor of 2.81 with each order. A perfectly symmetrical dichotomously branching system would have a branching ratio of 2.0; the more asymmetrical the system the higher the branching ratio when Strahler's method is used, and the lower the branching ratio when Horsfield's method is used. Thus for the bronchial tree the two branching ratios are 2.81 and 1.38 respectively, while for the more asymmetrical pulmonary arterial tree they are 3.0 and 1.33.

Table 2   Model of the bronchial tree using Strahler orders

Order	Number	Diameter (mm)	Length (mm)
1	2998	0.86	4.34
2	1160	1.31	7.16
3	400	1.96	11.62
4	137	2.54	18.33
5	51	3.13	17.17
6	18	4.56	21.68
7	5	6.88	28.04
8	2	11.55	49.00
9	1	16.00	100.00

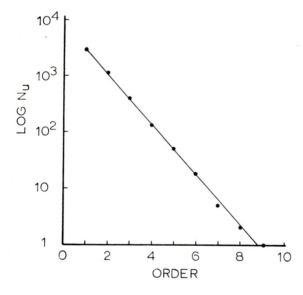

Figure 7   Number of branches (N_u) in each Strahler order of the bronchial tree

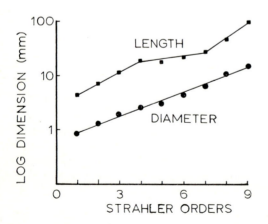

Figure 8   Mean diameter and length of branches in each Strahler order in the bronchial tree

Comparison of methods of ordering

The advantages and disadvantages of each method of ordering can now be discussed. In Horsfield's method each individual branch is counted, and if each parent branch is also uniquely identified it is possible to reconstruct the branching pattern from the data. When the branching system is one in which multiple side branches occur, as in the pulmonary vascular trees (Fig. 9) the number of Horsfield orders becomes too large to handle with ease. In this case Strahler's method is most appropriate. Many other systems have been analysed by Strahler's method, including hepatic arteries, veins

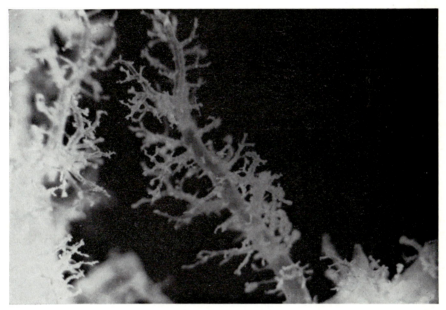

Figure 9   Resin cast of a pulmonary vein about 0.5 mm in diameter showing multiple supernumerary branches

and bile ducts (Woldenberg, 1968), Purkinje cells (Flinn, personal communication), rivers (Haggett and Chorley, 1969) and botanical trees (Barker, Cumming and Horsfield, 1973). Direct comparison of the branching patterns between these various systems is facilitated by the use of the same method of ordering. However, using Strahler's method it is not possible to reconstruct the exact branching pattern from a knowledge of the parent of every branch. The penalty paid for using the simpler Strahler method is that much detail is lost.

In summary, a system with well-developed dichotomous branching, such as the human bronchial tree, can be ordered by Horsfield's method to obtain a maximum of data. A system with multiple lateral branching is too complex for this method and can be more easily handled by Strahler's method. Comparison with other systems is then facilitated but detail is lost.

Morphology at a bifurcation

The patterns of airflow in the bronchial tree, which are of importance in determining aerosol deposition and energy losses from the flowing air, are profoundly influenced by the morphology at a bifurcation. This was studied by Sekihara, Olson and Filley (1968), who made silicone rubber casts of the airways and then cut serial sections of the casts in the region of a bifurcation. Horsfield et al (1971) described some of the details obtained by this method. Figure 10 shows how a branch is often curved at its origin before attaining

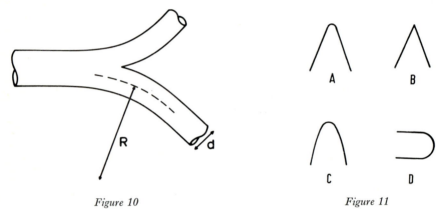

Figure 10   Figure 11

Figure 10   Radius of curvature *R* at the origin of a branch of diameter *d* in the bronchial tree. (From Horsfield et al (1971) by permission of the Editor of the *Journal of Applied Physiology*)

Figure 11   (A) The shape of a section through a typical flow divider at a bifurcation in the bronchial tree. (B and C) Sections which are respectively more pointed and more curved than that usually found. (D) The shape of the flow divider when sectioned along the direction of the arrow in Figure 12 at right angles to the plane of the daughter branches

its new line of direction. The radius of this curvature *R*, and the diameter of the branch, *d*, can be related as the ratio *R/d*. This ratio varies from 0.5 to 15 between the trachea and the bronchopulmonary segment branches. More peripherally, the range of values is less, being 3.5 to 7 down to branches 3 mm in diameter and 1 to 3 for branches below 1.5 mm diameter.

The dividing spur which lies between a pair of daughter branches, equivalent to the carina for the right and left main bronchi, is shown in section in Figure 11. The radius of curvature of its edge, *r*, and the diameter of a daughter branch, *d*, are related such that *r/d* is approximately 0.1. Successive sections taken from a bifurcating branch show the change in shape that occurs over the distal 20 per cent of the length of the parent branch (Fig. 12). The parent branch first becomes elliptical, then flattens, then indents and finally divides into nearly circular daughter branches.

The peripheral airways

The branching of the bronchioles from 0.7 mm diameter down to the distal end of the respiratory bronchioles has been studied by Parker, Horsfield and Cumming (1971). They analysed a sample of 272 structures broken off a bronchial tree cast and counted the branches in each order using Horsfield's method. A plot was made of log number of branches in each order (Fig. 13). The branching ratio obtained from the slope of the line is almost 2.0 which indicates that the branching pattern is close to symmetrical dichotomy. This change in pattern in the smaller airways is of interest, and probably reflects a change in function. It is in this region where molecular diffusion starts to become an important mechanism for the transport of oxygen and carbon dioxide, gradually taking over from mass flow which is of greatest importance

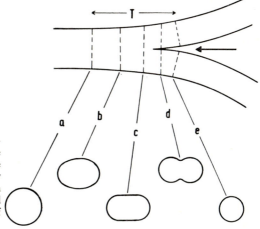

Figure 12 Sections through a dividing bronchus. T is the transition zone between the circular sections of the parent and daughter branches. Arrow shows the direction of section D in Figure 11. (From Horsfield et al (1971) by permission of the Editor of the *Journal of Applied Physiology*)

in the larger airways. The rapidly increasing cross sectional area down successive orders augments diffusion, this increase being brought about by the combination of the change to symmetrical dichotomy and the more gradual decrease in diameter peripherally.

The branching of the alveolar ducts is extremely difficult to study. Parker et al (1971) made a three-dimensional reconstruction from serial sections of half the branches arising from a respiratory bronchiole at a linear magnification of × 100. Branching was predominantly dichotomous, but trichotomy and irregular branching were common, especially towards the alveolar sacs. The number of divisions from distal respiratory bronchiole to alveolar sac varied from three to eight with a mean value of six. Estimates made from this study suggest that there are 224×10^3 distal respiratory bronchioles and 23×10^6 alveolar ducts and sacs. This is rather higher than the estimate of Weibel (1963) which was 13.8×10^6 ducts and sacs. If the commonly stated number of 300×10^6 alveoli is accepted, there are about 16 alveoli per duct and 10 per sac. The most detailed three-dimensional reconstructions of distal airways from serial sections have been made by Boyden (1971). He visualised the branching pattern of an entire acinus from the lung of a six year old child, at which age the branching pattern is probably fully developed. He found three orders of respiratory bronchiole and from two to five orders of alveolar ducts and sacs. His results confirm the findings of other workers (Ogawa, 1920; Willson, 1922; Pump, 1964, 1969) that the pattern of branching distal to the terminal bronchiole and the number of orders down to alveolar sacs are both extremely variable, and that this variability is both between acini and within them. Branching by dichotomy, trichotomy and polychotomy may be seen and there is also a marked variability of the lengths of respiratory bronchioles and alveolar ducts.

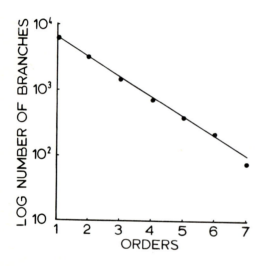

Figure 13   Number of branches in each order of a sample of bronchioles. In this case the distal respiratory bronchioles comprise order 1. (From Parker et al (1971) by permission of the Editor of the *Journal of Applied Physiology*)

Along with the marked variation in intra-acinar branching patterns there is also a wide range of shapes of the acinus as a whole (Pump, 1969). It may be nearly globular within the lung, pyramidal with the base outwards on a pleural surface, and fan-like on the edge of a lobe. Often it is symmetrical, but sometimes highly asymmetrical with one half quite a different shape to the other. Acini also vary in size, and must adapt to available space, both at the edge of the lung, and between bronchi and vessels within it. The alveolar ducts and sacs of adjacent alveoli may interlock and be quite difficult to separate when filled with casting material.

Dynamic changes in morphology during life

Up to this point airway morphology has been considered in the static state that necessarily exists in casts and fixed tissues. During life, however, the dimensions of the airways are constantly changing, and in addition similar structures situated at different points on the vertical axis of the lung have differing dimensions associated with the vertical gradient of pleural pressure (Glazier et al, 1967). An early study of the changes in diameter of the bronchi associated with expansion of the lung was made by Stutz (1949) using broncho-graphic techniques. He showed that the smaller bronchi, 1 to 2 mm in dia-meter, undergo the greatest percentage increase on inspiration. More recently tantalum bronchography has been used in animals and to a lesser extent in man (Nadel, Wolfe and Graf, 1968). This techniques involves insufflating the bronchial tree with finely powdered tantalum. This substance has the advantage of being very radiopaque, thereby permitting the bronchial wall to be visualised with x-rays when only a thin layer of dry powder has been deposited on them. The main disadvantage of tantalum is that it is highly inflammable so that its use in man has been limited.

Hughes, Hoppin and Mead (1972) used stereoscope pairs of x-ray photo-graphs of tantalum-insufflated excised dog lungs to obtain measurements of airway diameter and length. They showed that the percentage increase in bronchial dimensions with lung inflation did not differ between large bronchi and those down to 1 mm diameter. In most cases the changes in diameter and length were proportional to the changes in the cube root of lung volume.

An interesting analysis of the change of airway length associated with change of lung volume has been made by Hoppin and Hughes (personal communica-tion). The airways are attached peripherally to the lung substance and centrally to the trachea. When the lung expands the transpulmonary pressure is applied as a stretching force along those airways that have a peribronchial space. Some of the stress might be taken up by the surrounding lung tissues, but as there is considerable freedom of movement between a bronchus and its surrounding sheath this probably represents only a small part of the total. Considering one parent branch and its two daughter branches, the stretching force F acting on the parent is balanced by the sum of the forces acting in the opposite direction on the two daughter branches. Thus the axial force in one daughter branch is $0.5 \times \cos \theta \times F$ where θ is the branching angle.

This formula was applied to Weibel's model (1963) using the data of Horsfield and Cumming (1967) on branching angles and allowing for differ-ences in wall thickness in bronchi of different diameters. Passing from the trachea to the periphery of the lung the stretching force is distributed over an increasing number of branches so that the force per branch steadily diminishes. However, the branches decrease in diameter and their walls become thinner peripherally, so that the force per unit of cross-sectional area (longitudinal stress) on the wall remains almost constant. Given similar mechanical properties of bronchial wall tissue from bronchi of various diameters, strain would be similar in all airways if stress were. This is the case, which explains why the increase in length per unit length is the same for large and small airways.

Peripheral airway changes with age

With increasing age there is an increase in the average diameter of alveolar ducts. The connective tissue which makes up the wall of the ducts, and that which forms the mouths of their associated alveoli, are closely linked. Indeed, they are probably one and the same, an alveolar duct being likened to a tube of wire netting the holes in which are the mouths of the alveoli. Thus as the ducts expand the alveolar mouths stretch open, while the alveoli themselves become wider and shallower. They thus become more saucer shaped, just as they were at the start of their development. Alveolar ducts thus occupy an increasing proportion of total lung volume with increasing age.

Alveoli

Both the size and shape of the alveoli are very variable. This has been demonstrated by casting techniques (Pump, 1964, 1969), by reconstruction from serial sections (Parker et al, 1971; Boydon, 1971; Stelter, Hanson and Fairchild, 1966), measurement of microscopic sections (Weibel, 1963) and scanning electron microscopy (Kuhn and Finke, 1972). The general shape may be a shallow saucer-shaped depression, a hemisphere, or three-quarters of a sphere like a radar dome. The alveolar walls themselves are flat in an inflated lung, so that the shape is actually an irregular polyhedral one. During life, when there is a layer of fluid on the alveolar walls, the corners of the polyhedra may be rounded off, so that the airspace approximates in shape to part of a sphere (Kuhn and Finke, 1972).

Just as the bronchi change dimension in the living subject so do the alveoli. Furthermore, there is a wide difference in mean alveolar diameter between the top and bottom of an upright lung. Glazier et al (1967) showed that in upright dogs frozen intact the alveoli at the top of the lung have a mean diameter five times greater than those at the bottom. This is brought about by the complex distribution of stresses in the elastic tissues of the lung confined within the thorax (West and Matthews, 1972). The increase of stress towards the top of each lobe stretches the tissues here and it has been suggested by West (1971) that this might be a factor in the localisation of centrilobular emphysema predominantly in these areas.

The number of alveoli in an adult human lung can be found very approximately by dividing a 5 litre volume into spherical alveoli of 300 μm diameter, which gives an estimate of 300×10^6. Weibel (1963) measured the number of alveoli in five lungs and found a mean of 296×10^6 with a range of from 286×10^6 to 310×10^6. Dunnill (1963) found 286×10^6 alveoli in the lungs of one subject. More recently Angus and Thurlbeck (1972) showed a much wider range of values than had previously been noted. In 32 subjects the number of alveoli ranged from 212×10^6 to 605×10^6.

This observation raises the interesting point of the relation between lung volume on the one hand, and alveolar numbers and size on the other. In the series studied by Angus and Thurlbeck (1972) alveolar number was found to be positively correlated with body length, that is, bigger lungs contain more alveoli. Mean interalveolar wall distance (a function of alveolar diameter) shows, however, no correlation with height (Thurlbeck, personal communication) but is positively correlated with lung volume. Thus bigger lungs contain bigger alveoli as well as greater numbers, but not as a function of body length. Another interesting observation made by Matsuba and Thurlbeck (1971) is that the number of small airways (2.0 mm diameter down to terminal bronchioles) in unit volume of lung tissue varies inversely with lung volume. Put another way, the number of small airways is relatively constant between lungs, independent of their volumes. Since the pattern of branching of these airways is probably fairly constant too, it follows that the number of terminal bronchioles, and hence acini, is also constant between lungs. Now if bigger lungs contain more alveoli, but the same number of acini, as smaller lungs, they must have more alveoli per acinus. This is unlikely to be achieved by centripetal spread of alveolar growth because this could produce only a very small percentage increase in numbers, whereas large lungs may have three times as many alveoli as small lungs. Alveoli must therefore be added more distally, and it seems likely that this is brought about by budding from alveolar ducts and sacs.

Growth of the airways

This discussion of alveolar numbers has necessarily touched on the topic of airways' growth. Bucher and Reid (1961) showed that the full number of orders of airways is present in the fetus at 16 weeks, but true alveoli do not develop until after birth. Boyden (1969) studied an acinus from the lungs of a premature infant born at about 30 weeks gestation. His serial sections and three-dimensional reconstructions showed four orders of respiratory bronchioles and up to five orders of saccules. Respiratory bronchioles, which are smooth-walled at this stage, were recognised by the presence of flattened epithelium on part of their wall, especially that which lies away from the accompanying artery and later develops alveoli. Saccules are lined entirely by flattened epithelium and are irregularly shaped; later on they develop into alveolar ducts and sacs. The branching within this acinus corresponds to the branching of respiratory bronchioles and alveolar duct found in adult lungs, thus further confirming that the adult airway pattern is present in the fetus.

In the prenatal period the saccules develop shallow depressions which number about 20×10^6. After birth true alveoli form on the saccules and increase rapidly in number, but not size, over the first three years (Davies and Reid, 1970). The complexity of alveolar shape also increases from the age of four months, changing from saucer shaped depressions to polyhedra.

During this time additional alveoli are formed by a different process (Boyden, 1967). They result from a pouching, and then invagination, of the cuboidal epithelium on the distal bronchioles. This process spreads centri-petally, converting terminal bronchioles into respiratory bronchioles, and respiratory bronchioles into alveolar ducts. Probably not more than three orders of bronchi are thus converted from non-respiratory to respiratory structures. If the adult number of terminal bronchioles is fixed then this centripetal formation of alveoli must stop at a predefined point, since by definition terminal bronchioles are the most distal airways not to bear alveoli.

Peripherally, alveolar numbers also increase by budding, and the resulting 'fight for space' between adjacent structures inevitably results in a more irregular pattern of branching than is found elsewhere in the airways (Boyden, 1971). By the seventh year ductular processes, arising from terminal bronchi-oles or one or two orders proximal to them, are beginning to penetrate adjacent alveoli to form the canals of Lambert.

Dunnill (1962) counted the alveoli in lungs from children of various ages and found that the adult number of about 300×10^6 alveoli had been reached by the age of eight years in one subject, and had nearly been reached at the age of four years in another. He therefore concluded that growth of alveolar numbers ceases between four and eight years. However, the finding by Angus and Thurlbeck (1972) that the number of alveoli in adult lungs varies from 200×10^6 to 600×10^6 suggests that Dunnill's conclusion is not necessarily correct. Thus, referring to Dunnill's figures, the four year old may have reached his final number of alveoli and had already stopped growing, whereas the eight year old may have been due to have 500×10^6 alveoli and was there-fore some way from stopping growing. The age at which growth of numbers of alveoli ceases is thus not known and this problem awaits further study.

In summary, alveolar growth occurs by increase in numbers up to the age of three, by increase in both numbers and dimensions up to the age of eight or over, and probably by a final increase in size after the adult number has been attained. Alveolar number is a function of body length, and is possibly at least partly genetically determined (Angus and Thurlbeck, 1972). Alveolar size is a function of lung volume and may be determined by the dimensions of the chest wall (Davies and Reid, 1970).

The number of acini

The individual component parts of the acinus have been discussed, and we will now compare various authors' interpretations of the average total number of terminal bronchioles, and hence acini, that there are in the lungs. Rohrer (1915) used graduated bougies to measure the diameter of dissected bronchi and came to the conclusion that there are about 30×10^3 terminal bronchioles. Reid (1958) investigated the bronchographic patterns of branch-ing in the distal airways. She found clusters of terminal bronchioles arising at intervals of 1 to 2 mm, the whole grouping constituting a secondary lobule. The diameter of the lobule is about 10 mm and each has three, four or five terminal bronchioles within it, four being the commonest. In a lung of 5 litres volume there would be therefore 5000 lobules and 20 000 acini. The model of the airways devised by Weibel (1963), based partly on measurement and partly on mathematical concept, has approximately 66×10^3 terminal bronchioles. The method by which this figure was obtained depends absolutely on the assumption of symmetrical dichotomy throughout the lung, the terminal bronchioles constituting order 16. If there were an 'error' of only one order, such that terminal bronchioles are better represented by order 15, then the estimate would be 33×10^6, rather closer to those made by other workers.

From measurements of a cast of the bronchial tree Horsfield and Cumming (1968) estimated the number of distal respiratory bronchioles at 223 941. Assuming three orders of dichotomously dividing respiratory bronchioles, this would give $223\,941/2^3 = 27\,993$ terminal bronchioles.

A radiological study of the acinus was made by Gamsu et al (1971). They found the average diameter to be 7.4 mm, and assuming it to be spherical they calculated that there would be 24 700 acini in a lung of 5.25 litres. Matsuba and Thurlbeck (1972) counted the number of airways between 2.0 mm diameter and the terminal bronchioles. The technique involves firstly a count of the number of those airways per unit area in random histologic sections, and secondly, the calculation from this count of the numbers in unit volume. The second step was done in four different ways, yielding four different estimates, namely 55 000, 33 000, 12 000 and 19 000 in a mean lung volume of 5.25 litres. In a dichotomously branching system the number of end branches is equal to the sum of all the other branches plus one. Thus the terminal bronchioles would constitute about half of the above numbers, namely, 27 500, 16 500, 6000 and 9500. The first two estimates were thought to be more nearly correct.

These various studies suggest that the number of acini lies between 20 000 and 30 000. The fact that the various methods by which these estimates were obtained are based on such widely different techniques suggests that the above estimates are fairly reliable.

The Pulmonary Arterial Tree

The value of a detailed morphological analysis of the pulmonary arterial tree in understanding the physiology of the lesser circulation parallels the value of morphology in understanding the flow of air in the bronchial tree. As an example, from a knowledge of arterial diameters and the percentage of capillary bed supplied, flow rates and flow velocities can be calculated in every branch. The principles and methods of analysing and ordering branching structures already discussed can be equally well applied to the pulmonary arteries. In general the branches of the artery follow the airways closely, the two running side by side and branching together. Respiratory bronchioles have one side on which alveoli are not developed and this smooth surface is where the arteriole and bronchiole are in apposition. Alveolar ducts are completely surrounded by alveoli and it is therefore not possible for the arterioles to be in direct contact with the ducts themselves. Pump (1966) describes the arterioles as running between alveolar ducts, and this view is not incompatible with the description of Miller (1947) that they run with the ducts right out to the sacs. From these vessels of about 30 to 40 μm in diameter arise precapillary vessels which give rise to the capillary network. Von Hayek (1960) describes precapillary vessels as being three times the diameter of a capillary and having a length equal to half the diameter of an alveolus, say 18 and 150 μm respectively. Pump (1966) describes them as

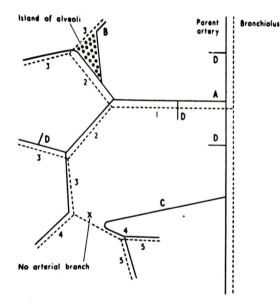

Figure 14   Mode of branching in the pulmonary arteries and the associated branches of the bronchial tree. (From Reid (1968) by permission of the Editor of *The Scientific Basis of Medicine Annual Reviews* and the Athlone Press)
——— Pulmonary artery; ········ bronchial tree; A, conventional artery; B, 'short-cut' artery; C, aberrant artery; D, accessory arteries. Generations of bronchial and arterial branching marked 1, 2, 3, 4 and 5

having a diameter of 30 μm and a length of 20 μm. The difference is so great that one wonders whether they are describing the same structure.

If the arterial tree (excluding the precapillary vessels) were as described above it would have the same branching ratio as the bronchial tree. Data acquired from measuring a cast of the pulmonary arteries give values of 3.0 (Singhal et al, 1973) and 3.4 (Woldenberg et al, 1970) for the branching ratio, depending on the method employed to correct for broken branches. Whatever the correct value, it seems to be greater than that for the bronchial tree, which is 2.8. The explanation for this is to be found in the work of Elliott and Reid (1965) who counted the supernumerary branches arising from the pulmonary arteries in addition to those following the airways (Fig. 14). These supernumerary vessels make it very difficult to order the pulmonary arterial tree by Horsfield's method because there would be so many orders. Elliott and Reid (1965) ignore the supernumerary vessels when counting generations, taking account only of those which branch with an airway, and thereby getting over the difficulty. This method has the merit of ascribing the same generation to adjacent segments of artery and airway.

A study of the pulmonary arterial tree based on measurement of a resin cast and using Strahler orders was made by Singhal et al (1973). The tree was arbitrarily divided into three zones: the proximal zone from the main pulmonary artery down to 0.8 mm diameter, the intermediate zone from 0.8 to 0.1 mm diameter, and the distal zone from 0.1 mm diameter to the precapillary arterioles. Apart from a few broken branches, all of the proximal zone branches were ordered, measured and counted. A sample of three intermediate zone casts, arising from vessels of 0.8 mm diameter, was also ordered, measured and counted. No measurements were made of the distal zone. Figure 15

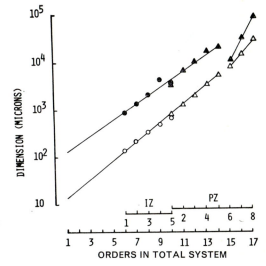

Figure 15 Mean dimensions of vessels in each Strahler order of the pulmonary arterial tree. ▲ = proximal zone, length; △ = proximal zone, diameter; ● = intermediate zone, length; ○ = intermediate zone, diameter; PZ = proximal zone orders; IZ = intermediate zone orders. (From Singhal et al (1973) by permission of the American Heart Association Inc.)

shows the plots of log mean diameter and log mean length for the proximal zone and intermediate zone. The lines are projected down to a diameter of 15 μm and a length of 150 μm (possible dimensions of first order of precapillary vessels) to give an estimate of 17 for the total number of orders. Figure 16 shows log number of vessels in each order plotted against order for the proximal and intermediate zones. The branching ratios for the two zones are similar (2.994 and 3.096 respectively) so it was considered justifiable to extrapolate the line for the proximal zone. This was done as far as order 2 where the slope probably changes because of the large number of precapillary vessels given off at this point. The number of these vessels was estimated to equal the number of alveoli, giving 3×10^8 first order vessels. From Figures 15 and 16 a table was constructed of arterial tree morphology (Table 3). The data in this for the proximal zone are well founded, but for the intermediate zone they are rather scanty, though in good continuity with the proximal zone data. For the distal zone the projections are no more than estimations which may in fact prove to be quite wrong. No data relating to Strahler orders are available for this part of the arterial tree.

The pattern of branching in the pulmonary arterial tree has been described by Elliott and Reid (1965). They injected the vessels of excised lungs with a mixture of chromopaque in gelatin and studied them using radiographs and serial sections. In general, the branching of the pulmonary artery follows that of the airways, and the branches which do this they termed 'conventional'. In addition there are many smaller branches which do not follow airway branching and these they termed 'supernumerary' (Fig. 14). The supernumerary branches are of two types. First the aberrant branches, which

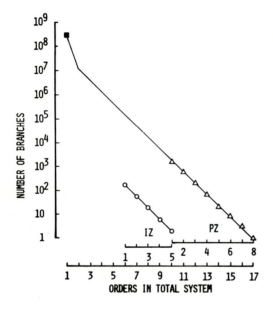

Figure 16   Number of vessels in each Strahler order of the pulmonary arterial tree. $\triangle$ = proximal zone; $\bigcirc$ = intermediate zone sample; $\blacksquare$ = assumed number (3×10^8) of order 1 branches; PZ = proximal zone orders; IZ = intermediate zone orders. (From Singhal et al (1973) by permission of the American Heart Association Inc.)

usually supply a distal or laterally placed portion of an acinus. They do not follow the recurrent course of the airways but take a direct short cut to the distal part of the airway and thereafter follow it in the normal manner. Second, the accessory branches, which are small in diameter, arise at right angles from the parent branch and run a short course to adjacent alveoli. These supernumerary branches offer the opportunity for collateral circulation to develop should the main artery to an acinus become blocked.

The number of branches arising along an arterial pathway were counted in the anterior bronchopulmonary segment of the lower lobe. There were 29 down to the lobule, of which 17 were supernumerary. Within a lobule, down to the distal respiratory bronchiole, there were 52 branches, 41 of which were supernumerary. Thus there would be 71 Horsfield orders in addition to the central branches and those along the alveolar ducts which were not counted. This amply illustrates the difficulty of using Horsfield's method of counting orders in vascular systems.

A considerable proportion of the total arterial cross sectional area at a given level is contributed by the supernumerary branches. In the prelobular region they contribute 17 per cent, in the lobular but pre-acinar region 43 per cent, and within the acinus 25 per cent (Reid, 1968).

Not very much is known regarding the range of variation in branching patterns in the population, between races, or between species. Hislop and Reid (1973a) were able to study the lungs of children from three sets of siblings who had died accidentally. Pulmonary arteriograms showed that the branching pattern of the larger branches had distinct intrafamilial similarities and interfamilial differences, such that the siblings could be grouped by families on the arteriographic patterns alone. Detailed studies of the smaller branches were not undertaken, so we do not know whether these also show familial similarities. Nor do we know whether an analysis based on Strahler orders would show interfamilial differences.

Table 3 Model of the pulmonary arterial tree using Strahler orders

Order	Number	Diameter (mm)	Length (mm)
1	1779	0.90	3.54
2	508	1.44	7.48
3	150	2.38	12.60
4	43	4.46	21.55
5	15	6.77	16.53
6	4	12.13	28.00
7	1	30.00	110.50

Structure of the arterial wall

The walls of the larger arteries down to about 3.2 mm in diameter are described as elastic or musculo-elastic. Below 2.0 mm in diameter they are muscular, and between the two they are transitional, showing histological features intermediate between the two types (Semmens, 1970).

Brenner (1935) stated that the walls of arteries 100 to 10 000 μm in diameter are muscular, but Elliott and Reid (1965) found the diameter range of muscular arteries to be from 30 to 2000 μm. Such vessels show a complete ring of muscle in section. More peripherally the complete muscle coat gives way to a spiral arrangement and this, on section, shows only segments of a circle in the walls of vessels which are therefore termed 'partially muscular arteries'. Finally the muscle coat peters out peripherally to give non-muscular arteries. The changes from wholly muscular, through partially muscular, to non-muscular arteries occur not at fixed diameters but over a range, so that any of the three types may be found in arteries from 30 to 150 μm in diameter. Furthermore, the relationship between arterial diameter and airway structure is very variable, so that the artery accompanying a respiratory bronchiole, for instance, may be from 100 to 1100 μm in diameter. Thus neither the diameter of an artery nor the nature of its accompanying airway characterises the structure of these smaller vessels. Because of this variability an 'arteriole' is a difficult structure to define anatomically, and further confusion is added if a functional definition is used. It is therefore probably better to avoid using the term altogether.

Growth of the pulmonary arteries

The development of the pulmonary arteries mirrors that of the airways. At 20 weeks gestation the pre-acinar airways, and the corresponding conventional and supernumerary arteries, are all present (Hislop and Reid, 1972). At birth there are few, if any, alveoli and correspondingly few acinar vessels. After birth there is a rapid increase in numbers of both the alveoli and the intra-acinar arteries supplying them, both of which apparently arise by peripheral budding from their parent structures.

The diameter range of the different types of artery varies with age (Davies and Reid, 1970). At birth, partially muscular arteries were found from 180 to 27 μm, non-muscular arteries up to 62 μm, and muscular arteries down to 42 μm, in diameter. With increasing age up to about 11 years the transition between different types appears at greater diameters, with partially muscular arteries appearing at 360 μm, and non-muscular arteries as large as 180 μm in diameter. In adults the situation again resembles that found in the newborn, the range over which the three types are found being from 30 to 150 μm in diameter. The least degree of muscularisation of the peripheral arteries is therefore found in late childhood.

Ageing of the pulmonary arteries

Semmens (1970) studied the lungs from six aged subjects. She found that elastic walled vessels went down only as far as 5 mm diameter, compared to the normal 3.2 mm, and that transitional vessels went down to 3 mm diameter, compared to the normal 2 mm. This could be due either to dilatation of the vessels or to a change in wall structure. Angiograms from these lungs showed that the dimensions of the arteries were similar to those found in young adults, so that a change in structure seemed to be the most likely explanation. This change consists of a loss of elastic tissue in vessels up to 5 mm in diameter. In addition, arteries of all diameters showed an increase in medial thickness, but this was greatest in vessels between 2 and 4 mm in diameter. The degree of this change did not correlate with age.

The Pulmonary Venous Tree

Very much less work has been done on the venous system and its branching pattern than on the arterial tree. The most detailed study is that of Hislop and Reid (1973b) based on vascular injections and serial sections of fetal and child lungs. They confirmed that the veins run independently of the airways and arteries, being situated in their own connective tissue sheath at the periphery of the lobules and acini, whilst the arteries run within them. Along a main venous pathway within a segment the general arrangement of the branching pattern is similar to that of the arteries. Conventional branches occur with branches of the airways and enter the parent vessel at an acute angle. Supernumerary vessels are of two types, both of which are smaller than the conventional branches and enter the parent vessel at right angles. The first type is smaller, has no collagen sheath, and drains only the immediately adjacent alveolar tissue. The second is larger, has a thin sheath and drains tissue further away. All three types of branch are found anywhere along the length of the main vessel.

The ratio of supernumerary to conventional branches is about 4:1 in all parts of the pathway, which is higher than that found in the arterial system. This finding confirms the impression that the veins branch more profusely than the arteries, as indicated by a fuller pattern seen on venography than on arteriography. Similarly, a resin venous cast shows many more branches than does an arterial cast (Horsfield, unpublished observations). It seems likely that the branching ratio of the veins, when analysed by Strahler's method, will prove to be higher than that of the arteries, but no one has as yet undertaken such a study. Five sites of origin of the venous tributaries were found. They are (1) alveolar walls, (2) points of division of alveolar ducts, (3) walls of bronchioli, (4) the pleura, and (5) connective tissue of septa and sheaths.

The structure of the vein wall may be muscular, partially muscular or non-muscular. The range of diameters of these three types overlap, the smallest wholly muscular vein being 200 μm in diameter and the smallest partially muscular vein being 70 μm in diameter. In general, the walls of the veins are thinner, expressed as a percentage of vessel diameter, than those of the arteries. The development of the veins parallels that of the arteries and airways so that at 20 weeks gestation all the branches are present down to the acinus. Within the acinus the saccules are drained by saccular veins, the veins from alveolar ducts and respiratory bronchioles only becoming distinguishable after birth when the airway structures differentiate.

The Pulmonary Lymphatic System

Until recently the lymphatics of the lung have been poorly understood. The work of Lauweryns (1970, 1971a) has added considerably to our detailed knowledge of this system, especially regarding the anatomical location of the finer branches within the lung. Lauweryns distinguishes between an alveolar wall, which consists of one layer of epithelial cells, a capillary net and connective tissue, and an interalveolar septum, which consists in essence of two contiguous alveolar walls. Where an alveolus is situated next to a non-alveolar structure only one alveolar wall is present. Lymphatics are found between an alveolar wall and the connective tissue of a bronchus, vessel, interlobular septum or pleura; they are not found in an interalveolar septum. Lauweryns states that a large percentage of alveoli are in fact situated next to a vessel, septum or pleura, and thus most alveoli have a direct lymphatic drainage, at least on one wall. The lymphatics drain back along the bronchi and vessels to the hilar nodes, or along septa and veins to the pleura. A dense network of lymphatics covers the pleura, and drainage proceeds over the pleural surface to the hilar lymph nodes.

Lymphatic valves have classically been thought to be bicuspid, as are those in the veins (Miller, 1947). Lauweryns (1971b) using a variety of techniques, has reconstructed the pulmonary lymphatic valves in three dimensions. He found that they are shaped like conical funnels, attached round the circumference of the larger opening to the inner wall of the lymph vessel. The rest of the valve hangs free in the lumen, the long axis of the valve lying along the axis of the vessel. Such an arrangement should form a very efficient one-way system, allowing the pumping action of adjacent vessels, and movement of the lung, to return lymph towards the heart.

THE AIRWAYS IN EMPHYSEMA AND CHRONIC OBSTRUCTIVE LUNG DISEASE

Morphologists who have studied the lungs of patients with emphysema hoping to find a simple anatomical explanation for respiratory failure have been largely disappointed. Whilst it is true that severe respiratory failure is likely if 90 per cent of alveolar tissue is lost, at lower values the correlation between loss of tissue and respiratory failure is poor. On the one hand 50 per cent tissue loss may be associated with only mild symptoms, and on the other patients may die with only 10 per cent loss. The problem becomes a little clearer when the two most important types of emphysema, namely panacinar and centrilobular, are considered separately from each other.

In panacinar emphysema there is a generalised destruction of the acinus, with loss of alveolar walls and their supplying blood vessels. The affected areas are distributed throughout the whole lung without a prediliction for any particular region. In common with other organs the lung has a considerable reserve of function so that provided the remaining alveoli are functioning normally blood gases can be maintained at normal levels in the face of greater than 50 per cent lung destruction (cf. the situation after pneumonectomy). The concurrent loss of blood vessels with alveolar destruction facilitates this by minimising perfusion to badly ventilated areas, though of course some ventilation is wasted in the emphysematous space. A poor correlation between destruction of lung tissue and function is thus found in panacinar emphysema, because in many cases it is something other than the simple loss of tissue which causes the poor function.

In centrilobular emphysema the lesion starts with dilatation and destruction of the first and second generations of the respiratory bronchioles, giving rise to a dilatation situated in series with the alveolar region of the acinus, as shown in Figure 17. The alveoli and their supplying blood vessels are preserved until late on in the progress of a lesion, which eventually may become large enough to destroy most or all of the acinus. Although the lesions are sometimes widespread throughout the lung, much more commonly they are situated at the apex of the upper lobe and to a lesser degree of the lower lobe. Functional changes, using right ventricular weight as an index of pulmonary hypertension, may correlate with the percentage of lung destruction in centrilobular emphysema. Lungs obtained postmortem from patients with centrilobular emphysema and respiratory failure usually show between 10 and 40 per cent of lung destruction, so that loss of alveolar tissue per se cannot be the cause of death in these cases. It was pointed out by Gomez (1965) and Staub (1965) that the centrilobular space is situated at the junction of two functional regions of the airways. These are the conducting airways proximally, in which mass flow predominates, and the acinus distally, in which molecular diffusion predominates. A dilatation in this situation, being in series with the alveoli, might produce a significant impairment of movement of gas in and out of the acinus. Since the circulation of the acinus is intact while ventilation is impaired, a low ventilation/perfusion ratio results giving rise to a low oxygen tension in the blood leaving the acinus. This hypothesis was used as the basis for a mathematical analysis of a model of centrilobular emphysema by Horsfield, Barer and Cumming (1973). They showed how centrilobular emphysema, if widely distributed, but occupying only 10 per cent of the lung volume, could result in severe blood gas disturbances.

When the lesions are not widely distributed other factors must come into play. Bignon et al (1969) studied the lungs from 40 patients with chronic obstructive lung disease and found that right ventricular weight correlated with the volume percentage of centrilobular emphysema, but not panacinar emphysema. They also counted the distribution of bronchiolar diameters per square centimeter of cross-sectional area, and found that there was an increase in the number of bronchioles less than 350 μm in diameter. The percentage of bronchioles less than 350 μm in diameter correlated well with right ventricular weight.

These findings were confirmed and extended in a subsequent paper by Bignon, Andre-Bougaran and Brouet (1970) who showed that in centrilobular emphysema the bronchiolar narrowings are widely distributed throughout the lung even when the emphysema is confined to the upper zones. The bronchiolar narrowing was found to be due to surrounding inflammation and fibrosis, and blockage by mucus.

Matsuba and Thurlbeck (1972) studied the lungs from 12 patients who had emphysema, chronic bronchitis and bronchiectasis. They too showed a change in the distribution of diameters of bronchioles, with an increase in

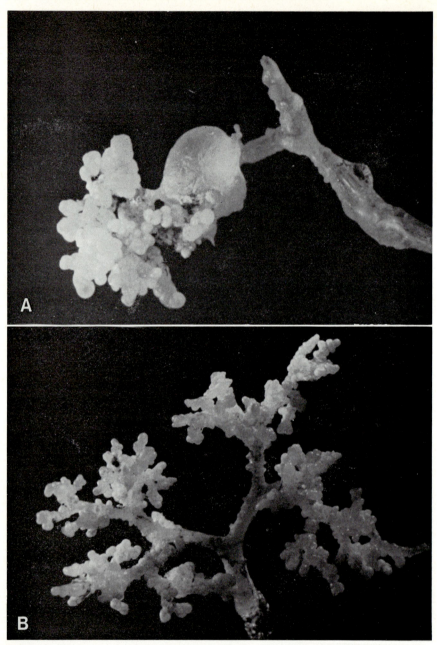

Figure 17   (A) A resin cast of the peripheral airways in centrilobular emphysema. A terminal bronchiole gives rise to a dilatation which is in series with relatively normal alveoli distally. (B) Incomplete resin cast of the normal airways. The bronchiole at the bottom of the picture gives rise to two terminal bronchioles. A first generation respiratory bronchiole passes vertically upwards from the right hand terminal bronchiole, some of its alveoli being seen in profile. More peripherally the alveoli on alveolar ducts show as rounded hemispherical structures

numbers of those of less than 400 μm in diameter, and a decrease in those of greater diameter. In the emphysematous lungs, the total number of small airways was reduced, presumably due to obliteration by inflammation.

A group of seven patients with chronic cough and airways obstruction clinically was studied by Macklem, Thurlbeck and Fraser (1971). In none was emphysema severe and morphologically they were a mixed group. The only common feature found in the lungs when examined postmortem was narrowing of the small bronchi and bronchioles, with inflammation, fibrosis and mucous plugging.

Taken together, these studies demonstrate the importance of disease of the small airways as a cause of respiratory failure and right ventricular hypertrophy, whatever the type, quantity or distribution of any associated emphysema. In the normal lung the peripheral airways less than 2.0 mm in diameter only contribute 10 per cent to the total airways resistance. Thus before there is any significant increase in airways resistance they must be severely damaged. More important are the changes produced in the distribution of ventilation. If circulation to an affected area is maintained in the presence of reduced ventilation, the ventilation/perfusion ratio will be low and the blood leaving that area will have a reduced oxygen saturation. This might be one factor contributing to pulmonary hypertension.

MODELS OF BRANCHING SYSTEMS

The main purpose in making detailed studies of branching systems in the lungs is to further our understanding of the factors influencing gas and blood flow in health and disease. Pulmonary physiologists are interested in studying flow rates, pressure drops, energy losses, fluid flow regimes, particle deposition and molecular diffusion in these branching structures. Apart from studying the structures themselves this is done by analysing these processes in a model.

Two kinds of model have been used in this way. Firstly, a physical replica, commonly enlarged, of part of the branching system may be used to study fluid flow directly. Secondly, a conceptual or mathematical model of the anatomy, combined with appropriate mathematical equations to represent the physiology, may be used to compute how fluid behaves within the system.

In the first method a very careful reproduction of the finer details of morphology of a limited part of the system is required. Examples of the kind of data which are useful for this are shown in Figures 10–12 (Horsfield et al, 1971). Studies of fluid flow in such models have been made by several groups of workers; for example Olson et al (1973) studied flow in positive casts of the airways from nose to segmental bronchi and Schroter and Sudlow (1969) studied the secondary motions set up by a bifurcation. In the second method the representation of very complex structure in mathematical form requires a great deal of simplification. This always leads to a difficult decision—whether to use a simple but unreal model from which it is easy to make calculations, or a complex more realistic model which is difficult to handle and expensive on computing time. The various methods employed in studying the movement of gas in the airways by mathematical modelling have been excellently reviewed by Chang and Farhi (1973) and will not be considered further. Probably the best known model of the human bronchial tree is Weibel's model A (1963). Less well known, although explicitly stated by Weibel, are the assumptions which went into it. He measured, incompletely, the first 10 generations of bronchi from a resin cast; measured the mean diameter of the alveolar ducts and counted them; assumed perfectly symmetrical dichotomous branching throughout and assumed four generations of alveolar ducts and sacs. From these measurements and assumptions he constructed a complete 23 generation branching system. Weibel's model has the great advantage of being easy to use, and it is probable that any one pathway down his model from trachea to alveolar sac is not too dissimilar from some kind of an average pathway in the lungs. For these reasons it has been much used. However, the real bronchial tree is quite asymmetrical, there being a threefold range of divisions down between the shortest and longest pathways and a corresponding range of asymmetry of branching.

In an attempt to meet this objection to Weibel's model Horsfield et al (1971) constructed two asymmetrical models based on their bronchial tree data. In principle the two models are the same, but the first and simpler model is based on the assumption that each lobe has a similar average branching pattern, whilst the second more complex model is based on an individual pattern of branching in each bronchopulmonary segment. These models are statements of the average degree of asymmetry in lobes or segments, but do not of course model the range of asymmetry of branching. Because these models represent the branching of the bronchial tree more closely than Weibel's model they are necessarily more complex and hence less easy to use.

The most recent developments in the utilisation of knowledge of airway and arterial morphology depends on access to modern computers with large core stores. Various workers are now using the actual data on branching patterns and dimensions of these structures instead of models in order to make calculations of various physiological processes. With this new approach to the study of morphology the days of the mathematical model of lung anatomy are numbered.

REFERENCES

Angus, G. E. & Thurlbeck, W. M. (1972) Number of alveoli in the human lung. *Journal of Applied Physiology*, **32**, 483–485.

Barker, S. B., Cumming, G. & Horsfield, K. (1973) Quantitative morphometry of the branching structure of trees. *Journal of Theoretical Biology*, **40**, 33–43.

Bignon, J., Khoury, F., Even, P., Andre, J. & Brouet, G. (1969) Morphometric study in chronic obstructive bronchopulmonary disease. Pathologic, clinical and physiologic correlations. *American Review of Respiratory Disease*, **99**, 669–695.

Bignon, J., Andre-Bougaran, J. & Brouet, G. (1970) Parenchymal, bronchiolar, and bronchial measurements in centrilobular emphysema. Relation to weight of right ventricle. *Thorax*, **25**, 556–567.

Boyden, E. A. (1967) Notes on the development of the lung in infancy and early childhood. *American Journal of Anatomy*, **121**, 749–762.

Boyden, E. A. (1969) The pattern of the terminal air spaces in a premature infant of 30–32 weeks that lived nineteen and a quarter hours. *American Journal of Anatomy*, **126**, 31–40.

Boyden, E. A. (1971) The structure of the pulmonary acinus in a child of six years and eight months. *American Journal of Anatomy*, **132**, 275–300.

Brenner, O. (1935) Pathology of the vessels of the pulmonary circulation. *Archives of Internal Medicine*, **56**, 211–237.

Bucher, U. & Reid, L. (1961) Development of the intrasegmental bronchial tree: the pattern of branching and development of cartilage at various stages of intra-uterine life. *Thorax*, **16**, 207–218.

Chang, H.-K. & Farhi, L. E. (1973) On mathematical analysis of gas transport in the lung. *Respiration Physiology*, **18**, 370–385.

Davies, G. & Reid, L. (1970) Growth of the alveoli and pulmonary arteries in childhood. *Thorax*, **25**, 669–681.

Dunnill, M. S. (1962) Postnatal growth of the lung. *Thorax*, **17**, 329–333.

Dunnill, M. S. (1964) Evaluation of a simple method of sampling the lung for quantitative histological analysis. *Thorax*, **19**, 443–448.

Elliott, F. M. & Reid, L. (1965) Some new facts about the pulmonary artery and its branching pattern. *Clinical Radiology*, **16**, 193–198.

Gamsu, G., Thurlbeck, W. M., Macklem, P. T. & Fraser, R. G. (1971) Roentgenographic appearance of the human pulmonary acinus. *Investigative Radiology*, **6**, 171–175.

Glazier, J. B., Hughes, J. M. B., Maloney, J. E. & West, J. B. (1967) Vertical gradient of alveolar size in lungs of dogs frozen intact. *Journal of Applied Physiology*, **23**, 694–705.

Gomez, D. M. (1965) A physico-mathematical study of lung function in normal subjects and in patients with obstructive pulmonary diseases. *Medicina Thoracalis*, **22**, 275–294.

Haggett, P. & Chorley, R. J. (1969) *Network Analysis in Geography*. London: Arnold.

Hislop, A. & Reid, L. (1972) Intra-pulmonary arterial development during foetal life—branching pattern and structure. *Journal of Anatomy*, **113**, 35–48.

Hislop, A. & Reid, L. (1973a) The similarity of the pulmonary artery branching system in siblings. *Forensic Science*, **2**, 37–52.

Hislop, A. & Reid, L. (1973b) Fetal and childhood development of the intrapulmonary veins in man—branching pattern and structure. *Thorax*, **28**, 313–319.

Horsfield, K. (1974) The relation between structure and function in the airways of the lung. *British Journal of Diseases of the Chest*, **68**, 145–160.

Horsfield, K. & Cumming, G. (1967) Angles of branching and diameters of branches in the human bronchial tree. *Bulletin of Mathematical Biophysics*, **29**, 245–259.

Horsfield, K. & Cumming, G. (1968) Morphology of the bronchial tree in man. *Journal of Applied Physiology*, **24**, 373–383.

Horsfield, K., Dart, G., Olson, D. E., Filley, G. F. & Cumming, G. (1971) Models of the human bronchial tree. *Journal of Applied Physiology*, **31**, 207–217.

Horsfield, K., Barer, D. H. & Cumming, G. (1973) Centrilobular emphysema studied with a mathematical model. *Scandinavian Journal of Respiratory Disease*, **54**, 53–64.

Hughes, J. M. B., Hoppin, F. G. & Mead, J. (1972) Effect of lung inflation on bronchial length and diameter in excised lungs. *Journal of Applied Physiology*, **32**, 25–35.

Kuhn, C. III & Finke, E. H. (1972) The topography of the pulmonary alveolus: scanning electron microscopy using different fixations. *Journal of Ultrastructure Research*, **38**, 161–173.

Lauweryns, J. M. (1970) The juxta-alveolar lymphatics in the human adult lung. Histologic studies in 15 cases of drowning. *American Review of Respiratory Disease*, **102**, 877–885.

Lauweryns, J. M. (1971a) The blood and lymphatic microcirculation of the lung. *Pathology Annual*, ed. Sheldon Summers, p. 365. New York: Appleton-Century-Crofts.

Lauweryns, J. M. (1971b) Stereomicroscopic funnel-like architecture of pulmonary lymphatic valves. *Lymphology*, **4**, 125–132.

Macklem, P. T., Thurlbeck, W. M. & Fraser, R. G. (1971) Chronic obstructive disease of small airways. *Annals of Internal Medicine*, **74**, 167–177.

Matsuba, K. & Thurlbeck, W. M. (1971) The number and dimensions of small airways in nonemphysematous lungs. *American Review of Respiratory Disease*, **104**, 516–524.

Matsuba, K. & Thurlbeck, W. M. (1972) The number and dimensions of small airways in emphysematous lungs. *American Journal of Pathology*, **67**, 265–275.

Miller, W. S. (1947) *The Lung*, 2nd edn. Springfield, Illinois: Thomas.

Nadel, J. A., Wolfe, W. G. & Graf, P. D. (1968) Powdered tantalum as a medium for bronchography in canine and human lungs. *Investigative Radiology*, **3**, 229–238.

Ogawa, C. (1920) The finer ramifications of the human lung. *American Journal of Anatomy*, **27**, 315–332.

Olson, D. E., Sudlow, M. F., Horsfield, K. & Filley, G. F. (1973) Convective patterns of flow during inspiration. *Archives of Internal Medicine*, **131**, 51–57.

Parker, H., Horsfield, K. & Cumming, G. (1971) Morphology of distal airways in the human lung. *Journal of Applied Physiology*, **31**, 386–391.

Pump, K. K. (1964) The morphology of the finer branches of the bronchial tree of the human lung. *Diseases of the Chest*, **46**, 379–398.

Pump, K. K. (1966) The circulation in the peripheral parts of the human lung. *Diseases of the Chest*, **49**, 119–129.

Pump, K. K. (1969) Morphology of the acinus of the human lung. *Diseases of the Chest*, **56**, 126–134.

Reid, L. (1958) The secondary lobule in the adult human lung, with special reference to its appearance in bronchograms. *Thorax*, **13**, 110–115.

Reid, L. (1968) Structural and functional reappraisal of the pulmonary artery system. In *The Scientific Basis of Medicine Annual Reviews*, pp. 289–307. London: Athlone Press.

Rohrer, R. (1915) Der Stromungs widerstand in den menschlichen Atemwegen und der Einfluss der unregelmassigen Verz weigung des Bronchial systems auf den Atmungsverlauf in vershiedenen Lungenbezinken. *Pflügers Archiv für die gesamte Physiologie*, **162**, 225–259.

Schroter, R. C. & Sudlow, M. F. (1969) Flow patterns in models of the human bronchial airways. *Respiration Physiology*, **7**, 341–355.

Sekihara, T., Olson, D. E. & Filley, G. F. (1968) Airflow regimes and geometrical factors in the human airway. In *Proceedings Eleventh Aspen Emphysema Conference*, pp. 103–113. Public Health Service Publication No. 1879, US Department of Health, Education and Welfare.

Semmens, M. (1970) The pulmonary artery in the normal aged lung. *British Journal of Diseases of the Chest*, **64**, 65–72.

Singhal, S., Henderson, R., Horsfield, K., Harding, K. & Cumming, G. (1973) Morphometry of the human pulmonary arterial tree. *Circulation Research*, **33**, 190–197.

Staub, N. C. (1965) Time-dependent factors in pulmonary gas exchange. *Medicina Thoracalis*, **22**, 132–145.

Stelter, G. P., Hanson, J. E. & Fairchild, D. G. (1966) A three-dimensional reconstruction of lung parenchyma. *American Review of Respiratory Disease*, **94**, 79–85.

Strahler, A. N. (1953) Revisions of Horton's quantitative factors in erosional terrain. *Transactions of the American Geophysical Union*, **34**, 345.

Strahler, A. N. (1957) Quantitative analysis of watershed geomorphology. *Transactions of the American Geophysical Union*, **38**, 913–920.

Stutz, E. (1949) Bronchographische Beitrage zus normalen und pathologischen Physiologie der Lungen. *Fortschritte auf dem Gebiete der Röntgenstrahlen*, **72**, 129–143, 309–338, 447–469.

Von Hayek, H. (1960) *The Human Lung*, p. 253. New York: Hafner.

Weibel, E. R. (1963) *Morphometry of the Human Lung*. Berlin: Springer-Verlag.

West, J. B. (1971) Distribution of mechanical stress in the lung, a possible factor in localisation of pulmonary disease. *Lancet*, **1**, 839–841.

West, J. B. & Matthews, F. L. (1972) Stresses, strains and surface pressures in the lung caused by its weight. *Journal of Applied Physiology*, **32**, 332–345.

Willson, H. G. (1922) The terminals of the human bronchiole. *American Journal of Anatomy*, **30**, 267–295.

Woldenberg, M. J. (1968) Hierarchical systems: cities, rivers, Alpine glaciers, bovine livers, and trees. *Geography and the Properties of Surfaces Series* No. 19. Cambridge, USA: Harvard University.

Woldenberg, M. J., Cumming, G., Harding, K., Horsfield, K., Prowse, K. & Singhal, S. (1970) Law and order in the human lung. *Geography and the Properties of Surfaces Series*, No. 41. Cambridge, USA: Harvard University.

6

AIRWAYS OBSTRUCTION

J. B. L. Howell

This review is organised in two parts. Firstly, the definition and nature of airway obstruction is considered together with the basic pathological processes affecting lung parenchyma and airways; secondly, the clinical presentation of the different types of airway obstruction is described including their pathophysiology and therapy.

Breathlessness on exertion in patients with chronic bronchitis, emphysema or 'chronic asthma' usually indicates that airways obstruction has complicated the underlying disorder. Without airways obstruction, chronic bronchitis (Ciba Foundation, 1959) presents only the nuisance of sputum expectoration and increased tendency to episodes of purulent bronchitis in winter. Emphysema may be quite extensive but until it is associated with airways obstruction, it is not symptomatic.

Definition of Airways Obstruction

Airways obstruction is essentially a slowing of forced expiration which sets an upper limit to the ability to ventilate the lungs. If demand for ventilation exceeds the capacity to respond, severe dyspnoea results. At lower levels of exercise, even though ventilatory capacity has not been reached, ventilatory response to demand is reduced and this mismatch is associated with breathlessness.

In view of the importance of airway obstruction it may seem surprising that, unlike chronic bronchitis or emphysema, there is no formally agreed definition. Indeed, some would disagree even with the term, preferring instead airflow obstruction. Either term implies some increased resistance to flow through bronchi, but as we shall see, airway obstruction may occur even though resistance to airflow measured during quiet breathing is not increased.

Airflow obstruction may be defined operationally in terms of the forced expiratory volume in 1 s (FEV_1), often expressed as a percentage of the vital capacity (VC). Normally, 70 to 80 per cent of the vital capacity can be expired in the first second, a smaller proportion implying airways obstruction. An absolute reduction in the FEV_1 below the predicted normal for the subject's height, age and sex may occur simply because of a reduction or effective reduction in lung volume due to such conditions as pneumonectomy, pulmonary fibrosis or infiltration, pleural effusion, etc, but in these conditions the vital capacity is also reduced and the FEV_1/VC ratio tends to be preserved.

Airways obstruction may therefore be defined as an 'inability to expel a normal proportion of the actual total lung capacity (TLC) in a given time'. Because there is no simple method of measuring TLC the vital capacity is usually used as an indirect index even though it is itself often reduced by airway obstruction, and therefore tends to make the ratio FEV_1/VC a less sensitive index of airways obstruction. It is even possible for the ratio FEV_1/VC to be virtually normal in the presence of severe airway obstruction if the vital capacity is also correspondingly reduced; clinical or radiological recognition of an increased volume of the lungs will usually allow this situation to be recognised.

Another commonly used index of airway obstruction is the peak expiratory flow rate delivered after full inspiration to TLC, usually measured using Wright's Peak Flow Meter, which records the maximum rate of expiratory airflow sustained for 10 ms (Wright and McKerrow, 1959).

Forced maximal expiratory flow rates are remarkable for their reproducibility and their independence of expiratory effort once maximum flow has been reached. The responsible factors will now be considered.

Limitation of Maximum Expiratory Airflow (the 'Starling Resistor')

Air flowing in a tube is hindered by resistance which is inversely related to the calibre of the tube. This is analogous to Ohm's law in electricity. In the tracheobronchial tree, this relationship holds only for flows below a certain value. Even in normal subjects, flow rates are readily reached above which no further flow is achieved no matter how much additional expiratory effort is made; a 'flow-limiting' mechanism must then be operating. An understanding of the mechanism of flow limitation is of fundamental importance as this mechanism underlies airway obstruction.

An adequate model of the mechanical relationships within and surrounding the bronchial tree must first be developed. The simplest model is illustrated in Figure 1 where the airspaces are shown as a single space and the tracheobronchial tree as a single airway leading from it, the whole being enclosed within the thorax. During inspiration, alveolar pressure is lowered by the action of inspiratory muscles and air flows through the bronchi at a rate which depends upon the alveolar-mouth pressure difference and the resistance of the airways; note that there is no intrathoracic limitation of inspiratory airflow. At the end of inspiration, intrapleural (intrathoracic) pressure is lower than atmospheric because of the elastic recoil of the lungs. During quiet expiration, the inspiratory muscles slowly relax allowing the lungs slowly to recoil, raising alveolar and intrabronchial pressure above atmospheric (Fig. 1a) thereby driving air from alveoli to mouth. It is important to realise that the pressure within the bronchi is higher than that surrounding them *solely* because of the recoil of the elastic elements of the lungs. If expiratory muscles contract and raise intrathoracic pressure, this pressure is added to the recoil pressure of the lungs and raises alveolar pressure further, causing increased expiratory airflow along the bronchi. If this increased flow causes a drop of pressure greater than that contributed by elastic recoil, the pressure

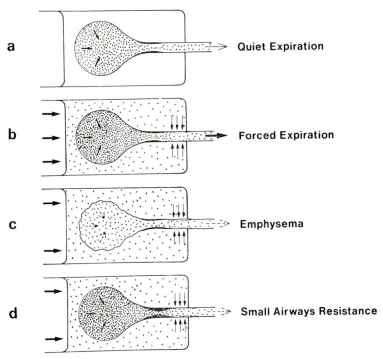

Figure 1 Diagrammatic representation of factors influencing maximum expiratory airflow. (a) Passive recoil of the lungs raises alveolar and intrabronchial pressure above intrathoracic pressure; no compression occurs. (b) During forced expiration rapid airflow results in pressure within the airway falling below the raised intrathoracic pressure and compression occurs. (c) With emphysema recoil pressure is diminished; compression occurs at lower rates of airflow. (d) With increased small airways resistance, e.g. associated with chronic bronchitis, even though recoil pressure is normal, the more rapid fall in pressure along the airway resulting in compression at lower flow rates

within the airways will fall below the intrathoracic pressure and compression of the bronchi will occur (Fig. 1b). This will happen more readily, i.e. at lower flow rates, firstly if the elastic recoil of the lungs is reduced by, for instance, breathing at low lung volumes, or by pulmonary emphysema (Fig. 1c); and, secondly if there is increased resistance to airflow through the smaller bronchi (Fig. 1d).

The site within the tracheobronchial tree at which extra- and intrabronchial pressures become equal has been termed the equal pressure point (EPP)

(Mead et al, 1967), and must occur first in the trachea close to the thoracic outlet. The trachea is normally prevented from collapsing because of its cartilaginous hoops and musculomembranous posterior wall. If expiratory flow rate is increased by further expiratory effort, the EPP will move upstream, i.e. lower down the trachea into the major bronchi and perhaps beyond, depending upon their ability to resist compression. The whole of the intra-thoracic tracheobronchial tree downstream (mouthwards) of the EPP is subject to a compressive force; actual compression will occur first at the weakest, proximal point along this section. According to Macklem and Wilson (1965) this is usually in the main or segmental bronchi or possibly the lower trachea, but data on this are scanty. Once compression of the weakest segment has occurred, flow is limited to that flow rate because further expiratory effort, while raising alveolar pressure, also raises intrathoracic pressure so that the driving pressure between alveoli and compressed segment is not increased. When compression first occurs, the increased resistance to flow which it causes slows the flow rate, reduces the degree of compression and allows the segment to dilate. But in so doing it permits an increase in flow rate, thereby restoring the compression. Unless the compressed segment of the tracheo-bronchial wall is highly damped it will oscillate rapidly, and be responsible for the expiratory wheeze which a normal person may induce by forced expiration and which a patient with chronic airways obstruction exhibits more markedly. This flow limiting mechanism is commonly called a 'Starling resistor'.

Although the intrinsic rigidity of the intrapulmonary airways becomes progressively less as they branch into smaller divisions, they receive consider-able support from the surrounding lung parenchyma and can resist very great compressing forces. In emphysematous regions this support may be lost; nevertheless, these individual unsupported segments do not cause flow limitation because two Starling resistors cannot operate in series; in these circumstances the downstream resistor will dominate and the intrabronchial pressure in the upstream airway will not fall low enough for a Starling resistor to develop. Eventually, as expiration proceeds, and lung volume diminishes, the alveolar driving pressure is reduced, as well as the parenchymal support for the small bronchi; Starling resistors may appear in parallel in progressively more peripheral generations of bronchi. This is presumably the mechanism of the sibilant rhonchi which appear towards the end of expiration especially at the bases, in patients with bronchitis and emphysema.

In summary, the three main factors influencing maximum expiratory flow rate are:

(a) resistance of the airways, especially upstream of the flow limiting segment
(b) elastic recoil pressure of the lungs
(c) rigidity or collapsibility of the larger airways.

These will now be considered in more detail.

Resistance to Airflow Through the Bronchial Tree

In estimating the resistance to airflow at different sites in the bronchial tree two types of approach have been made. Using a retrograde catheter technique, Macklem and Mead (1967) measured pressures during airflow in bronchi of about 2 mm diameter (i.e. about the eighth generation of branching from the trachea), and showed that approximately 75 per cent of the pressure drop between trachea and alveolus occurred in these larger airways, only

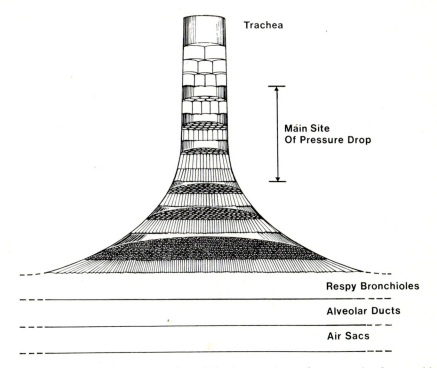

Figure 2 Diagrammatic representation of the increase in total cross-sectional area with branching of the tracheobronchial tree

25 per cent occurring in the more numerous smaller peripheral branches. In the second, anatomical approach, Weibel (1963), and Horsfield and Cumming (1968), made careful detailed measurements of the dimensions of the branches of the tracheobronchial tree of normal subjects and, using the number of airways and their diameters, calculated the total cross-sectional area and hence the relative linear velocity of airflow at any level and the resistance to airflow. Their conclusions are illustrated schematically (Fig. 2). Note that although the bronchi branch repeatedly, there is only a small change in the total cross-sectional area until the eighth or ninth generation when individual bronchi have a diameter of approximately 2 mm.

It is in this region of the fifth to ninth generations that the greatest pressure drop occurs during airflow; the increased resistance produced by the many small bronchi is not outweighed by an increase in cross-sectional area and therefore lower linear velocity of airflow. It is also of interest that in animal studies these airways showed the greatest reduction in calibre on vagal stimulation.

The total cross-sectional area then increases more rapidly but is still only about four-fold by the twelfth generation at which level the bronchioles are less than 1 mm diameter. The greatest increase in cross-sectional area occurs beyond the terminal bronchioles when, although branching continues, no further reduction in the calibre of the airways occurs.

Site of Increased Resistance in Disease

Chronic irreversible airway obstruction

Using the retrograde catheter technique in autopsy specimens of lungs from patients with chronic airway obstruction Hogg, Macklem and Thurlbeck (1968) showed that the normal situation was reversed; most of the pressure drop between the larynx and alveoli now occurred in airways smaller than 2 mm diameter. These are not necessarily the same generation of 2 mm bronchi as in the normal as they themselves may have undergone narrowing.

Since normally only 25 per cent of the total resistance resides in the small airways, major changes may occur here with only a small effect upon the total airway resistance. For example, a doubling of peripheral resistance (100 per cent increase) would, in simple terms, only increase the resistance of this region from 25 to 50, and the total resistance from 100 to 125, i.e. a 25 per cent increase. Airflow measurements including spirometry are therefore relatively insensitive methods of detecting small to moderate changes in the small airways in disease. Alternative attempts at detection of small changes in the peripheral bronchi have been by measurement of the frequency dependence of compliance (p. 167) and by measurement of closing volumes (p. 166). In a recent study in which a wide range of measurements directed at detecting deviations from normality in smokers compared with non-smokers, the most sensitive measurement was the arterial P_{O_2}. Closing volume was no more sensitive than the FEV_1.

The nature of this increased small airways resistance is still uncertain and is the subject of investigation at various centres at present. Matshuba and Thurlbeck (1973) showed that in chronic bronchitis, there was narrowing of the airways together with excess mucus, but there was no loss of airways; with emphysema, there was loss of airways as well. Depierre et al (1972) demonstrated multiple inflammatory bronchial stenoses in association with centrilobular emphysema. In panlobular emphysema, no bronchiolar stenoses were present.

Reversible airway obstruction

In asthma, the distribution of the changes within the bronchial tree is not known. It is generally assumed that increased bronchomotor tone, mucosal oedema, and increased secretions affect all levels of the bronchial tree, but the effects of such changes upon airways resistance are probably greatest in small airways. Mucosal oedema and secretions have a greater effect upon the resistance of small than large airways, especially since resistance varies inversely as the fourth power of the radius. Increased bronchomotor tone produces a greater tendency to airway narrowing in bronchi of small diameter, due to Laplace's law (the inward acting pressure due to tension in the wall of a tube varies inversely with the radius of curvature).

Most pathological studies of the lungs in asthma have been made perforce in patients dying with presumed allergic asthma, and are unlikely to represent fairly the changes occurring in the moderately severe cases. The most striking feature is mucous plugging in both large and small bronchi, even extending to terminal bronchioles. In addition, eosinophilia and desquamated epithelial cells commonly occur in this exudate. In the mucosa, there is thickening of the basement membrane, oedematous submucosa with dilated capillaries, enlarged mucous glands are seen and infiltration with eosinophils. The smooth muscle in the bronchial wall is hypertrophied (Dunnill, Massarella and Anderson, 1969).

Currently, a number of centres are studying mucosal biopsy specimens from asthmatic subjects taken with a fibreoptic bronchoscope, but no results have yet been reported.

Lung Elastic Recoil

It is not always appreciated that the elastin/collagen framework of the lungs is relatively inextensible; distensibility of the lungs is conferred not only by stretching of the elastin/collagen framework but also by a geometric reorganisation like the uncoiling of a spring. This is responsible for approximately two-thirds of the total elastic recoil, the remainder being due to surface tension forces. Apart from the respiratory distress syndrome of the newborn, oxygen toxicity and 'shock lung', there is no firm evidence that disturbance of surface tension forces plays an important role in the genesis of disease, and in particular airways obstruction.

The most important cause of diminished elastic recoil is emphysema which is characterised by increased volume of terminal lung units and destruction of alveolar walls.

Types of Emphysema

Three main types of emphysema are recognised:

1. Centrilobular (or centri-acinar) affecting respiratory bronchioles;
2. Panlobular (or panacinar) affecting the whole acinus or secondary lobule;

3. Paraseptal—adjacent to septa. This is probably of no clinical significance and will not be discussed further.

A detailed monograph has been prepared by Reid (1967).

Centri-acinar (centrilobular) emphysema

Centri-acinar emphysema is most commonly found in the upper part of the upper and lower lobes. West and Matthews (1972) have drawn attention to the fact that the tension within the lung parenchyma is greatest at these sites in erect man, due to gravitational effects. A model of the causation of centri-acinar emphysema is that of some destructive process occurring in the central part of the lobule, weakening the respiratory bronchiolar walls; tension within the lung parenchyma then causes the weakened bronchial walls to rupture, causing centri-acinar emphysema. Centri acinar emphysema probably involves two different types of lesion, according to the type of precipitating factor, dust inhalation or inflammatory lesion including smoking (Heppleston, 1974).

The mechanisms of the destructive processes affecting respiratory bronchioles remains uncertain; but the extension of purulent bronchitis to these bronchioles causing respiratory bronchiolitis and release of lysosomal proteases is one possibility. Another possibility is the deposition of inhaled irritants (tobacco smoke, air pollutants) in this region; this is quite likely in view of the calculations by Cumming (1973) that the 'interface' of the normal inspired breath and alveolar gas probably occurs in alveolar ducts. Although deposition would tend to occur at a number of sites within the bronchial tree, the larger bronchi have powerful protective mechanisms, including the mucus blanket, which is not present at the level of respiratory bronchioles and beyond.

With destruction of centrilobular regions, penetration of inspired gas towards alveolar ducts will be reduced, increasing the length and altering the geometry of the diffusion pathways for gases, thereby decreasing the concentration of oxygen and increasing the P_{CO_2} in the peripheral parts of the lobule. This 'stratified inhomogeneity' is probably an important mechanism of arterial unsaturation (venous admixture) in patients with centrilobular emphysema.

Panacinar (panlobular) emphysema

The mechanism of panlobular emphysema is uncertain in the majority of cases but there is a group of younger patients with predominantly basal emphysema in whom a probable mechanism has been revealed.

Clues to a possible mechanism followed the observation in 1963 by Laurell and Eriksson that the alpha$_1$ globulin electrophoretic peak was absent in a number of patients with emphysema. This was shown to be associated with deficiency of serum protease inhibitory activity, largely due to deficiency of alpha₁ antitrypsin (AAT). Severe AAT deficiency has been estimated to occur in approximately 0.06 per cent of the population (Eriksson, 1965).

Since then, there have been extensive studies of AAT showing that it is a plasma protein which can exist in a number of different phenotypic forms, due to the occurrence in the population of different autosomal genes; these have been labelled M, S, Z, etc, including a completely 'silent' gene, O. In the UK about 86 per cent of people are of the homozygous MM phenotype. Of the heterozygotes approximately 5 per cent are of the heterozygous MS type, and 3 per cent of the MZ type, both of which are associated with normal or near normal levels of AAT. The homozygous ZZ is uncommon (0.29 per cent) as is the heterozygote SZ but are important because both are associated with low levels of serum AAT, and hence low levels of protease inhibitory function.

The significance of AAT deficiency has been extensively investigated and although the picture is not entirely clear, some features seem to have been established.

1. Subjects homozygous for the Z or O genes, types ZZ, or OO or heterozygous SZ or OZ, have severe deficiency of serum AAT with severe deficiency of serum protease inhibitory activity. These individuals are especially prone to develop pulmonary emphysema characterised by: (a) panlobular type, (b) onset at an earlier than usual age, i.e. usually in the fourth or fifth decades, though it has even been recorded in homozygous deficient children, and (c) predominantly basal distribution.
2. The onset is about a decade earlier in smokers than non-smokers.
3. Females with AAT are affected with emphysema almost as frequently as males.

Hutchison et al (1971) have studied a large group of patients of all ages with emphysema and found that 13 per cent had evidence of AAT deficiency. In another series (Thomas and Jones, 1961) 16 per cent of 87 cases of emphysema were deficient in AAT.

While the significance of severe reduction in serum protease levels associated with the ZZ, ZO, ZS, OO phenotypes in the genesis of lower zone emphysema is established, the clinical importance of the heterozygous state remains uncertain. There is some evidence to support the view that a relative deficiency state may exist in heterozygotes which in the presence of inhaled irritants such as tobacco smoke leads to an increased liability to emphysema (Cooper et al, 1974). The implications of this 'model' of emphysema is that until some means is discovered of increasing serum protease inhibitor levels the logical approach to preventing or delaying the onset of emphysema is by avoidance of situations leading to inflammatory reactions in the lungs, i.e. avoidance of the irritation of inhaled tobacco smoke, SO_2 and other pollutants and the prompt treatment of infections. If an individual is known to have

AAT deficiency he should be urged strongly not to smoke and it would seem reasonable to recommend avoidance of dusty occupations.

In 1969 it was shown that certain cases of neonatal hepatitis were associated with AAT deficiency (Sharp et al, 1969). Cases have since been described in adults associated with chronic airways obstruction. The AAT occurs as PAS positive granules in the liver, and is associated with cirrhosis and its complications. It is suggested that in these cases, the defect is in AAT release rather than formation, but attempts to induce release with enzyme inducing agents have not been successful.

Rigidity or Collapsibility of Tracheobronchial Tree

Diminished rigidity

When expiratory airflow is rapid, the rigidity of the intrathoracic airways determines whether significant flow limitation occurs or not. In patients with markedly diminished rigidity of the trachea, for example due to polychondritis but with otherwise normal lungs, flow limitation will occur at somewhat lower rates of airflow than if the tracheal rigidity were normal. Although no direct measurements have been reported in this condition, the flow limiting segment would be expected to lie within the trachea close to the thoracic outlet. Diminished rigidity of the trachea has also been described in patients with chronic bronchitis and airways obstruction (Wright, 1960).

Increased collapsibility

Airways have a tendency to collapse due to surface tension forces unless there is an opposing distending force. At normal resting lung volumes, this is provided for extrapulmonary airways by the subatmospheric intrathoracic (pleural) pressure and for the intrapulmonary airways by the tension in the surrounding lung parenchyma in addition.

Where there is inherent 'collapsibility' of the airways due to increased bronchomotor tone, the situation is complex.

During forced expiration 'compression' of airways occurs when broncho-motor tone plus intrathoracic pressure is sufficient to overcome the support of the bronchi. Because the pressure due to increased bronchomotor tone is inversely related to the calibre of the airways (Laplace's law) the effect is greater in small calibre airways, and will tend to cause flow limitation to occur in smaller intrapulmonary bronchi.

Where bronchomotor tone is high, collapse of small bronchi may occur even at high lung volume (Howell, 1969) accounting for the expiratory wheezing throughout tidal breathing but it is not known which generations of bronchi are involved. Increased tone in tracheal muscle leads to increased rigidity by strengthening the segment between the posterior ends of the cartilaginous loops. These theoretical considerations lead to the conclusion that in conditions of increased bronchomotor tone, e.g. asthma, flow limitation is likely to occur more peripherally in smaller airways. Evidence in support of this deduction has been obtained by Hertzog et al (1968) but this difficult work has not been repeated.

Measurement and Display of the Factors Influencing Airway Obstruction

Diminished elastic recoil

This requires the determination of the static volume–pressure relationships of the lung and involves measurement of transpulmonary pressure, i.e. oesophageal pressure relative to mouth pressure throughout the vital capacity and preferably displayed in relation to absolute lung volume. This measurement is not made routinely, but may be necessary in the investigation of obscure airways obstruction (Leaver, Tattersfield and Pride, 1974).

Airways resistance

This may be measured from pressure-flow loops by the method of Mead and Whittenberger (1954), by the multiple interruptor method of Clements and Elam (1955), or by the body plethysmograph (Dubois, Botelho and Comroe, 1956). The last is probably the most widely used at present especially as the lung volume at which measurements of airway resistance are made is also measured. This is important because airways resistance is affected by changes in lung volume. The reciprocal of resistance, airways conductance, is an alternative method of expressing the results, often favoured because the relationship between conductance and lung volume is more linear; it is therefore possible to describe changing airways conductance–lung volume relationships by a single figure; conductance/lung volume, which is termed 'specific conductance'. However, this only applies when the conductance–lung volume relationship extrapolates to zero.

Large airway rigidity or collapsibility

There is no easy way at present available of measuring this factor independently. Crofton et al (1963) have measured the 'squeeze pressure' of bronchi which is probably related to bronchomotor tone, though it is likely to be influenced by other factors as well.

Expiratory Airflow

The resultant of the interaction of these three factors is reflected by measurements of expiratory flow rates during forced expiration sufficient to induce flow limitation. The best known are the FEV_1 and the peak expiratory flow rate (PEFR), but the maximal mid-expiratory flow rate may be more sensitive in detecting small changes (McFadden and Linden, 1972). Another more recently introduced measurement is the flow–volume diagram (see

Pride, 1971) in which the maximum expiratory flow rate is displayed (y axis) against the volume expired (x axis). This display shows the maximum flow rates which can be achieved throughout the vital capacity. There is no additional information in the flow–volume diagram compared with the FEV_1 but it is a more revealing display of some aspects of these relationships. Other indirect measures of factors influencing airway obstruction include closing volumes, frequency dependent compliance and regional ventilation perfusion relationships using radioactive xenon (see Chapter 1).

Closing volume and closing capacity

One of the most interesting recent advances in understanding of pulmonary function in health and disease has been the development of the concept of 'closing volume' or 'closing capacity'. A review of this topic has been published as a report of an International Symposium (see Milic-Emili, 1974) where extensive references may be found for further reading.

In healthy young adults virtually all of the bronchi and bronchioles are patent at the end of normal expiration. With deeper expiration the reduction in lung elastic retractive force allows closure of airways, first in the most dependent parts of the lung where, because of gravitational effects, elastic recoil is least, and then gradually airway closure occurs in the upper parts as residual volume is approached. The volume of air in the lungs when airway closure begins to occur is known as the 'closing capacity' and the volume of air which can still be expired the 'closing volume' (i.e. closing capacity = closing volume + residual volume). It was once thought that at residual volume in normal individuals, closure occurred in all airways, completely isolating the alveolar gas from the larger airways, but more recent studies with radioactive xenon have demonstrated closure only in the lower parts of the lungs. In normal non-smoking young men airways closure begins when expiration is continued below FRC and increases steadily down to RV when near 50 per cent of lung units have closed airways, trapping about 700 ml of alveolar gas. The site of airway closure was suggested on indirect evidence based on transpulmonary pressure and surface tension measurements in man to be in terminal or respiratory bronchioles (Howell, 1957) and this location has recently been demonstrated directly in dogs (Hughes, Rosenzweig and Kivitz, 1970).

Closing capacity is proportionally larger in children and also in older people in whom it increases linearly with age, presumably because of progressive lowering of elastic recoil pressures. In these two groups airway closure may thus occur during tidal breathing, especially in the supine position, and may result in some venous admixture.

Closing volume is increased in a number of clinical disorders: hepatic cirrhosis, pulmonary oedema, smokers, obesity, asthma, patients having undergone upper abdominal surgery.

Because closing volume and closing capacity are influenced by the behaviour of small airways, it has been suggested as a means of detecting changes in the peripheral airways too small to affect spirometric results (McCarthy et al, 1972). But, to date, its value as a screening procedure for early disease has not been established.

Frequency-dependent compliance

This is another special test directed at detecting early changes in the peripheral airways (Woolcock, Vincent and Macklem, 1969). The compliance of the lungs is normally measured under static conditions when elastic forces within the lungs are in equilibrium. If lung compliance is measured during cyclic breathing using the points of no airflow to indicate static conditions, and if some airways offer a greater resistance than others, a reduction in lung compliance will occur with increasing frequency of breathing. Alveoli distal to the wider airways will receive more air than those distal to narrower airways, and hence will contribute a greater recoil pressure. Thus, reduction in lung compliance with increasing frequency of breathing should indicate disease in smaller airways. In practice, this is technically a very difficult measurement, the results are equivocal, and it is not recommended at present as a practical test.

Regional ventilation/perfusion relationships

Regional differences in the distribution of pulmonary blood flow and of inspired gas, using radioactive xenon have been demonstrated in patients with chronic bronchitis, airways obstruction, and even in asthmatic subjects apparently fully recovered from an attack. This technique is described in more detail in Chapter 1.

CLINICAL SYNDROMES OF AIRWAYS OBSTRUCTION

The majority of patients with airways obstruction show some degree of improvement in response to bronchodilator therapy; in this sense most cases are partly reversible. However, some patients show very large degrees of reversibility both objectively and subjectively. It is in the situation where the subject may be restored virtually to normal that we usually use the term 'reversible'. There is, however, a wide range of reversibility and more precise categorisation would need to be based on arbitrary quantitative criteria not yet agreed.

Chronic Airways Obstruction

The clinical syndromes associated with chronic airways obstruction are often termed 'chronic bronchitis and emphysema' or just 'emphysema' because these features are commonly present. A more accurate description would, therefore, be chronic airways obstruction with chronic bronchitis, chronic bronchitis and emphysema, or emphysema as the case may be. Note that emphysema is strictly a pathological diagnosis and can only be diagnosed in life by physiological and radiological evidence of lung parenchymal destruction. There are also a small number of patients with chronic airways obstruction who apparently have neither chronic bronchitis nor emphysema and who have evidence only of increased airway resistance.

Clinical Presentation

In 1956, Dornhorst drew attention to two extreme clinical presentations of patients with chronic airways obstruction. One was characterised by severe breathlessness but no cyanosis, i.e. they were pink and puffing (pink puffers), while the other type was cyanosed and oedematous, i.e. blue and bloated (blue bloaters).

Pink puffers

These subjects are characteristically middle-aged men, of thin build who have developed increasing shortness of breath on exertion. They may or may not have evidence of chronic bronchitis, but are usually long-standing smokers. As they progress to severe incapacity, they show signs of marked overinflation of the chest with loss of cardiac and hepatic dullness, quiet breath sounds and prolonged expiration. Fine, sibilant expiratory rhonchi may be present on quiet breathing but, if not, they can usually be induced by forced expiration. There is no clinical evidence of disturbed gas exchange at rest though some cyanosis may be induced by exercise. Both the FEV_1, VC and FEV_1/VC are reduced. TLC is usually increased. The resting P_aO_2 may be slightly reduced but further falls may occur on exertion. The P_aCO_2 is normal. Indices of gas mixing are abnormal and the transfer factor for carbon monoxide (CO) is markedly reduced, consistent with extensive reduction in the alveolar capillary bed. There is no evidence of 'heart failure' until the terminal stages. At autopsy the lungs show extensive panacinar and sometimes patchy centrilobular emphysema and there may be right ventricular hypertrophy.

MANAGEMENT

The nature of flow-limitation which is responsible for most of their symptoms should be explained in very simple terms; the use of the term emphysema is best avoided as it often causes grave anxiety. The subject must be urged to stop smoking and instructed in the recognition of bronchial infections which must be treated promptly. Self-medication with an antibiotic (e.g. with tetracycline, cotrimoxazole, ampicillin or amoxycillin) at the earliest sign of purulence of the sputum should be encouraged by providing the patient with a home supply to start without delay. Bronchodilator aerosol and/or tablets should be prescribed, if they are found to be symptomatically helpful. Physical work load should ideally be adjusted to be well within the patient's capacity. Unfortunately this cannot always be done, especially as so many patients are in social class IV or V where manual labour predominates. In very severe cases, the use of portable oxygen may enable the patient to remain more mobile but it seldom has a major effect upon physical capacity. This therapy is expensive and is best prescribed after a full evaluation of lung function and the objective response to O_2 in a specialised Pulmonary Function Unit. The value of measures to reduce sputum volume and aid expectoration, e.g. bromhexine, or carboxymethylcysteine, must be critically assessed individually on patients, lest this expensive therapy is continued unnecessarily.

Blue bloaters

By contrast to pink puffers, blue bloaters are characteristically of heavier build, with a long history of chronic mucopurulent bronchitis. Their breathlessness is usually less severe, and they may sometimes present first with evidence of congestive heart failure, especially ankle oedema. On examination, they are cyanosed with a plethoric appearance, and may have less severe airways obstruction and overinflation of the chest. Breath sounds may be well preserved. There is often clinical and electrocardiographic evidence of right ventricular hypertrophy, raised right atrial pressure, hepatomegaly and oedema. Laboratory investigation may show polycythaemia, the haematocrit sometimes exceeding 70 per cent, but even if normal, the red cell mass is usually raised. Arterial saturation is reduced to varying degrees, sometimes as low as 75 per cent but much lower values may be seen during an acute exacerbation. The $P\mathrm{co}_2$ is elevated, e.g. 55 to 60 mmHg, but the respiratory acidosis is usually well compensated. The FEV_1, VC and FEV_1/VC are reduced but the TLC may be little increased. The transfer factor for CO may sometimes be normal.

Radiographically, the heart is enlarged and pulmonary vessels may be congested. There is usually no radiographic evidence of emphysema, although at autopsy, extensive centri-acinar and panacinar emphysema is often seen.

Earlier observations suggested a reduced sensitivity to CO_2 proportional to the severity of the disturbance of gas exchange (Lane, Howell and Giblin, 1968) but there is recent evidence that any elevation of $P\mathrm{co}_2$ in association with chronic airways obstruction indicates a severe loss of CO_2 sensitivity (Matthews and Howell, 1975). The mechanisms of this loss of CO_2 sensitivity is unknown.

MANAGEMENT

This is basically the same as for pink puffers except that for most patients long-term diuretic therapy is needed once oedema has occurred; digitalis is usually not required. There is no evidence that so-called respiratory stimulants have any role in this situation. Sedatives, including even the benzodiazepines, are contraindicated as they may induce severe hypoventilation. Occasionally, a carbonic anhydrase inhibitor—acetazoleamide (250 mg b.d.) or dichlorphenamide (50–100 mg b.d.) may be helpful in both types of clinical presentation but there is no way of judging other than by therapeutic trial.

Acute respiratory failure in association with chronic airways obstruction

Hypoxaemia may occur in either type of case but severe ventilatory failure is much more likely in the blue bloater, because of the loss of CO_2 sensitivity. There may also be left ventricular failure leading to pulmonary oedema.

The usual precipitating factors are infection, smog (now rare in Britain), and inadvertent use of sedation. The increased mechanical load imposed by increased secretions and increased airways obstruction are not matched by increased ventilatory drive and hypoventilation therefore occurs. These factors also increase venous admixture causing hypoxaemia which may become very severe. The physician, in assessing this situation, must decide on two things. First, does the patient need oxygen? The patient may be deeply cyanosed but there may be no evidence of serious tissue hypoxaemia. In patients with severe respiratory failure, and using increase in lactate/pyruvate ratios as evidence of tissue hypoxia, it has been found that even an arterial Po_2 as low as 17 mmHg is not necessarily associated with tissue hypoxia, unless there is evidence of circulatory failure as well, viz. low volume pulse, low blood pressure, cold clammy skin. By contrast, circulatory failure even with high P_aO_2 is frequently associated with evidence of tissue hypoxia. The practical lesson is that patients with evidence of circulatory failure require high concentrations of O_2 immediately, while those with a good volume pulse, blood pressure and warm extremities are unlikely to be suffering from serious tissue hypoxia and immediate O_2 therapy is not mandatory. But the margin of safety will not be known and it is therefore advisable to move the patient further from 'the brink of hypoxia' by the administration of a small supplement of inspired O_2. The most practical way of achieving this is via a Ventimask designed to delivery 24 per cent O_2 which adds about 20 mmHg Po_2 to the inspired air, and which will not induce severe hypoventilation. A further measurement of arterial blood gases after 1 to 2 h will show whether any significant hypoventilation has been induced, and whether any reduction in hypoxaemia has been obtained.

The second question is: can the patient cough up secretions? This is a most valuable physical sign in this situation; if the patient cannot raise secretions, it may be because (i) his airway obstruction is too severe or (ii) he is too drowsy to cooperate. This situation requires an intravenous injection of aminophylline 250 to 500 mg given slowly over 3 to 5 min to try to induce some bronchodilatation, and if the patient is drowsy an analeptic, e.g. nikethamide 2 ml i.v., to rouse the patient to cooperate. Removal of even a small amount of sputum may so improve the patient that further expectoration becomes much easier. There is no doubt that a trained physiotherapist may be more successful at this than a nurse or physician. Inability to raise secretions, despite all efforts, indicates a grave situation and requires a decision about tracheal intubation for bronchial toilet and assisted ventilation. Such a decision requires accurate knowledge about the patient's state prior to the exacerbation, including an assessment of the quality of his life. If this information is lacking and doubt exists, the writer believes that this active and somewhat unpleasant therapy should be undertaken. Prolonged intubation with plastic endotracheal tubes has greatly reduced the need for tracheostomy in this situation.

Reversible Airways Obstruction (Asthma)

In the following discussion the term 'asthma' will be used to denote the clinical syndrome of reversible airways obstruction of a severity and a degree of reversibility such as to be clinically unequivocally recognised as such. It is not intended to denote a well-defined disorder, pathologically distinct or otherwise.

Some would seek a precise operational definition of asthma in terms of the degree of reversibility, but there is no agreement about how reversibility is to be measured, how it is to be expressed, and the extent of the change which would qualify. This aim presupposes that there is some advantage in defining 'asthma' with this degree of precision. An international symposium (Ciba Symposium, 1971) failed to agree on a definition of asthma. There was, however, complete agreement that in reporting studies on patients with any form of airways obstruction full information about clinical, functional, pathological, and immunological aspects should be described whenever possible.

The clinical syndromes associated with 'reversible airways obstruction', i.e. asthma, include:

1. Extrinsic asthma, usually associated with type I allergic reaction, but sometimes with type III and occasionally both (Pepys, 1968);
2. Exercise induced asthma (McNeill et al, 1966);
3. 'Intrinsic' or non-atopic (sometimes called 'infective') asthma in which no antigen can be identified and which may sometimes progress rapidly to chronic irreversible airways obstruction.

There are some patients with reversible airways obstruction who do not fall into any of these categories.

Allergy and asthma

The majority of patients with 'asthma' have associated allergic reactions and this has resulted in asthma being considered always to have an allergic aetiology. Conversely, patients with poorly reversible airways obstruction especially if associated with chronic bronchitis are usually considered not to have allergic disorders. Such views are not consistent with the evidence. Some patients with asthma have no evidence of allergic disorder, while many patients with chronic airways obstruction have evidence of atopy, sputum and blood eosinophilia, and a good clinical but often poor objective response to sodium cromoglycate and corticosteroids. Patients with airways obstruction presenting as asthma are likely to be investigated for an allergic aetiology and treated as such. By contrast, allergic bronchial reactions in association with chronic poorly reversible airways obstruction are often overlooked and hence may not receive effective therapy.

Certain clinical features should alert the physician to the possible presence of allergic reactions. These include recurrent chest tightness, episodes of nocturnal dyspnoea (in older patients often mistaken for left ventricular failure), the presence of eczema, or vasomotor rhinitis, and a family history of allergy. In these cases, sputum or blood eosinophilia is strong supporting evidence, but even if absent a therapeutic trial with sodium cromoglycate and/or corticosteroids may result in unexpected benefit.

Even when associated with allergic reactions the concept of asthma as an acute reaction to inhaled antigen is deficient in other respects. While this is an acceptable explanation of classical extrinsic asthma, i.e. asthma on exposure to a specific antigen, the majority of the problem cases of asthma have no such clear relationship to an allergen. Attacks may occur with bronchial infections, emotional stress, following exercise, or during sleep, and occasionally during coughing or even hearty laughing. How is asthma associated with such diverse precipitants to be explained? The answer lies in the phenomenon of bronchial hyperreactivity.

Bronchial hyperreactivity

Normal subjects may inhale a variety of irritants such as smoke, SO_2, dusts and, in certain concentrations, aerosols of pharmacological agents such as histamine, carbachol or methacholine with little or no change in airways resistance. By contrast, subjects exist in whom inhalation of these agents promptly provoke bronchoconstriction with tightness, breathlessness, and often coughing, i.e. they exhibit bronchial hyperreactivity. The most sensitive individuals are usually patients with the clinical syndrome of asthma, but some patients with chronic bronchitis and airway obstruction in whom there is no evidence of allergy are also hyperreactive. Some patients with diffuse pulmonary fibrosis may also exhibit this phenomenon.

The mechanism of hyperreactivity is uncertain but the ability of iso-prenaline to reverse rapidly the changes strongly suggests that constriction of bronchial muscle is the dominant reaction. Whether bronchoconstriction is due to direct effect of the agent upon the tissues or due to a reflex response mediated by the vagi is also uncertain and there is evidence that either or both mechanisms may exist. A striking example of reflex bronchoconstriction has been reported by Gold (1973) in dogs sensitised to intestinal parasites;

the relevant antigen instilled intrabronchially into one lung resulted in generalised bilateral bronchoconstriction. Vagotomy prevented this development. On the other hand, direct hyperreactivity has been shown on isolated tracheal rings from patients with chronic airway obstruction in which vagal reflexes (other than axon reflexes) could not possibly have been involved. Benson (1975) in a review of this phenomenon has adduced evidence that at least a part of bronchial hyperreactivity is a consequence of bronchoconstriction and of increased bronchomotor tone.

If one accepts that hyperreactivity of the bronchi is a central abnormality in patients with asthma, one can hypothesise about the different situations in which asthmatic (i.e. episodic bronchoconstriction) reactions occur. Thus infections and other irritants may well stimulate these hyperreactive bronchi directly or reflexly; emotional reactions act by increasing autonomic vagal discharge; and the same mechanism may account for nocturnal attacks of asthma (Howell, 1971).

Allergic states associated with asthma

IMMEDIATE ALLERGIC REACTION (ANAPHYLACTIC, TYPE I)

This is responsible for the best recognised form of asthma yet this does not usually present a serious clinical problem. The mechanism of this reaction has become better understood since the identification of the class of responsible immunoglobulins (IgE) by the Ishizakas (1966) and by the introduction of sodium cromoglycate (Altounyan, 1967).

The highly active IgE both circulates and is bound to mast cells. It is a reagin, i.e. it has a long persistence of tissue sensitisation. At one time it could only be identified by its biological effect and because of its low serum concentration it was thought to be largely bound to tissue cells. It can now be measured in serum by a radioimmunoassay and is known to be reversibly bound to receptor sites with only a minor proportion attached to mast cells.

When the appropriate antigen is inhaled, it first has to penetrate the epithelium to reach the antibody on mast cells. The union of antigen, probably with two adjacent antibodies, is thought to set up stresses at the cell membrane which trigger the mast cell to discharge its granules. There is evidence that a sequence of events, including a calcium-ion dependent process, results in the release of preformed histamine and eosinophil chemotactic factor (ECF-A) (Kay, Stechschulte and Austen, 1971) and also of slow reacting substance of anaphylaxis (SRS-A) which must be formed as well as released. Histamine is responsible for a part of the response of the bronchi to acute anaphylactic reactions through its action on capillary permeability and smooth muscle; it may well be the dominant mediator in allergic rhinitis which responds so well to antihistamine. However, antihistamines do not block the asthmatic reaction to inhaled antigen; this may be partly because insufficient concentration of the drug is achieved at the site of histamine release, but more likely because other mediators are involved. Using the response of guinea-pig ileum to the products of challenging sensitised lung tissue, antihistamines will prevent the rapid response but a more slowly developing contraction persists due to SRS-A (Brocklehurst, 1960). At present there is no clinically applicable inhibitor of SRS-A. Prostaglandin $F_{2\alpha}$ which exists in high concentration in lung tissue, and which is a potent bronchoconstrictor, has been suggested as a mediator; there is no direct evidence of its involvement, and administration of inhibitors of prostaglandin synthesis, indomethacin and aspirin, have no consistent effect in clinical asthma (Smith, 1975). At the present time there is insufficient evidence to discuss the role of other possible constrictor agents following bronchial challenge; these include serotonin, bradykinin, kallikrein, kallinen, and platelet-activating factor. There is also evidence that in certain circumstances not only IgE but some IgG will trigger off mast cell degranulation.

Evidence is accumulating that a number of factors affect the release of mediators. Mast cells possess alpha and beta adrenergic and cholinergic receptors which can modulate their secretory activity. Agents capable of increasing tissue cyclic AMP (e.g. isoprenaline) suppress histamine release from sensitised human and monkey lung; the reverse occurs with alpha stimulation. Stimulation of cholinergic receptors enhances mediator release but does so by increasing the levels of intracellular cyclic GMP (cyclic guanosine monophosphate) (see review by Austen, 1973).

PSYCHOLOGICAL FACTORS AND THE RESPONSE TO INHALED ANTIGEN

The mental state of subjects has long been known to influence the response to inhaled antigen. In a relaxed subject there might be no response to inhaled antigen, but if agitated and anxious, an asthmatic response readily occurs. A possible basis for this phenomenon is now seen in the effect of cholinergic receptors on mast cells. Cholinergic stimulation, for example, by increasing cyclic GMP may potentiate the release of mediators and set off a chain of events including further reflex cholinergic stimulation (Gold, 1973).

Conditioned reflexes have also been shown to be capable of inducing and perpetuating asthma (Moore, 1965). Verbal deconditioning reduces the number of attacks and improves peak expiratory flow rates.

The beneficial effect of reassurance and relaxation in the management of patients with asthma now becomes explicable in organic terms.

DELAYED ALLERGIC REACTION

Mainly due to the studies of Pepys (1968) it is now recognised that broncho-constriction, wheezing, chest tightness and breathlessness may develop by a different mechanism from the IgE mediated response, viz. precipitating antibodies mediating the Arthus reaction. This reaction is better known in relation to extrinsic alveolitis, e.g. farmer's lung, but in certain instances of bronchial allergy, e.g. to house dust or *Aspergillus fumigatus*, a delayed asthmatic reaction may occur. In the last two instances cited there may also be an immediate IgE mediated response occurring within the first 30 min, followed by a symptom-free interval before the delayed response occurs more slowly after 6 to 8 h. The clinical frequency of this type of response is uncertain—it is theoretically of great importance as the relationship between the exposure to antigen and the reaction may be overlooked because of their dissociation in time.

It must be emphasised that the quantitative importance of this kind of allergic response presenting as asthma is not known at present, and therefore all who are involved in the management of patients with asthma, especially with occupational hazards, should be alert to the possibility. This type of reaction, particularly if associated with alveolitis, can lead to irreversible and disabling pulmonary fibrosis. It should respond to corticosteroid therapy and some patients at least may respond to sodium cromoglycate.

Rational management of 'asthma'

IDENTIFICATION OF PRECIPITATING FACTORS

Careful attention to detail in the history is required to provide this information. Particular attention should be paid to external precipitants, and in adults an influence from industrial exposure should be carefully excluded. Psychological factors should be discussed openly. A vital rapport with the patient is unlikely to be achieved unless the patient has had the opportunity to present his or her problems in detail.

INVESTIGATION OF ALLERGIC STATUS

There are two main investigations: skin tests and provocation tests.

Skin testing indicates whether the individual has a single sensitivity or is highly atopic with multiple sensitivities, and enables the constituents of a potential hyposensitisation vaccine to be decided. The value of such therapy remains uncertain, but in the opinion of the writer since success cannot be predicted, a trial of hyposensitisation is indicated in skin-test positive individuals in whom pharmacological therapy is inadequate to maintain good control.

The most notable innovation in recent years has been the recognition of house-dust mite (*Dermatophagoides pteronyssinus* or *farinae*) as the main antigen in house dust, and the introduction of this antigen in hyposensitising programmes. However, there is no clear evidence that this has been effective (British Thoracic and Tuberculosis Association, 1968). In the UK approximately 80 per cent of asthmatics have positive skin tests to house-dust mite antigen, i.e. have increased amounts of specific IgE in skin mast cells.

Provocation tests by aerosol inhalation are potentially dangerous, and should be performed only by an experienced investigator, and when this is the only effective way of identifying an allergen (usually in the case of industrial exposures).

THERAPY

Reassurance and establishment of confidence is a basic requirement. Advice on the avoidance of known precipitants, especially house dust, should be given. An aerosol bronchodilator (isoprenaline, salbutamol, orciprenaline, terbutaline) is sufficient to control the symptoms in many patients. Persisting nocturnal symptoms, or reluctance to use an inhaler is an indication for oral therapy with one of the wide range of bronchodilator preparations now available. Because of the rarity of significant side-effects a therapeutic trial of sodium cromoglycate (20 mg q.i.d.) via a Spinhaler for two to three weeks should be given, preferably using a diary record to assess response. Failure to achieve adequate control is an indication for corticosteroid therapy; this is best done initially with an oral course of prednisone (or its equivalent) in a dose, for example, of 30 to 45 mg daily for three days reducing thereafter by 5 mg daily. A good response may induce remission for a long period in which case intermittent courses (perhaps with lower doses) may suffice. If long-term therapy is needed, the minimum suppressive dose can be found by a much slower reduction in steroid dosage, e.g. 1 mg in the daily dose weekly. If this dosage is below 10 to 15 mg daily, an aerosol preparation, beclomethasone dipropionate, or betamethasone 17-valerate, may be substituted. With higher oral dose requirement, a combination of aerosol and oral therapy may be the most effective.

Status Asthmaticus

This is an ill-defined term which denotes an attack of severe airways obstruction which has persisted for many hours and which has not responded to therapy. The condition is serious because dyspnoea is so distressing and contrary to earlier beliefs the patient may die in the attack.

There have been a number of studies of the mechanical and blood gas changes during severe asthma attacks in recent years (Rees, Millar and Donald, 1968; McFadden, Kiser and deGroot, 1973) and a number of clinical indices of their severity are recognised.

1. Severe reduction in FEV_1, e.g. < 1.0 litre/s.
2. Elevation of P_{CO_2}. This is of grave significance for it indicates that all reserves of ventilatory capacity have been exhausted, unless ventilation has been depressed by the incautious use of sedative drugs.
3. A pulse frequency of more than 130/min indicates severe hypoxaemia.
4. An absence of wheezing indicates very severe airways obstruction. During recovery from an attack wheezing persists until the FEV_1 has returned to more than 65 per cent of its optimal value and hence loss of this sign in an ill patient indicates extreme severity.
5. McFadden et al claim that the only constant accompaniment of severe airways obstruction is inspiratory contraction of the sternomastoid muscle.

Because the severity of the airways obstruction during an attack of asthma is so often underestimated, the writer considers that spirometry should be performed or attempted serially in *every* case as a routine, and blood gas measurement, P_{O_2}, P_{CO_2}, made whenever the FEV_1 is severely reduced.

Management of status asthmaticus

The essentials of management are:

1. The instilling of confidence in the patient;
2. Adequate corticosteroid and bronchodilator therapy;
3. Humidification of the inspired air.

Oxygen may be given freely in most cases because CO_2 sensitivity is not lost. Sedatives are contraindicated. Progressive ventilatory failure is an indication for intubation and artificial ventilation.

ADEQUATE CORTICOSTEROID THERAPY

This will vary according to the severity of the case, and will be found by therapeutic trial. Thus hydrocortisone 500 mg intravenously (or its equivalent) may be given initially and 200 to 400 mg repeated hourly or two-hourly during the first 24 to 48 h until relief is obtained. The majority of cases will improve before very large total doses are given but occasionally severe airway obstruction will persist despite this therapy.

HUMIDIFICATION

This may be achieved using heated water bath humidifiers or ultrasonic nebulisers. Care must be taken with the latter lest the cold supersaturated air induces further bronchospasm.

Effective humidification should be associated with physiotherapy to try and remove the inspissated mucous plugs which are usually present.

INTUBATION AND IPPV

If the patient becomes exhausted, if the pulse frequency continues to rise despite adequate oxygenation, or if the P_{CO_2} continues to rise, endotracheal intubation and IPPV is indicated. Muscle relaxants will probably be necessary to achieve adequate ventilation; even so, very high inspiratory pressures (e.g. $60\ cmH_2O$) may be required. Removal of inspissated secretions may be helped by instilling 5 to 10 ml warm saline or weak bicarbonate solution into the trachea via the endotracheal tube. This is followed by a few breaths of IPPV and then removal of the liquefied mucus by suction through a soft catheter. Some advocate actual bronchial lavage; this involves catheterising each main bronchus separately and introducing a large volume of saline into the bronchial tree of one lung and literally washing out the bronchial secretions. The writer is not convinced that this approach is required if the former repeated small volume instillations are used. Intravenous salbutamol

(5–15 μg/min) by slow intravenous infusion has been reported to be of benefit but, to date, experience with this approach is limited. Intravenous alpha blocking drugs, e.g. thymoxamine and intravenous antihistamines, have induced small degrees of improvement in an extremely severe case (personal observations).

New Bronchodilator Drugs

There have been considerable advances in bronchodilator drugs in the past decade; for a fuller account the excellent review by Paterson and Shenfield (1974) is recommended. This account will attempt to summarise the main properties and usage of these drugs.

Adrenoceptor drugs

Bronchial smooth muscle, tissue mast cells, myocardium and vascular smooth muscle possess receptor sites enabling them to respond to adrenergic drugs. These drugs are believed to exert their effects through increasing the formation of cyclic AMP from ATP by enhancing the activity of the enzyme, adenylate cyclase. The actions of cyclic AMP are numerous but in the lung two are most beneficial.

1. Relaxation of bronchial smooth muscle;
2. Decreased degranulation of mast cells.

In 1948, two different types of adrenoceptor alpha and beta were postulated by Ahlquist to explain the different responses to adrenaline which caused either stimulation or inhibition depending upon the tissue. Thus it caused bronchial smooth muscle to relax (beta stimulation) and vascular smooth muscle to contract (alpha stimulation). Subsequently, noradrenaline was found to stimulate only alpha receptors while the synthetic isopropyl-noradrenaline (isoprenaline, isoproterenol) was a pure beta receptor stimulator. In the bronchi, beta stimulation resulted in dilatation; in the heart it caused tachycardia (chronotropic effect) and increased force of contraction (inotropic effect).

Adverse effects of beta-adrenoceptor drugs upon the heart and circulation include tachycardia and increased excitability of the myocardium leading to an increased incidence of arrhythmias. In some patients increased physiological tremor is prominent and is due to direct beta stimulation of skeletal muscle.

Selective beta-adrenoceptor drugs

Further synthetic analogues were later synthesised. Iseotharine was the first compound with the ability to stimulate beta receptors in the bronchi to produce bronchodilatation without also stimulating beta receptors in the heart to produce tachycardia. Subsequently salbutamol and terbutaline were shown to be even more highly selective in this respect. These observations suggested that two different types of beta receptor existed in different tissues (Lands et al, 1967). Support for this concept was gained from the development of drugs capable of selectively blocking the beta receptors of the heart without affecting those of bronchi, e.g. practolol (Barrett, 1971). Beta receptors in the heart, causing tachycardia and increased force of contraction, are termed $beta_1$ receptors, while those in the bronchial smooth muscle are $beta_2$ receptors. An alternative model to the presence of two distinct types of beta receptor is that of a single receptor with different accessibility in different tissues depending upon the molecular configuration of the drug.

Beta receptors and mast cells

More recently, a previously unsuspected effect of beta stimulation (? $beta_2$ receptors) has been demonstrated in its ability to inhibit the release of bronchoconstrictor and inflammatory mediators from sensitised mast cells challenged with the appropriate reaginic antibody. Therefore, beta stimulant drugs may induce bronchodilatation either directly by their action on beta receptors in bronchial muscle, or indirectly by inhibiting the release of bronchoconstrictor mediators (cf. sodium cromoglycate).

Duration of action

Further modification of a different part of the molecular structure of beta stimulant drugs has resulted in differences in their metabolic fate when compared with adrenaline.

Adrenaline is removed by a number of mechanisms:

1. Uptake by sympathetic nerve endings (uptake 1);
2. Uptake by adrenergically innervated tissues (uptake 2);
3. Metabolic transformation by the enzyme catechol-O-methyl transferase (COMT) in the tissues, to the inactive, possibly beta-blocking product.

Isoprenaline is also rapidly removed by mechanisms (b) and (c) listed above. When taken into the mouth, isoprenaline is absorbed through the buccal mucosa into the blood stream to induce bronchodilatation ($beta_2$ effect) and tachycardia ($beta_1$ effect). However, the bulk of ingested isoprenaline is converted to an ethereal sulphate by the enzyme sulphatase in the gut; oral therapy with isoprenaline is therefore largely ineffective.

Orciprenaline in which an OH group has been transposed is not metabolised by COMT; likewise terbutaline in which this OH group is similarly placed. Salbutamol which has an alkyl substitution is similarly unaffected by COMT. All three are largely unaffected by sulphatase in the gut. For these reasons these three compounds are effective in inducing bronchodilatation when given both by aerosol and in higher dosage orally and the last two, terbutaline and salbutamol, are also largely selective $beta_2$ stimulants.

Clinical significance of non-cardiac selective beta-adrenergic drugs

In 1968 Speizer, Doll and Heaf recorded an increase in deaths from asthma, especially an eight-fold increase in the 10 to 14 age group in the United Kingdom between 1960 and 1967. Inman and Adelstein (1969) noted that it correlated with the introduction of pressurised aerosols of isoprenaline. Subsequently, further epidemiological studies showed a similar correlation in different countries. In 1972 Stolley attempted to explain this discrepancy by correlating deaths in asthma not with the usual isoprenaline aerosol but with a concentrated form of isoprenaline aerosol. Further studies of this relationship were prevented by an abrupt reduction in asthma deaths, possibly due to either more caution on the part of doctors and patients in the use of isoprenaline, or to the disappearance of the real but unidentified cause of the increased deaths in the first place. A special MRC working party set up to investigate this relationship was unable to come to firm conclusions because of the reduction in numbers of deaths. In addition to the possibility of death being due to cardiac arrhythmia through excessive use of isoprenaline an alternative explanation is that by obtaining even short periods of relief, patients delayed seeking medical advice until the severity of the airways obstruction became extreme.

Awareness of the potential danger of overdosage with isoprenaline in patients with severe asthma heightened interest in those selective drugs with an effect predominantly on the bronchi rather than upon the heart. Also, in addition to safety, some patients prefer the longer duration of action and the virtual absence of tachycardia when these drugs are taken as an aerosol. However, the dose by this route is normally small and apart from duration of action there is little clinical difference between the response to isoprenaline and the newer drugs. Blood concentrations are usually too low to be measurable. Taken orally, blood levels of the new drugs are quite high and the relatively high incidence of muscle tremor may limit their use in certain patients.

Sodium Cromoglycate (SCG)

This novel compound, a derivative of khellin, was shown by Altounyan (1967) to possess the unique property of inhibiting the immediate asthmatic reaction to inhaled antigen in a sensitised subject. Corticosteroids do not possess this property. Sodium cromoglycate is virtually inactive when swallowed and has to be administered by inhalation. In order to inhale sufficient quantities to ensure a prolonged duration of protection, a special device called a Spinhaler was developed.

Subsequently SCG (Intal) was shown to be effective in improving patients with allergic bronchial disease and airway obstruction. An extensive, authoritative review and bibliography of the drug has recently been published (Brogden, Speight and Avery, 1974). Briefly, the drug acts by preventing the discharge from mast cells of granules which contain or release mediators of the allergic reaction but the mechanism by which it exerts this effect is uncertain.

As might be expected from this action, sodium cromoglycate is most consistently effective in preventing asthmatic reactions to known specific antigens, but its ability to effect improvement in 60 to 75 per cent of patients with chronic symptoms when continuous exposure to antigen is unlikely suggests that through its protective effect on mast cells it may gradually diminish bronchial hyperreactivity.

Clinical use of sodium cromoglycate

The drug is prepared dispersed with lactose alone (Intal), or with 0.1 mg isoprenaline in addition (Intal Co.). Whereas initial therapeutic trials should be made with Intal alone, certain patients prefer Intal Co. for their long-term management. Dosage: it is usual to start with one capsule (20 mg) six-hourly for two to three weeks, and to review the response using clinical assessment aided if possible by records of symptoms on diary cards. If benefit has been gained, the dose may be progressively reduced, e.g. by one capsule a day at weekly intervals until benefit begins to be lost. If symptoms persist on four capsules a day, a trial of up to six capsules a day may be found to be helpful.

Relation to corticosteroid therapy

Because of the virtual lack of side-effects, sodium cromoglycate should be used whenever possible in preference to corticosteroids. Unfortunately, many patients receive either no or only partial benefit from sodium cromoglycate alone and combination therapy with corticosteroids is required. The following routine has been found effective. First, the effect of sodium cromoglycate alone as outlined above should be observed. If the response is insufficient prednisone (or its equivalent) 10 to 15 mg t.d.s. for five days should be added. The prednisone dosage should then be reduced by 5 mg in the daily dose twice weekly until down to 15 mg a day or until symptoms being to recur; finally the daily dose should be reduced by 1 mg once or twice weekly to the minimum required to maintain benefit. The patient should be carefully instructed in adjustment of dosage according to need; slow reduction to the minimum suppressive dose with prompt increase for a few days to 20 to 30 mg at the earliest sign of an exacerbation followed by rapid reduction to the previous low levels. These dosages and their timing are given only as a guide—they need to be modified in the light of experience with individual patients.

Corticosteroid Aerosol Therapy

The incidence of troublesome side-effects with systemic corticosteroid therapy in a daily dosage greater than 5 to 8 mg prednisone, or its equivalent, led to a search for topically active preparations suitable for inhalation directly into the bronchial tree. Early studies showed that systemic effects, usually assessed as hypothalamic-pituitary adrenal (HPA) suppression were similar whether aerosol or oral dosage was used, leading to the conclusion that aerosols were effective solely through their systemic action.

It was not fully appreciated at that time that only about 10 per cent of an inhaled dose remained in the lungs and that about 90 per cent was ingested. Consequently, any absorbable corticosteroid preparation given in aerosol form was in effect largely taken into the gut and absorbed.

It was not until beclomethasone dipropionate and betamethasone valerate, highly topically active steroids poorly absorbed from the gut, were studied that an aerosol form which produced little HPA suppression was found. These preparations permit a local action in the bronchi with little or no systemic effect when given in recommended dosage. Thus two 'puffs' of either drug taken six-hourly produce local effects which appear to be equivalent to those of low-dosage systemic maintenance therapy but without any measurable evidence of HPA suppression; a single metered dose of beclomethasone delivers 50 μg and a betamethasone inhaler delivers 100 μg per 'puff'.

There have been many clinical studies to evaluate the use of these compounds (Brown, Storey and George, 1972) and the following conclusions appear to have been established:

1. With a dosage of 400 μg beclomethasone dipropionate and 800 μg betamethasone valerate daily, there is usually no evidence of HPA suppression.
2. Aerosol therapy in these dosages can often substitute for systemic therapy when the latter is less than 15 mg prednisone (or its equivalent) daily. When higher systemic dosage is needed to achieve the desired clinical response, it is unusual in aerosol therapy to substitute completely for systemic therapy though it often permits a reduction in the daily requirement of prednisone.
3. In patients on moderate to high doses of systemic corticosteroids, HPA suppression may have developed and care must be taken not to reduce systemic therapy too rapidly when aerosol therapy is being initiated lest hypocorticism develops.
4. It is common for symptoms of fatigue, irritability and arthralgia (pseudorheumatism) to develop during the substitution but these are usually of short duration.
5. Oral and laryngeal candidiasis occurs in about 10 per cent of patients on this therapy though it is often possible to control this by antimonilial therapy.
6. In some patients, better control of the asthmatic symptoms is obtained than with oral therapy alone.

LARGE AIRWAY OBSTRUCTION

Obstruction of the trachea may be caused by tumours, stricture following prolonged tracheal intubation, or external compression from enlarged mediastinal glands, retrosternal thyroid, thymoma, etc. There are four types of tumour: (a) carcinoma, sometimes originating in a bronchus, and extending to occlude the trachea; (b) adenocystic carcinoma (cylindroma); (c) tracheal polyp; (d) amyloid tumours.

Obstruction of the intrathoracic trachea may simulate diffuse generalised airway obstruction closely, even the spirometric tracing being similar since a flow limiting mechanism is induced. Features strongly suggesting a localised upper airway constriction are: prominent inspiratory stridor; a 'straight' forced expirogram, i.e. forced expiratory airflow remains virtually constant instead of becoming progressively slower, over the reduced vital capacity. Forced inspiratory volume measurements may be misleading. Bronchoscopy with biopsy is essential to establish the tissue diagnosis. Failure to recognise the localised nature of the obstruction is tragic, because in some instances surgical 'cure' is possible and considerable relief is usual.

Treatment

Multiple amyloid tumours may be curetted but regular bronchoscopic follow-up is required. Advances in surgical technique involving extensive mobilising of the trachea have permitted major resections to be undertaken, with end to end anastomosis of the trachea.

REFERENCES

Altounyan, R. E. C. (1967) Inhibition of experimental asthma by a new compound—disodium chromoglycate 'Intal'. *Acta Allergologica*, **22**, 487.

Austen, K. F. (1973) A review of immunological, biochemical and pharmacological factors in the release of chemical mediators from human lung. In *Asthma, Physiology, Immunopharmacology and Treatment*, ed. Austen, K. F. & Lichtenstein, L. M., pp. 109–122. New York and London: Academic Press.

Barrett, A. M. (1971) The pharmacology of practolol. *Postgraduate Medical Journal*, **47**, Suppl. Jan., 7.

Benson, M. K. (1975) Bronchial hyperreactivity. *British Journal of Diseases of the Chest*, **69**, 227–239.

British Thoracic and Tuberculosis Association (1968) Treatment of house-dust allergy. A report from the Research Committee. *British Medical Journal*, **3**, 774–777.

Brocklehurst, W. E. (1960) The release of histamine and formation of a slow-reacting substance (SRS-A) during anaphylactic shock. *Journal of Physiology (London)*, **151**, 416–435.

Brogden, R. N., Speight, T. M. & Avery, G. S. (1974) Sodium cromoglycate (cromolyn sodium): a review of its mode of action, pharmacology, therapeutic efficacy and use. Part I: asthma. *Drugs*, **7**, 164–282.

Brown, H. M., Storey, G. & George, W. H. S. (1972) Beclomethasone dipropionate: a new steroid aerosol for the treatment of allergic asthma. *British Medical Journal*, **1**, 585–590.

Ciba Guest Symposium (1959) Terminology, definitions, and classification of chronic pulmonary emphysema and related conditions. *Thorax*, **14**, 286–299.

Ciba Foundation Study Group No. 38 (1971) *Identification of Asthma*, eds. Porter, R. & Birch, J. Edinburgh and London: Churchill Livingstone.

Clements, J. A. & Elam, J. O. (1955) Estimation of lung-airway resistance by repetitive interruption of air flow. *American Journal of Physiology*, **183**, 604.

Cooper, D. M., Hoeppner, V., Cox, D., Zamel, N., Bryan, A. C. & Levison, H. (1974) Lung function in alpha₁-antitrypsin heterozygotes (Pi Type MZ). *American Review of Respiratory Disease*, **110**, 708–715.

Crofton, J., Douglas, A., Simpson, D. & Merchant, S. (1963) The measurement of bronchial andomural or 'squeeze' pressure. *Thorax*, **18**, 68–76.

Cumming, G. (1973) In *Disorders of the Respiratory System*, ed. Cumming, G. & Semple, S. J. G., p. 13. Oxford: Blackwell Scientific Publications.

Depierre, A., Bignon, J., Lebeau, A. & Brovet, G. (1972) Quantitative study of parenchyma and small conductive airways in chronic non-specific lung disease. *Chest*, **62**, 699–708.

Dubois, A. B., Botelho, S. Y. & Comroe, J. H. Jr (1956) A new method for measuring airway resistance in man, using a body plethysmograph: values in normal subjects and in patients with respiratory disease. *Journal of Clinical Investigation*, **35**, 327–335.

Dunnill, M. S., Massarella, G. R. & Anderson, J. A. (1969) A comparison of the quantitative anatomy of the bronchi in normal subjects, in status asthmaticus, in chronic bronchitis and in emphysema. *Thorax*, **24**, 176–179.

Eriksson, S. (1965) Studies in alpha₁-antitrypsin deficiency. *Acta Medica Scandinavica*, **177**, Suppl., 432.

Gold, W. M. (1973) Cholinergic pharmacology in asthma. In *Asthma, Physiology, Immunopharmacology and Treatment*, ed. Austen, K. F. & Lichtenstein, L. M., Ch. 11. New York, San Francisco and London: Academic Press.

Heppleston, A. G. (1974) Correspondence: types of emphysema. *British Medical Journal*, **3**, 253–254.

Herzog, H., Keller, R., Maurer, W., Baumann, H. R. & Nadjafi, A. (1968) Distribution of bronchial resistance in obstructive pulmonary diseases and in dogs with artificially induced tracheal collapse. *Respiration*, **25**, 381–394.

Hogg, J. C., Macklem, P. T. & Thurlbeck, W. M. (1968) Site and nature of airway obstruction in chronic obstructive lung disease. *New England Journal of Medicine*, **278**, 1355–1360.

Horsfield, K. & Cumming, G. (1968) Functional consequences of airway morphology. *Journal of Applied Physiology*, **24**, 384–390.

Howell, J. B. L. (1957) Mechanics of respiration in man. Ph.D. Thesis, University of London.

Howell, J. B. L. (1969) In *A Symposium on Reversible Airways Obstruction*, ed. Marsh, B. T., p. 34. London: Allen and Hanburys Ltd.

Howell, J. B. L. (1971) In *Identification of Asthma*, Ciba Symposium Study Group No. 38, ed. Porter, R. & Birch, J. Edinburgh and London: Churchill Livingstone.

Hughes, J. M. B., Rosenzweig, D. Y. & Kivitz, P. B. (1970) Site of airway closure in excised dog lungs: histologic demonstration. *Journal of Applied Physiology*, **29**, 340–344.

Hutchison, D. C. S., Cook, P. J. L., Martelli, N. A. & Hugh-Jones, P. (1971) Alpha-antitrypsin deficiency and emphysema. *Thorax*, **26**, 488.

Inman, W. H. W. & Adelstein, A. M. (1969) Rise and fall of asthma mortality in England and Wales in relation to use of pressurised aerosols. *Lancet*, **2**, 279–285.

Ishizaka, K., Ishizaka, T. & Hornbrook, M. M. (1966) Physicochemical properties of reaginic antibody. V. Correlation of reginic activity with γE-globulin antibody. *Journal of Immunology*, **97**, 840–853.

Kay, A. B., Stechschulte, D. J. & Austem, K. F. (1971) An eosinophil leukocyte chemotactic factor of anaphylaxis. *Journal of Experimental Medicine*, **133**, 602–619.

Lands, A. M., Arnold, A., McAuliff, J. P., Luduena, F. P. & Brown, T. G. (1967) Letter: Differentiation of receptor systems activated by sympathomimetic amines. *Nature (London)*, **214**, 597–598.

Lane, D. J., Howell, J. B. L. & Giblin, B. (1968) Relation between airways obstruction and CO_2 tension in chronic obstructive airways disease. *British Medical Journal*, **3**, 707–709.

Laurell, C. B. & Eriksson, S. (1963) The electrophoretic alpha₁-globulin pattern of serum in alpha₁-antitrypsin deficiency. *Scandinavian Journal of Clinical and Laboratory Investigation*, **15**, 132–140.

Leaver, D. G., Tattersfield, A. E. & Pride, N. B. (1974) Bronchial and extrabronchial factors in chronic airflow obstruction. *Thorax*, **29**, 394–400.

Macklem, P. T. & Wilson, N. J. (1965) Measurement of intrabronchial pressure in man. *Journal of Applied Physiology*, **20**, 653–663.

Macklem, P. T. & Mead, J. (1967) Resistance of central and peripheral airways measured by a retrograde catheter. *Journal of Applied Physiology*, **22**, 395–401.

McCarthy, D. S., Spencer, R., Greene, R. & Milic-Emili, J. (1972) Measurement of 'closing volume' as a simple and sensitive test for early detection of small airway disease. *American Journal of Medicine*, **52**, 747–753.

McFadden, E. R. Jr, Kiser, R. & deGroot, W. J. (1973) Acute bronchial asthma. *New England Journal of Medicine*, **288**, 221–225.

McFadden, E. R. Jr & Linden, D. A. (1972) A reduction in maximum mid-expiratory flow rate. A spirographic manifestation of small airway disease. *American Journal of Medicine*, **52**, 725–737.

McNeill, R. S., Nairn, J. R., Millar, J. S. & Ingram, C. G. (1966) Exercise-induced asthma. *Quarterly Journal of Medicine*, **35**, 55–67.

Matthews, A. W. & Howell, J. B. L. (1975) The rate of isometric inspiratory pressure development as a measure of responsiveness to carbon dioxide in man. *Clinical Science and Molecular Medicine*, **49**, 57–68.

Matsuba, K. & Thurlbeck, W. M. (1973) Disease of the small airways in chronic bronchitis. *American Review of Respiratory Disease*, **107**, 552–558.

Mead, J. & Whittenberger, J. L. (1954) Evaluation of airway interruption technique as a method for measuring pulmonary airflow resistance. *Journal of Applied Physiology*, **6**, 408–416.

Mead, J., Turner, J. M., Macklem, P. T. & Little, J. B. (1967) Significance of the relationship between lung recoil and maximal expiratory flow. *Journal of Applied Physiology*, **22**, 95–108.

Milic-Emili, J. (1974) Small airway closure and its physiological significance. *Scandinavian Journal of Respiratory Diseases*, Suppl. 85, 181–189.

Moore, N. (1965) Behaviour therapy in bronchial asthma: a controlled study. *Journal of Psychosomatic Research*, **9**, 257–276.

Paterson, J. W. & Shenfield, G. M. (1974) Bronchodilators. *British Thoracic and Tuberculosis Association Review*, **4**, Part I, 25–40; Part II, 61–74.

Pepys, J. (1968) Hypersensitivity diseases of the lungs due to fungi and organic dusts. *Monographs in Allergy*, **4**, pp. 147. Basel: Karger.

Pride, N. B. (1971) The assessment of airflow obstruction. *British Journal of Diseases of the Chest*, **65**, 135–169.

Rees, H. A., Millar, J. S. & Donald, K. W. (1968) A study of the clinical course and arterial blood gas tensions of patients in status asthmaticus. *Quarterly Journal of Medicine*, **37**, 541–561.

Reid, Lynne (1967) *The Pathology of Emphysema*. London: Lloyd-Luke Medical Books.

Sharp, H. L., Bridges, R. A., Krivit, W. & Freier, E. F. (1969) Cirrhosis associated with alpha$_1$-antitrypsin deficiency: a previously unrecognised inherited disorder. *Journal of Laboratory and Clinical Medicine*, **73**, 934–939.

Smith, A. P. (1975) Prostaglandins and the bronchus. *Thorax*, **30**, 236–237.

Speizer, F. E., Doll, R. & Heaf, P. (1968) Observations on recent increase in mortality from asthma. *British Medical Journal*, **1**, 335–339.

Stolley, P. D. (1972) Asthma mortality. *American Review of Respiratory Disease*, **105**, 883–890.

Thomas, G. O. & Jones, M. C. (1971) Alpha$_1$-antitrypsin deficiency and pulmonary emphysema. *Thorax*, **26**, 488–489.

Weibel, E. R. (1963) *Morphometry of the Human Lung*. Berlin: Springer-Verlag.

West, J. B. & Matthews, F. L. (1972) Stresses, strains and surface pressures in the lung caused by its weight. *Journal of Applied Physiology*, **32**, 332–345.

Woolcock, A. J., Vincent, N. J. & Macklem, P. T. (1969) Frequency dependence of compliance as a test for obstruction in the small airways. *Journal of Clinical Investigation*, **48**, 1097–1106.

Wright, B. M. & McKerrow, C. B. (1959) Maximum forced expiratory flow rate as a measure of ventilatory capacity. *British Medical Journal*, **2**, 1041–1047.

Wright, R. R. (1960) Bronchial atrophy and collapse in chronic obstructive pulmonary emphysema. *American Journal of Pathology*, **37**, 63–78.

7
DIFFUSE INTERSTITIAL DISEASE OF THE LUNGS

Margaret Turner-Warwick

Broadly speaking, the lung diseases to be considered in this chapter are those which present with widespread shadowing on the chest radiograph and which histologically are characterised by predominant involvement of the 'peripheral' gas exchanging parts of the lung. It should be recognised at the outset that it is unrealistic to make a strict division of diseases involving the bronchial tree from those involving the alveolar walls. It is also unrealistic to divide sharply those diseases characterised by intra-alveolar inflammatory exudates and those in which involvement of alveolar walls predominate: virtually no intra-alveolar exudate occurs in the absence of wall changes and many diseases affecting predominantly the alveolar walls have, to a greater or lesser extent, an intra-alveolar exudative component.

As this chapter is to focus upon disorders affecting the interstitial parts of the lung, then the 'interstitium' must be defined. In organs containing a specialised cell, such as the hepatocyte of the liver lobule or the nephron of the kidney, the interstitium must be defined as the connective tissue framework supporting these organ-specific units. In the case of the lung the specific elements are the cells of the bronchial and bronchiolar walls, extending peripherally to the alveolar lining cells. The interstitium can then be regarded as the connective tissue and capillary network within the alveolar walls, the alveolar septa and the perivascular and peribronchial supporting tissues. The fact that the interstitium of the lung defined in this way occupies (in the more peripheral parts of the lung) a far greater volume than the specific elements is immaterial. The use of the word interstitium in relation to the gas exchanging parts of the lung has been criticised in that the basement membranes of the alveolar lining and that of the pulmonary capillary endothelium fuse, but it is of considerable interest that studies using the electron microscope have demonstrated that the basement membranes of these two structures separate when collagen tissue and inflammatory cells infiltrate between them in various disease states.

In many organs, diseases of the interstitium are of minor importance because the specific function of the organs are not at all, or only slightly modified. In the case of the lung its functional integrity is in large part dependent on the preservation of the connective tissue and capillary structure of the gas exchanging parts; thus interstitial diseases of the lung have major physiological implications.

In a discussion of the pathogenesis and causation of widespread radiographic shadowing, Scadding (1952) listed more than 80 possibilities. Attempts at classification have not been very satisfactory because in many instances the pathology is characteristic but the cause is unknown (e.g. sarcoidosis) and in others several different causal agents result in the same pathology (e.g. fibrosing alveolitis (Turner-Warwick, 1974).

In the present chapter a classification based on histological features seen especially in the early stages of disease will be used, because so often the 'diagnosis' ultimately depends upon the histological characteristics. This system has some logical advantages but has practical clinical limitations which have to be recognised.

The histological features observed in any given case depend largely on the stage in the natural history of the disease at which the material is studied. Many widespread interstitial diseases of the lung heal by fibrosis rather than resolution and the pathological appearances during the acute stages may differ widely depending upon the cause, whereas in the later stages an indistinguishable pattern of widespread alveolar wall fibrosis may be the sole residuum.

Largely excluded from this chapter are disorders where the pathological changes are predominantly intra-alveolar, e.g. pneumonic consolidation and pulmonary oedema. However they cannot be excluded altogether because interstitial exudate virtually always accompanies intra-alveolar exudate and where the causes are long standing or persisting, the interstitial changes may predominate in the later stages.

Although the classification used here will be based on pathology, clinical prediction of this can often be achieved with considerable accuracy by integrating the total body of clinical information. Diagnostic clues may be derived from the following:

History
1. The nature and order of appearance of respiratory symptoms, particularly the predominance of breathlessness, cough, sputum or wheezing episodes.
2. The duration of these symptoms and their progression.
3. History of occupational or environmental exposure to noxious fumes or gases, organic or inorganic dusts.
4. History of associated symptoms in organs other than the lungs, especially the joints, and evidence of other systemic disorders.

Physical signs
The presence or absence of adventitious sounds in the lungs, and finger clubbing. Pulmonary granulomas tend to have fewer adventitious sounds, especially in the acute stages, and contrast with widespread interstitial

exudates, where crepitations are very common. Finger clubbing is most common in cryptogenic fibrosing alveolitis, asbestosis and widespread bronchiectasis; it is also quite common in alveolar proteinosis.

Radiograph
1. The characteristics of the widespread shadows: the shape and size of the individual lesions, their density and distribution, e.g. upper or lower zone predominance.
2. Associated radiographic features, e.g. hilar gland or pleural involvement, oesophageal abnormalities or bony lesions.

Laboratory investigations
Especially serology, bacteriology, virological and haematological studies.

A CLASSIFICATION OF DIFFUSE INTERSTITIAL LUNG DISEASE

The following scheme is suggested as a useful guide but of course cannot be interpreted too rigidly. It is based essentially on the acute and active component and not the fibrotic healing stages of disease. Many disorders listed as granulomas may have in addition a substantial and important cellular infiltrate in the alveolar wall, or an exudative component. The extent to which these changes are found in any individual case will depend not only on the stage and the severity of the disease but on the responsiveness of the individual patient. For example, it is generally agreed that the immunological behaviour of the host (including ethnic group as well as nutrition) will have a profound influence on the histological appearances of lung lesions caused by mycobacteria. Host factors are probably equally important in many other widespread lung diseases.

Widespread Granulomas

A detailed and systematic review of each disorder mentioned in this classification is quite outside the scope of this chapter. The object here will be to emphasise points of particular histological importance and to relate these to the radiographic and clinical features which aid clinical diagnosis, particularly when histological verification is considered undesirable or is not feasible. Emphasis will also be laid on the natural history because, depending on the state of evolution or resolution of the disease so the clinical and radiographic features vary. Understanding of these is particularly important when planning therapy because treatment too early exposes the patient to unnecessary iatrogenic hazards and if given too late deprives the patient of his chance of recovery and may thus shorten his life.

Table 1   Classification of diffuse interstitial lung disease associated with widespread radiographic shadows

---

1. *Widespread granulomas*

   i. Sarcoidosis.
   ii. Beryllium disease.
   iii. Tuberculosis, histoplasmosis, coccidioidomycosis, blastomycosis.
   iv. Extrinsic allergic alveolitis, caused by various organic dusts.
   v. Rare granulomas associated with immune deficiency or eosinophilic infiltrates.

2. *Interstitial exudates* (of variable fluid and cellular composition)

Many pulmonary exudates have an important intra-alveolar component in the most acute stages but also develop more chronic changes in the alveolar walls, either because of the severity of the initial insult or because of persisting exudation over prolonged periods.

  (a) Non-inflammatory

    i. Persistently high left atrial pressure, as in long-standing mitral valve disease.
    ii. Persisting uraemic oedema.

  (b) Inflammatory

    i. Infective viral pneumonia, e.g. influenza.
    ii. Chronic interstitial pneumonia associated with bronchiectasis, e.g. from childhood infections, *A. fumigatus* hypersensitivity, immune deficiency, cystic fibrosis.
    iii. Non-infective chronic inhalation pneumonia, e.g. associated with megaoesophagus, following Mendelson's syndrome, inhalation of lipids, fumes and gases. Chronic primary or secondary haemosiderosis.
    iv. Cytotoxic or hypersensitivity responses to drugs, e.g. busulphan, bleomycin, nitrofurantoin, salazopyrine.
    v. Lone cryptogenic fibrosing alveolitis and its variants:
    Desquamative interstitial pneumonia.
    Lymphocytic interstitial pneumonia.
    Plasma cell pneumonia.
    Giant cell interstitial pneumonia.
    vi. Cryptogenic fibrosing alveolitis associated with mixed or other systemic connective tissue disease, e.g. rheumatoid arthritis, SLE, Sjögren's syndrome, systemic sclerosis, dermatomyositis, polymyositis, chronic active hepatitis, renal tubular acidosis.

3. *Disorders related to inorganic particulate inhalants*

   i. Non-fibrogenic: coal, tin, iron.
   ii. Fibrogenic: silica, asbestos, talc and occasionally coal.

4. *Tumours*

   i. Lymphangitis carcinomatosa.
   ii. Haematogenous secondary tumours.
   iii. Reticuloses and lymphosarcoma.
   iv. Pulmonary adenomatosis.

5. *Congenital dysplasias*

   i. Tuberose sclerosis.
   ii. Eosinophilic granuloma.
   iii. Leimyomatosis.

N.B. This classification is intended as a practical scheme and most disorders can be fitted under these five major headings. No attempt has been made to mention every conceivable condition.

Sarcoidosis

This condition affects particularly young adults but may occur for the first time in late adult life. In the acute stages the widespread shadows are very variable, having the appearance of 'miliary mottling', 'ground glass' opacity occasionally, and rounded or irregular reticular shadows in many; their density is also variable. Often the shadows of whatever pattern are very diffuse, extending up to the apices and, as in so many granulomatous lesions, the radiographic lung volumes are often well maintained. Pleural shadows

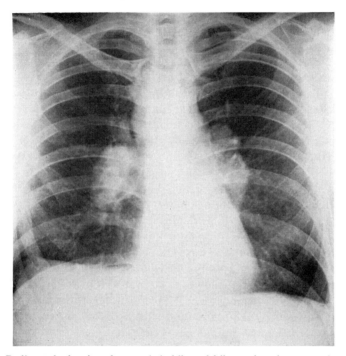

Figure 1   Radiograph showing characteristic bilateral hilar node enlargement in sarcoidosis

are very uncommon and occurred in only two instances amongst 275 cases reported by Scadding (1967). When widespread pulmonary shadows are associated with bilateral hilar node enlargement and particularly when these are set out from the hilar regions in such a way as to show transradient lung between the enlarged glands and the mediastinum (see Fig. 1) then the features are virtually pathognomonic.

At this acute stage, while the radiographic appearances are prominent the patient is usually in good health, without systemic symptoms, and the radiographic appearances are disproportionately severe compared with the trivial or absent breathlessness. Many cases are thus picked up on routine radiographic examination. This comment applies particularly to Caucasians developing sarcoidosis; a much more florid clinical disorder may be seen in other races, particularly African Negroes.

Clinical signs in the chest are also minimal or absent and in particular crepitations are usually absent. The presence of characteristic lesions in other organs, such as erythema nodosum or skin nodules, uveitis, lymphadenopathy, or splenomegaly also greatly increase the likelihood of sarcoidosis.

Intracutaneous skin tests showing impaired delayed hypersensitivity to antigens such as purified protein derivative or *Candida albicans* will provide further support for the diagnosis. Hypercalciuria or hypercalcaemia, although only present in a minority of cases, is very suggestive when present. Kveim tests with validated antigens are positive in some 74 per cent of cases with peripheral shadows on the chest radiograph (Siltzbach, 1961) but the exact frequency varies considerably in different reports depending upon the particular extract used and on the stage of the disease.

Scadding has shown that about half (36/71) of the patients presenting with 'prefibrotic' sarcoid infiltrates resolve spontaneously; all but seven observed for over two years resolved without treatment. Six persisted for longer than two years. Of the 71 cases, 21 showed evidence of fibrosis and this was severe in six. That some cases, albeit a minority, progress is important because prevention of irreversible changes in this group is the challenge of sarcoidosis. As fibrosis develops the radiographic shadows become more irregular and tend to predominate in the upper lobes, resulting in their contraction with consequent elevation of the hilar shadows. Emphysematous distortion of the over expanded lower lobes may occur. With these changes breathlessness increases and, because of the airways distortion, changes of infective chronic bronchitis with airways obstruction may occur (Smellie and Hoyle, 1960). At this stage a mixed physiological pattern of restrictive and obstructive ventilatory defect is demonstrated. Treatment at this stage is too late; progressive deterioration occurs and death from respiratory infection, respiratory failure or cor pulmonale occurs in 5 per cent of those having persisting shadows at anything from 3 to 22 years (Smellie and Hoyle, 1960).

The physical signs in the later stages depend on the extent of fibrosis, emphysema and bronchial involvement; finger clubbing is almost exclusively limited to those with substantial bronchial involvement (Smellie and Hoyle, 1960). Widespread crepitations are unusual except in cases with extensive bronchial damage.

Chronic beryllium disease

The radiological and clinical features are identical with those described for sarcoidosis and follow the acute disease in about 6 per cent of cases (Hardy, Rabe and Lorch, 1967). Recent evidence suggests that the immunopathogenesis of the granuloma is dependent upon cell sensitisation to beryllium (Marx and Burrell, 1973), though tests of delayed hypersensitivity with other allergens are normal.

The natural history is very variable, as in sarcoidosis. There is some evidence that the prognosis is worse in patients whose lungs show marked interstitial cellular infiltration and fewer granulomas (Freiman and Hardy, 1970) and they appear to respond less well to corticosteroids.

Infections by mycobacteria and fungi

Widespread shadowing due to *Mycobacterium tuberculosis* is most typically seen in miliary tuberculosis. Here the shadows of 'miliary mottling' are so characteristic that virtually no other cause simulates them. The shadows on the radiograph are fine and discrete and appear as if they might be 'plucked with tweezers', as described by Dr George Simon, and they extend from the base of the lungs to the extreme apices. Breathlessness is usually slight compared to the severity of the radiological abnormality, though systemic illness is often prominent, with fever and weight loss.

Relatively 'silent' miliary tuberculosis occurs particularly when systemic symptoms have been suppressed in patients receiving corticosteroids, and the tuberculin tests may also be negative. Diagnosis is vital because miliary tuberculosis is curable with antituberculous drugs. When isolation of mycobacteria from sputum, gastric washings or urine fails but the characteristic radiographic features are present, it is usually reasonable to give a therapeutic trial of antituberculous drugs such as ethambutol, isoniazid and PAS (drugs affecting *M. tuberculosis* selectively) and observe the clinical and radiographic response. In some very sick patients it is wise to add rifampicin although it has a wider spectrum of antibacterial activity.

Similar clinical and radiographic appearances may be seen in haematogenous dissemination of histoplasmosis or coccidioidomycosis. These infections are frequent in endemic areas of the world and the diagnosis will be supported by appropriate serological tests such as complement fixation tests. If the diagnosis is suspected in non-endemic areas, intracutaneous skin tests will also be helpful.

A number of diagnostically difficult cases occur in certain racial groups especially Indian and African Negroes. In some, the histology shows non-caseating inflammatory lesions with scanty lymphocytes but with large numbers of mycobacteria found on fluorescence or culture ('non-reactive' tuberculosis) (Ball, Joules and Pagel, 1951; Forbes, 1961). In others the lesions show minimal caseation and the distinction between sarcoidosis and tuberculosis is then difficult. Some cases respond to antituberculous drugs and others in addition require corticosteroids. In this difficult intermediate group treatment with a combination of corticosteroids and antituberculous drugs is a sensible practical policy.

When a lung biopsy is undertaken for diagnosis, a portion must always be sent for culture, or at least kept unfixed, and frozen until the routine histological report is available so that culture is possible at a later date.

Extrinsic allergic alveolitis (see Chapter 3)

The radiographic appearances and clinical features vary greatly depending on the stage in the natural history and the pattern of exposure (intermittent or continuous). The commonest causes in the UK are exposure to mouldy hay and cereal (farmer's lung) and avian protein hypersensitivity (bird fancier's lung) in pigeon racers or those keeping budgerigars (parakeets) in their homes. In the acute stages, and particularly with intermittent exposure, systemic and respiratory symptoms are prominent and characteristic. Some hours after exposure (often during the evening or night following a day's work with mouldy grain) influenza-like symptoms appear with malaise, mild fever and limb pains; some breathlessness with a dry cough without sputum or wheeze is typical. These symptoms resolve spontaneously over the next 24 h or so. Examination at this time shows occasional scattered crepitations in the chest; finger clubbing is usually absent. The chest radiograph may show, particularly after heavy and repeated exposure, widespread nodular shadowing, prominent in the mid-zones or scattered very widely throughout the lung fields, often without reduction of the lung volume. The appearances frequently resolve spontaneously with time, if antigen exposure is avoided. The physiological defect is well defined. There is a transient, usually slight fall in vital capacity and transfer factor for carbon monoxide, but no evidence of airways obstruction. During the acute episode the sedimentation rate may be increased slightly, together with a moderate polymorphonuclear leucocytosis but eosinophilia does not develop. A few cases, however, have an asthmatic component either occurring immediately on contact with the mouldy grain (regarded as reflecting a type I anaphylactic response) or occurring at the same time as the 'late' restrictive reaction just described.

It has been suggested on the basis of the timing of these late responses and the presence of precipitating antibody, that the immunopathogenesis of both the late asthma and the late restrictive defect may depend upon a type III 'Arthus' reaction. Two difficulties about this attractive hypothesis have to be faced. So far most workers have failed to find evidence of immune complexes in the lesions either in human biopsy material or in experimental animals; to date one report alone (Wenzel, Emanuel and Gray, 1971) has detected these. The second difficulty is that the characteristic pathological appearance in these cases is that of non-caseating 'sarcoid-like' granulomas. This appearance is not typical of the experimental Arthus response, although it has been produced experimentally under very special conditions where preformed antigen–antibody immune complexes are injected in equivalence (Spector and Heesom, 1969).

In the *chronic stages*, due either to often-repeated acute episodes or where exposure has been slight but continuous, as with budgerigar fanciers, the clinical and radiographic characteristics are entirely different. Symptoms are those of insidious breathlessness, often developing over many months or even years, without noticeable systemic symptoms. On examination, mild finger clubbing is seen in some cases but this is less severe and much less common than in patients with cryptogenic fibrosing alveolitis; it is found in only 14 per cent (Hargreaves, 1970) of the former compared with about 60 per cent of the latter (Livingstone et al, 1964; Turner-Warwick and Doniach, 1965). Crepitations are also absent or far less prominent than in cryptogenic fibrosing alveolitis. They are observed in some 14 per cent of patients with extrinsic allergic alveolitis and 90 per cent of those with cryptogenic fibrosing alveolitis. The most characteristic radiographic appearance is bilateral contraction of the upper lobes with elevation of the hilar shadows, associated with variable shadowing extending towards the bases. This upper zone predominance stands in striking contract to the basal predominance of cryptogenic fibrosing alveolitis and many other interstitial fibroses resulting from long-standing exudates of various types.

The natural history of extrinsic allergic alveolitis depends on the conditions of continuing exposure and upon the extent of irreversible fibrosis. Many cases resolve spontaneously if removed from exposure at the stage of widespread nodular shadowing, but this does not occur in all (Hapke et al, 1968). It is therefore important to follow patients with the acute condition both physiologically and radiographically to establish that spontaneous and *complete* resolution has in fact occurred. If this does not happen within four to eight weeks of cessation of exposure to antigen, it is probably wise to give a short course of corticosteroid therapy at this stage. This is done to encourage a complete return to normal rather than to risk slower healing by fibrosis; once the latter has occurred there is permanent impairment of lung function. A few cases have been seen recently who, despite apparent antigen elimination and high dosage corticosteroid and immunosuppressant therapy, have suffered progressive deterioration with death from cor pulmonale and respiratory failure in as little as four to six years from first hospital attendance. It is uncertain whether this progression is due to: persistence of insoluble antigen; continuing active inflammation which is no longer dependent upon the presence of antigen (the consequence, perhaps, of continuing intravascular coagulation); or to progressive healing by fibrosis which nevertheless results in progressive functional impairment of ventilation. Postmortem studies in one such case support the suggestion of progressive fibrotic healing. This case also showed very severe endarteritis of small pulmonary vessels.

While the typical histological pattern of acute extrinsic allergic alveolitis is that of non-caseating granulomas there is in addition a variable and sometimes extensive non-granulomatous infiltrate of lymphocytes and plasma cells in the alveolar walls. Dr R. M. E. Seal (personal communication) has suggested that the functional impairment of the lung is more dependent upon the non-granulomatous inflammatory infiltrates than the visually more striking granulomas; the extent of the former may in large part determine the amount of irreversibility in untreated cases. This suggestion is in accordance with other observations by Freiman and Hardy in cases of chronic beryllium disease. Hapke et al (1968) have shown that in more chronic cases of allergic alveolitis nearly 40 per cent have in addition bronchial wall involvement. For this reason they have very reasonably objected to the term 'alveolitis' and have emphasised the frequency of irreversible airways obstruction as part of the pathology of organic dust hypersensitivity and not necessarily attributable, as is often done, to the individual's smoking habits.

Rare granulomas

Localised granulomas may be found in various types of lung pathology, including bronchial carcinoma, but these are not relevant to this chapter. Uncommonly, however, widespread granulomas may be found in the lungs which give rise to much clinical controversy.

Cases have been described (Bronsky and Dunn, 1965) showing many features of sarcoidosis in patients with immune deficiency, especially in those with a predominant antibody deficiency. The suggestion has been made that the host response to inhaled antigen occurring in antigen excess (because of antibody depletion), augmented by an intact cellular immunity, may determine the granuloma formation in these cases. However, this remains an hypothesis. One case at least has been described where the Kveim test was positive, and it seems possible that the alteration in immunological balance between cellular and humoral systems predisposed to the development of sarcoid-like granulomas secondary to some unestablished initiating agent(s).

An even greater rarity is the condition described by Churg and Strauss (1951) and termed by them 'allergic eosinophilic granuloma'. This has to be distinguished from eosinophilic granuloma or histiocytosis X, which, using terminology correctly, should not be regarded as a 'granuloma' at all.

Interstitial Exudates

It is difficult to limit the terms for discussion here, because virtually all intra-alveolar exudates, occurring in all forms of pneumonia and in frank pulmonary oedemas from many causes, have to some degree an associated interstitial exudation of fluid and inflammatory cells into the supporting tissue of the alveolar walls. This statement is not merely of academic importance since it is the interstitial changes which often form the basis of the more long-standing changes in the lung. Indeed these changes determine the irreversible component of alveolar wall fibrosis which can be found in many cases. For this reason it is the interstitial component that must be assessed and treated if irreversible changes are to be prevented.

Because the distribution and pattern of alveolar wall fibrosis is relatively uniform it is not surprising that exudates from a wide variety of causes result in a common clinical syndrome of 'fibrosing alveolitis', when the alveolar wall changes become established. Not only are the pathological and radiographic features similar but the clinical and physiological features are also indistinguishable. Understanding of these basic facts about the evolution of alveolar wall fibrosis does much to clarify the basic concept of 'fibrosing alveolitis' as a tissue response to many different initiating factors (Turner-Warwick, 1974; Scadding, 1974).

On the basis of this approach it is possible to subdivide cases of widespread pulmonary fibrosis. First there are those due to a pulmonary exudate and the cause of this is known. When these have been defined there remains a group where no cause has yet been specified but which nevertheless form a fairly well-defined clinical syndrome. These cases can be termed 'cryptogenic fibrosing alveolitis'. When more causes are known then further subdivision is likely to be possible in the future.

Non-inflammatory Interstitial Exudates

The best examples of non-inflammatory interstitial exudates are persisting pulmonary congestion, usually related to long-standing elevation of the left atrial pressure as in mitral valve disease, left atrial myxoma and non-critical cor triatriatum, and the now increasingly recognised cases of chronic pulmonary oedema relating to uraemia. Whether the latter is entirely accounted for by hypertension and fluid retention, or whether increased capillary permeability also plays an important role, remains controversial, but it is well established that increased alveolar wall fibrosis with normal alveolar architecture occurs in uraemia (Figs. 2, 3).

When such fibrosis has occurred, whatever the cause, the clinical features are similar. Breathlessness depends on the severity and extent of the changes; widespread crepitations are characteristic and clubbing is also a common but unexplained characteristic. The physiological pattern is that of a restrictive defect with a ventilation/perfusion abnormality causing a fall in Po_2 and Pco_2. The radiograph shows predominantly basal shadows which may be accompanied by lymphatic lines (Kerley A and B lines) and, in cardiac cases, the additional presence of prominent upper lobe pulmonary veins. In the latter cases the radiographic shadows may be further increased if there is additional secondary haemosiderosis due to leakage of red cells. Whether such leakage in itself causes a further fibrogenic stimulus is unresolved, but cases of both primary and secondary pulmonary haemosiderosis are characterised by the presence of alveolar wall fibrosis in addition to the obvious deposition of iron inside as well as outside alveolar macrophages.

Inflammatory Exudates

Many acute and short-lived inflammatory exudates resolve completely without leaving long-standing changes in the alveolar walls. There are, however, an increasing number of instances where, either because of the initial severity of injury or because of persistence, chronic interstitial changes develop. A comprehensive list cannot be given but a number of examples can be cited. For instance, cases of persistent radiographic shadowing are now being recognised after established episodes of influenza. A group of patients has recently been described in Johannesburg (Webster, 1972), where, following recovery from unexceptional Hong Kong A_2 influenza, progressive breathlessness developed after two or three weeks and extensive patchy shadowing was observed on the radiograph. Crepitations without finger clubbing were found on examination and lung biopsy revealed patchy changes

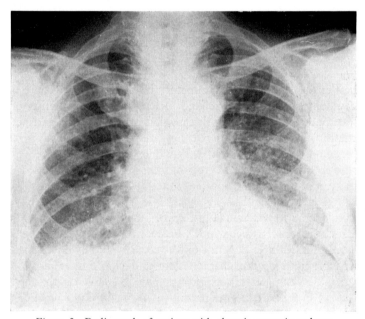

Figure 2   Radiograph of patient with chronic uraemic oedema

typical of desquamative interstitial pneumonia with alveolar wall infiltration by mononuclear cells. Resolution was obtained by early treatment with corticosteroids. In one patient, treatment was withheld for three months and the shadows progressed over this time but resolved rapidly when treatment was started. Other similar cases are now being seen throughout the world. So far the majority have been identified within influenzal epidemics; if cases occur sporadically their viral origin could easily be overlooked.

Cases of bronchiectasis may also be associated with widespread inflammatory exudates due to peribronchial pneumonic changes which lead to persisting extensive shadowing on the chest radiograph. The true nature of these cases is easily overlooked because substantial radiographic abnormality is not a feature of the majority of bronchial wall diseases. However, when

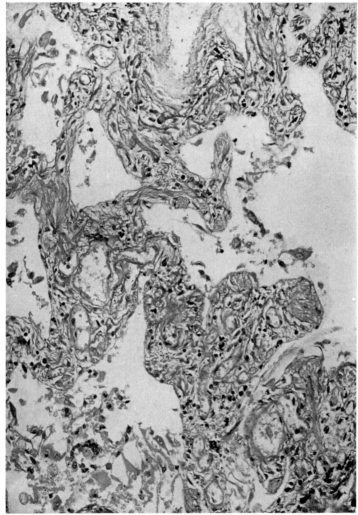

Figure 3 Histological section to demonstrate increased collagen in alveolar walls in uraemic oedema (same case as Fig. 2). × 235

bronchial wall damage is the primary cause of widespread shadowing the symptoms are often characteristic, with large amounts of purulent sputum. Evidence of bronchial wall dilatation and peribronchial thickening may be observed on the plain chest radiograph if sought carefully, and a bronchogram is sometimes justifiable to confirm the diagnosis.

Why some cases of bronchiectasis are associated with extensive alveolar involvement and not others is not entirely clear. Cases particularly liable to extensive alveolar wall damage seem to be those related to *A. fumigatus* hypersensitivity in extrinsic asthmatic patients (Figs. 4, 5). A rather different but predominantly upper-zone pattern of shadowing is seen in cases of cystic fibrosis. Extensive alveolar involvement is perhaps rather less common in cases of bronchiectasis resulting from early childhood infections such as measles or whopping cough. There are, however, many exceptions to these general statements.

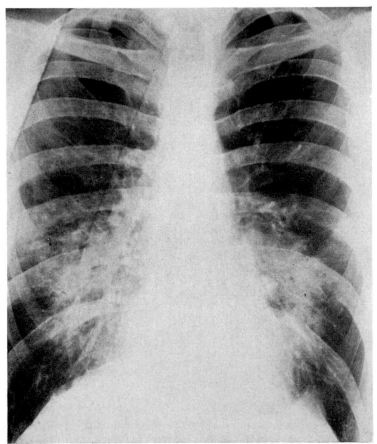

Figure 4 Chest radiograph from a patient with long-standing bronchopulmonary aspergillosis showing 'fixed' bilateral shadows

Drugs are now recognised as causes of chronic interstitial exudates. They include hexamethonium, busulphan (Heard and Cooke, 1968; see also Chapter 3), bleomycin (De Lena et al, 1972), nitrofurantoin (Nicklaus and Snyder, 1968) and salazopyrine. The immunopathogenesis probably varies with different drugs. Lung changes accompanying hexamethonium therapy may be more related to the long-standing associated increase in left atrial pressure than to the drug itself. Cytotoxicity may be important with busulphan and bleomycin. Hypersensitivity responses may be especially important in lung damage due to nitrofurantoin and salazopyrine; blood eosinophilia is prominent in the acute stages of nitrofurantoin pneumonitis (Nicklaus and Snyder, 1968). A number of irritant gases and fumes which are capable of producing florid pulmonary oedema in the acute stages are now also recog-

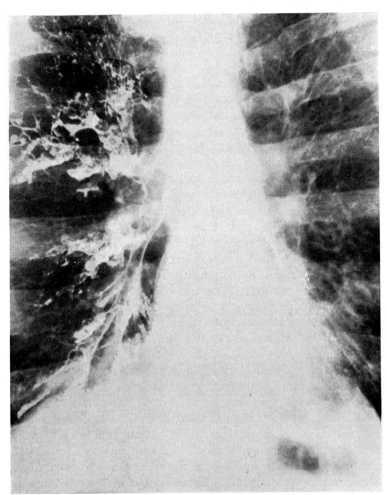

Figure 5 Bronchogram from the same cases showing extensive, especially proximal, bronchiectasis

nised as causing long-standing interstitial changes. These include cadmium fumes, ozone and nitrogen dioxide.

Cryptogenic fibrosing alveolitis
In the early stages there is an inflammatory exudate with mononuclear cell infiltration of the alveolar walls. With progression, an increasing amount of

reticulin and then collagen are laid down in the alveolar walls, with little disturbance of the normal architecture.

With increasing fibrotic contraction and more extensive involvement of the lung, whole tracts of the alveoli disappear and are replaced by fibrotic scarring. There is increasing distortion and destruction until finally widespread honeycombing results with bronchiolar dilation and cyst formation.

The natural history of cryptogenic fibrosing alveolitis is very variable. The cases first reported as acute Hamman–Rich syndrome (1944) ran their complete course to death from respiratory failure in less than a year. At the other extreme, cases have survived for more than 25 years. In two large series the mean survival times from the onset of symptoms were four and six years respectively (Stack, Choo-Kang and Heard, 1972; Turner-Warwick, personal series). Only a small number of cases respond substantially to corticosteroids (11 per cent, Stack et al, 1972; 14 per cent, Turner-Warwick). This is explained, at least in part, by the insidious nature of the majority of cases, so that there is much irreversible fibrosis before symptoms of breathlessness become apparent and medical aid is sought. Many cases show radiographic and physiological progression in spite of corticosteroid or immunosuppressant therapy.

The physical signs are typical, with showers of crepitations in more than 90 per cent of the proven cases and finger clubbing in about 60 per cent. Radiographically, bilateral, predominantly basal, shadowing is typical; with progression the shadows extend upwards to affect all zones. In a minority, upper-zone predominance is seen. The reason for the basal shadowing in cases of fibrosing alveolitis, compared with the upper-zone predominance in many essentially granulomatous diseases, has not been adequately explained.

Scadding and Hinson (1967) showed that, within the group of patients with clinical features characteristic of fibrosing alveolitis, some showed extensive desquamative changes within the alveoli similar to the description of desquamative interstitial pneumonia (Liebow, Steer and Billingsley, 1965; see also Chapter 3). Others showed virtually no intra-alveolar exudate but a progressive alveolar wall fibrosis which they termed the 'mural type'. Many showed both appearances simultaneously. Desquamative interstitial pneumonia has other additional histological characteristics, particularly lymphoid collections containing germinal follicles and numerous scattered plasma cells. Immunofluorescence studies have shown antibody production within these lymphocytic collections and this, together with the frequent finding of non-organ specific autoantibodies (antinuclear antibodies and rheumatoid factor), suggests that the pathogenesis depends upon some form of immunological response (Turner-Warwick and Haslam, 1971; Turner-Warwick, Haslam and Weeks, 1971).

More recently, Liebow has identified cases presenting with clinical features similar to cryptogenic fibrosing alveolitis but with other types of histological appearances. These include dense infiltration by mature lymphocytes (interstitial lymphocytic pneumonia) (Liebow, Carrington Friedman, 1972), plasma cells (plasma cell pneumonia) or giant cells (giant cell pneumonia) (Liebow, 1968). It has yet to be resolved whether these are varied tissue responses to the same initiating agent or whether they reflect different trigger factors. In the meantime it is convenient to group these different cell types of interstitial pneumonia together because of their similar clinical presentation.

Cryptogenic fibrosing alveolitis with associated connective tissue disorders

A further reason for suspecting that many cases of cryptogenic fibrosing alveolitis have an underlying immunological abnormality is that, in addition to the associated presence of circulating tissue antibodies, many have now been described with other systemic connective tissue disorders, which in their own right are characterised by a similar type of non-organ specific auto-antibody. Approximately 20 per cent of the patients with fibrosing alveolitis seen at the Brompton Hospital had associated rheumatoid arthritis, and others have been associated with Sjögren's syndrome, systemic sclerosis, dermatomyositis, polymyositis and chronic active hepatitis. Although no case in this series had renal tubular acidosis, the association has been reported by other workers (Hood and Mason, 1970).

The immunopathogenesis of the pulmonary changes is not certain. Immuno-fluorescent evidence of immune complexes has been demonstrated in eight cases (all of whom had circulating antinuclear antibody) but none could be identified in 25 other lung biopsies studied (Turner-Warwick et al, 1971). Serum C_3 complement levels are not reduced and no other positive evidence of circulating immune complexes has yet been identified using the Laurell crossed immunoelectrophoresis technique. In some cases lymphocyte sensitisation to tissue antigens, notably nuclear components, has been demonstrated (Haslam and Turner-Warwick, 1975), suggesting that delayed hypersensitivity responses may account for some of the changes seen in the lung. Whether these autoallergic features are primary, or secondary to viral or other agents, has not been resolved. However, there is increasing evidence that many other autoallergic syndromes, particularly those of the non-organ specific group, are virus determined and it seems possible that this will be the case in lung disease. The finding of very similar histological changes in cases following influenza pneumonia is further supporting evidence.

Disorders Relating to Inorganic Particles

Although a detailed description of all forms of pneumoconiosis is not appropriate here, some of the interstitial changes observed following exposure to certain dusts should be mentioned because they form further illustrative examples of patterns of widespread pulmonary response to various inhaled agents.

Of the common inorganic dusts in the United Kingdom giving rise to widespread changes in the lung, two broad groups can be identified: those agents resulting in dust deposition with little or no tissue response, and those initiating a substantial fibrogenic reaction. A number of mixed patterns are also seen.

Coal miners' pneumoconiosis

It is important to distinguish simple coal dust deposition in the lung from complex fibrogenic reactions resulting in progressive massive fibrosis. In simple coal pneumoconiosis dust is taken up by alveolar macrophages and carried through the lymphatics into the alveolar septa and deposited in the lymphoid tissues. Coal deposits are therefore found particularly in the inter-lobular septa and in lymphoid tissue peripherally, and in the lymph nodes centrally. Dust is also deposited in a centrilobular position around respiratory bronchioles; this presumably reflects the migration of macrophages centrally up the bronchial pathways on their way to the ciliary escalator. Although dust deposition is extensive, little associated fibrosis occurs. This, however, depends in part on the nature of the coal-bearing rock; where there is com-bined coal and silica exposure, extensive fibrosis may occur.

The tissue response to coal also seems to be modified by the host capacity to respond, because in those individuals with sero-positive rheumatoid arthritis (Caplan, Payne and Withey, 1962), the histology in the lungs is altered and necrobiotic lesions of small or larger size similar in structure to subcutaneous rheumatoid nodules are found.

The cause of progressive massive fibrosis (PMF) lesions is not certain. In part it seems to be dose-dependent. Although some have suggested that the frequency of PMF amongst any group of miners is influenced by the type of coal, being more common where the coal-bearing rock has a high silica con-tent, others have challenged this. It also seems to depend upon the host response because an increasing number of PMF cases have antinuclear anti-bodies and rheumatoid factor when compared with those who have simple pneumoconiosis (Soutar, Simon and Turner-Warwick, 1974; Lippmann et al, 1973).

The radiographic opacities in simple coal miners' pneumoconiosis tend to be rounded lesions particularly concentrated in the upper lobes; the pleura is rarely involved. When PMF shadows occur these too have an upper-zone predominance, as do Caplan's nodules. Occasionally, irregular basal shadows similar to fibrosing alveolitis are seen in coal miners; these are associated with extensive alveolar wall fibrosis (Parkes, 1974). The conditions for their development and the immunological responses, if any, have not yet been defined but certainly deserve further study.

Silica

The lesions of silicosis stand in sharp contrast to those of coal miners. Here, characteristic whorls of fibrosis are found particularly in alveolar septa but separated by well-preserved normal non-fibrotic alveoli. Much work has been done on the fibrogenesis of silica dust (Heppleston, 1969). Macrophage handling of the dust seems to play a central role; soluble products from macrophages cultured with silica have resulted in increased collagen production from fibroblasts on the one hand, and increase of macrophage accumulation from reticuloendothelial tissues on the other.

Asbestosis

The fibrogenic response, typically in the lower lobes, caused by asbestos dust and talc contrasts in turn with the whorled fibrotic nodules often predominantly in the upper zones due to silica. In asbestosis the appearances are those of fibrosing alveolitis with widespread alveolar wall thickening and destruction. The clinical signs, with crepitations and finger clubbing, are also identical, as are the radiographic features in the lungs. However, in contrast to cryptogenic fibrosing alveolitis, the pleura is involved in about 60 per cent of cases with evidence of intrapulmonary involvement (Soutar, Turner-Warwick and Parkes, 1974). The explanation for the different pattern of fibrogenic response in silicosis on the one hand and asbestosis upon the other is evidently of fundamental importance. The difference may depend upon the cytotoxic capacity of the two dusts as well as the particular ways in which they are handled and react with macrophages.

In experimental asbestosis, early capillary wall damage has been demonstrated at the initial site of deposition, with diapedesis of red cells and inflammatory exudates (Holt, Mills and Young, 1966). These initial changes in the alveolar walls presumably directly depend upon cytotoxic properties of asbestos fibre and may determine the characteristic widespread alveolar wall fibrosis. Further evidence of subtle cytotoxic capacity of asbestos fibre has been demonstrated by in vitro studies on lymphocytes (Maini and Turner-Warwick, 1974) and macrophages (Allison, 1973).

Tumours

Common in the differential diagnosis of widespread shadows in the lung are various types of disseminated tumour, and certain of these might be considered within the context of interstitial disease of the lungs, in so far as tumour occupies vascular or lymphatic spaces within the connective tissue framework.

Lymphangitis carcinomatosa

Patients with lymphangitis carcinomatosa frequently present with progressive breathlessness, though an established case is sometimes seen where this symptom is absent or only slight. There may be no abnormal physical signs and finger clubbing is uncommon.

The radiographic appearances in their most characteristic form show streaky shadowing extending from the hilar regions which are often enlarged by infiltrated lymph nodes. However, the radiograph may show a more nodular appearance and only on histological examination will the extensive involvement of lymphatics be confirmed.

Haematogenous dissemination

A number of primary carcinomas may be disseminated very widely through the blood stream to the lungs and give a generalised nodular shadowing. These are often, but not always, larger in size than lesions due to inorganic or organic dusts. Common primary tumours are those of breast, stomach and thyroid. Many rare tumours such as chorionepithelioma may on occasion be distributed widely throughout the lung.

Lymphomas

Rarely, various reticuloses may infiltrate the lungs extensively (Peckham, 1972) and their diagnosis is important because with modern regimens of cytotoxic drugs their response to treatment can be dramatic. Of the reticuloses, cases of Hodgkin's, lymphosarcoma and reticulum cell sarcoma have been seen most frequently, but many other cell variants have also been described. Clinically, adventitious sounds and finger clubbing are usually absent and the diagnosis is frequently made only by lung biopsy.

Rare Congenital Dysplasias

There remains a group of cases that may be regarded as dysplasias of pulmonary tissue although their certain origin has not been confirmed. All are characterised by very extensive cystic formation in the lungs and are frequently complicated by pneumothorax resulting from their rupture.

Tuberose sclerosis (Dawson, 1954)

This condition is characterised not only by extensive fibrosis and honeycombing in the lung but with associated fibrotic nodules under the nails (subungual fibromata) and in the kidney and brain. Most of these patients are mentally retarded. The condition is generally regarded as an autosomal recessive.

Eosinophilic granuloma—histiocytosis X (Lewis, 1964)

Histologically the cellular elements are characterised by an infiltration of foamy histiocytic cells, eosinophils and fibroblasts; as the condition extends, larger or smaller cysts appear (Fig. 6) and there is very extensive honeycombing. In the later stages physiological changes of severe airways obstruction may be seen in addition to the more typical restrictive defect. Osteoporotic areas in bones may be found and the combination of changes in the lungs and bones are then pathognomonic. There is no blood eosinophilia.

In the earlier stages some arrest of the process may be obtained with corti-costeroids but many cases progress relentlessly to an early death. The origin of this disorder is quite unknown and it is only by its similarity to lipoid storage disease (Letterer–Siwe and Hand–Schuller–Christian) that it has been perhaps prematurely grouped with these forms of tissue dysplasias.

Leiomyomatosis

This rare disorder is only diagnosed by lung biopsy, and it presents with all the characteristics of fibrosing alveolitis. Histologically, a vast increase in

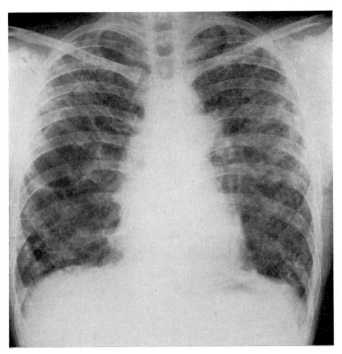

Figure 6   Widespread honeycombing with bullous formation in advanced eosinophilic granuloma

smooth muscle and fibrous tissue is seen. This is quite in excess of the amount of muscle that may be found in fibrotic lungs, where a *relative* predominance of smooth muscle of normal bronchial wall occurs pari passu with contracted alveolar tissue. No form of treatment is of any value in leiomyomatosis.

Conclusion

In this chapter no attempt has been made to review in detail every indivi-dual disorder known to affect the peripheral parts of the lung; for this, reference must be made to comprehensive textbooks and individual articles.

An attempt has, however, been made to group together special radiographic features, histological patterns and clinical findings to help the physician in his approach to diagnosis. Identification of cases at an early and treatable stage is emphasised because, so often, when the changes are reversible symptoms are relatively slight, and patients are allowed to continue untreated until extensive fibrous destruction has occurred; at this late stage therapy will be useless. The correct decision about when to wait and when to treat is likely to become easier as better methods are found to monitor more accurately the changes occurring in these chronic interstitial lung diseases.

REFERENCES

Allison, A. C. (1973) Experimental methods—cell and tissue culture effects of asbestos particles on macrophages, mesothelial cells and fibroblasts. In *Biological Effects of Asbestos*, ed. Bogovski, P. et al. IARC Scientific Publication No. 8. WHO International Agency for Research on Cancer.

Ball, K., Joules, H. & Pagel, W. (1951) Acute tuberculous septicaemia with leucopenia. *British Medical Journal*, 2, 869–873.

Bronsky, D. & Dunn, Y. O. L. (1965) Sarcoidosis with hypogammaglobulinaemia. *American Journal of the Medical Sciences*, 250, 11–18.

Caplan, A., Payne, R. B. & Withey, J. L. (1962) A broader concept of Caplan's syndrome related to rheumatoid factors. *Thorax*, 17, 205–212.

Churg, J. & Strauss, L. (1951) Allergic granulomatosis, allergic angiitis and periarteritis nodosa. *American Journal of Pathology*, 27, 277–301.

Dawson, J. (1954) Pulmonary tuberose sclerosis and its relationship to other forms of disease. *Quarterly Journal of Medicine*, 23, 113–145.

De Lena, M., Guzzan, A., Monfardin, S. & Bonadonna, G. (1972) Clinical radiographic and histopathogenic studies on pulmonary toxicity induced by treatment with bleomycin. *Cancer Chemotherapy Reports*, 56, 343.

Forbes, G. B. (1961) Non reactive tuberculosis in a cortisone-treated patient. *Tubercle*, 42, 233–240.

Freiman, D. G. & Hardy, H. L. (1970) Beryllium disease. *Human Pathology*, 1, 25–44.

Hamman, L. & Rich, A. R. (1944) Acute diffuse interstitial fibrosis of the lungs. *Bulletin of the Johns Hopkins Hospital*, 74, 177–212.

Hapke, E. J., Seal, R. M. E., Thomas, G. O., Hayes, M. & Meek, J. C. (1968) Farmer's lung: a clinical radiographic functional and serological correlation of acute and chronic stages. *Thorax*, 23, 451–468.

Hardy, H. L., Rabe, E. W. & Lorch, S. (1967) United States Beryllium Case Registry (1952–1966). *Journal of Occupational Medicine*, 9, 271–276.

Hargreaves, F. E. (1970) M.D. Thesis, Leeds University.

Haslam, P. & Turner-Warwick, M. (1975) Lymphocyte sensitisation to nuclear antigens in lung diseases associated with circulating antinuclear antibodies. *Clinical and Experimental Immunology*, 20, 379–395.

Heard, B. E. & Cooke, R. A. (1968) Busulphan lung. *Thorax*, 23, 187–193.

Heppleston, A. G. (1969) The fibrogenic action of silica. *British Medical Bulletin*, 25, 282–287.

Holt, P. F., Mills, J. & Young, D. K. (1966) Experimental asbestosis in the guinea-pig. *Journal of Pathology and Bacteriology*, 92, 185–195.

Hood, J. & Mason, A. M. S. (1970) Diffuse pulmonary disease with transfer defect occurring with coeliac disease. *Lancet*, 1, 445–447.

Lewis, J. G. (1964) Eosinophilic granuloma and its variants with special reference to lung involvement. *Quarterly Journal of Medicine*, 33, 337–359.

Liebow, A. A. (1968) New concepts and entities in pulmonary disease. *The Lung*, ed. Liebow, A. A. & Smith, D. E. Baltimore: Williams & Wilkins.

Leibow, A. A., Steer, A. & Billingsley, J. G. (1965) Desquamative interstitial pneumonia. *American Journal of Medicine*, **39**, 369–404.

Liebow, A. A., Carrington, C. R. B. & Friedman, P. J. (1972) Lymphomatoid granulomatosis. *Human Pathology*, **3**, 457–558.

Lippmann, M., Eckert, H. L., Hahon, N. & Morgan, W. K. C. (1973) Circulating antinuclear and rheumatoid factors in coal miners. *Annals of Internal Medicine*, **79**, 807–811.

Livingstone, J. L., Lewis, J. G., Reid, L. & Jefferson, K. E. (1964) Diffuse interstitial pulmonary fibrosis. *Quarterly Journal of Medicine*, **33**, 71–103.

Maini, T. & Turner-Warwick, M. (1974) Lymphocyte toxicity due to asbestos dusts. Unpublished.

Marx, J. J. & Burrell, R. (1973) Delayed hypersensitivity to beryllium compounds. *Journal of Immunology*, **111**, 590–598.

Nicklaus, T. M. & Snyder, A. B. (1968) Nitrofurantoin pulmonary reaction. *Archives of Internal Medicine*, **121**, 151–155.

Parkes, W. R. (1974) *Occupational Lung Disorders*. London: Butterworths.

Peckham, M. J. (1972) Lymphomas and the lung. Current concepts of the management of Hodgkin's disease with particular reference to intrathoracic involvement. *British Tuberculosis and Thoracic Association Review*, **2**, 1–18.

Scadding, J. G. (1952) Chronic lung diseases with diffuse nodular or reticular radiographic shadows. *Tubercle*, **33**, 352–365.

Scadding, J. G. (1967) *Sarcoidosis*. London: Eyre and Spottiswoode.

Scadding, J. G. (1974) Diffuse pulmonary alveolar fibrosis. *Thorax*, **29**, 271–281.

Scadding, J. G. & Hinson, K. F. W. (1967) Diffuse fibrosing alveolitis. *Thorax*, **22**, 291–304.

Seal, R. Personal communication.

Siltzbach, L. E. (1961) The Kveim test in sarcoidosis: a study of 750 patients. *Journal of the American Medical Association*, **178**, 476–482.

Smellie, H. & Hoyle, C. (1960) The natural history of pulmonary sarcoidosis. *Quarterly Journal of Medicine*, **29**, 539–558.

Soutar, C. A., Simon, G. & Turner-Warwick, M. (1974) The radiology of asbestos-induced disease of the lungs. *British Journal of Diseases of the Chest*, **68**, 235–252.

Soutar, C. A., Turner-Warwick, M. & Parkes, W. R. (1974) Circulating antinuclear antibody and rheumatoid factor in coal pneumoconiosis. *British Medical Journal*, **3**, 145–147.

Spector, W. G. & Heesom, N. (1969) The production of granulomata by antigen–antibody complexes. *Journal of Pathology*, **98**, 31–39.

Stack, B. H. R., Choo-Kang, F. J. & Heard, B. E. (1972) The prognosis of cryptogenic fibrosing alveolitis. *Thorax*, **27**, 535–542.

Turner-Warwick, M. (1974) A perspective view on widespread pulmonary fibrosis. *British Medical Journal*, **2**, 371–376.

Turner-Warwick, M. & Doniach, D. (1965) Autoantibody studies in interstitial pulmonary fibrosis. *British Medical Journal*, **1**, 886–891.

Turner-Warwick, M. & Haslam, P. (1971) Antibodies in some chronic fibrosing lung diseases. I. Non-organ-specific autoantibodies. *Clinical Allergy*, **1**, 83–95.

Turner-Warwick, M., Haslam, P. & Weeks, J. (1971) Antibodies in some chronic fibrosing lung diseases. II. Immunofluorescent studies. *Clinical Allergy*, **1**, 209–219.

Webster, I. (1972) Desquamative pneumonia following A_2 influenza. Personal communication.

Wenzel, F. J., Emanuel, D. A. & Gray, R. G. (1971) Immunofluorescent studies in patients with farmer's lung. *Journal of Allergy and Clinical Immunology*, **48**, 224–229.

8
RESPIRATORY DISEASE IN EARLY LIFE

N. R. C. Roberton

Nearly half the children who die between birth and 14 years of age do so in the first week of life. In 1970 the major causes of death among live-born infants during these first seven days (early neonatal death rate) were pulmonary diseases (Table 1). Despite this high mortality rate, many of the pulmonary diseases are treatable, with good pulmonary function (Bryan et al, 1973), normal intelligence and normal life expectancy among survivors. These critically ill neonates in cardiorespiratory failure require the facilities of an

Table 1 Causes of death in childhood (Registrar General's Report for England and Wales, 1970)

Total deaths <14 years		18 997
Early neonatal deaths <7 days		8 326
Early neonatal deaths excluding malformations		6 960
Hyaline membrane disease	1340	
Immaturity[a]	1513	
Pneumonia	195	
Asphyxia[b]	1267	
	4315	

[a] Most of these infants would have hyaline membrane disease.

[b] Most of these infants would have aspiration syndromes, pulmonary haemorrhage, etc.

intensive care unit. It seems difficult to believe that there has been a need to justify such services even to the extent of controlled trials (Schlesinger, 1973). However, it is now widely accepted that such units are essential in maternity hospitals, and that they result in a considerable reduction in the neonatal mortality (Table 2).

This review deals with some of the major advances which have been made in the past few years in the understanding and management of these severe respiratory diseases.

I. DISEASES OF THE NEWBORN

The majority of admissions to a special care nursery for reasons other than low birth weight or intrapartum asphyxia are for some form of pulmonary disease (Table 3).

Table 2 Neonatal deaths in the United Oxford Hospitals

	A Total neonatal deaths	B Lethal congenital malformation	A–B	IPPV survivors
1971	57	16	41	1
1972	44	16	28	9
1973	37	16	21	21

The birth weight distribution of all deliveries was constant during this period.

A–B can be regarded as 'preventable' neonatal deaths. The satisfactory application of intensive care and IPPV has halved this neonatal mortality

Table 3 Major causes of admission to special care baby unit, United Oxford Hospitals July 1972 to December 1973

Total admissions		1150
Low birth weight (uncomplicated)		321
Intrapartum asphyxia		242
Severe	37	
Mild	205	
Pulmonary disease		320
HMD (Classical)	134	
(Transient)	47	
Apnoeic attacks	55[a]	
Aspiration pneumonia	39	
Pneumomediastinum/pneumothorax	23	
Pulmonary haemorrhage	11	
Pneumonia	11	

[a] These were often single apnoeic attacks.

Respiratory Distress

This label is applied to all infants who have at least two of the following three signs for more than 1 h before the age of 4 h: tachypnoea greater than 60/min; subcostal and intercostal retraction; a characteristic grunt due to expiration against a closed glottis.

In infants who survive respiratory distress, a precise diagnosis cannot be made in the absence of histological confirmation. However, in premature infants, the major cause of respiratory distress is hyaline membrane disease.

HYALINE MEMBRANE DISEASE (HMD), IDIOPATHIC
RESPIRATORY DISTRESS SYNDROME (IRDS)

This is the major life-threatening disease in the newborn infant and develops within the first 4 h of life. Respiratory illness which begins more than 4 h after birth is not HMD. The incidence increases with decreasing duration of gestation, though the mortality rate remains remarkably constant below 36 weeks, but the more premature infants frequently require assisted ventilation (Table 4).

The diagnosis of HMD is made *clinically* when a newborn infant develops respiratory distress, and congenital heart disease and the other types of pulmonary disease discussed below have been excluded on clinical or radio-

Table 4   Incidence of HMD United Oxford Hospitals, 1973

Gestation weeks	No. infants born	% with HMD[a]	% Survival[a] of HMD	% HMD survivors[a] who had needed treatment by CDP or IPPV
25–26	2	100 (2)	—	—
27–28	10	100 (10)	80 (8)	87.5 (7)
29–30	9	88.9 (8)	75 (6)	66.6 (4)
31–32	22	54.5 (12)	83.3 (10)	40 (4)
33–34	52	30.8 (16)	87.5 (14)	50 (7)
35–36	132	12.1 (16)	81.3 (13)	23.1 (3)
37+	4210	0.57 (24)	100 (24)	25 (6)
Total		88	85.2 (75)	41.3 (31)

[a] Actual number of cases in brackets.

logical grounds. The chest x-ray often shows a reticulogranular pattern (Donald and Steiner, 1953). However, this may be minimal or absent particularly in the early stages of the disease, and in a study of chest x-rays of infants suffering from HMD born at the Royal Postgraduate Medical School at Hammersmith, Gupta (unpublished data) found that the only radiological feature correlating with severity of HMD, was the failure of intestinal gas to pass beyond the second part of the duodenum. Nevertheless, an AP and lateral chest x-ray must always be obtained in infants with respiratory distress to exclude diseases other than HMD from the diagnosis.

Aetiology

In an established case of HMD, pulmonary surfactant is grossly diminished, and the lungs are unstable and tend to collapse. Pulmonary hypoperfusion, increased right to left shunting of the cardiac output, hypoxaemia and hypercapnia, are all secondary to this.

Although it is primarily a disease of prematurity, many premature infants survive without developing HMD, and occasionally a term infant may develop the typical disease (Roberton, Hallidie-Smith and Davis, 1967). In some premature infants pulmonary stability may be abnormal at the moment of birth (Hey and Hull, 1971). In other cases of HMD lung function deteriorates during the first few hours of life (Reynolds, Roberton and Wigglesworth, 1968). Indeed, four of Hey and Hull's infants who developed fatal HMD had normal lung function at birth. Gluck et al (1972) have shown that surface active lecithins disappear from tracheal aspirate during the period when an infant is developing HMD.

It therefore appears that several different factors are involved in the aetiology of HMD.

Prematurity (Table 4)

The major surface tension lowering lecithin present in the normal fetal lung is dipalmitoyl lecithin, synthesised by the choline incorporation pathway. Myristoyl-palmitoyl lecithin, synthesised by the methylation pathway, in which myristic acid (14:0) is substituted for palmitic acid (16:0) at the beta position of the glycerol molecule (Gluck et al, 1972) is less effective than dipalmitoyl lecithin at lowering surface tension and is present in small amounts. Both synthetic pathways are sensitive to changes in pH, oxygenation and temperature. The synthetic pathway for dipalmitoyl lecithin—the choline incorporation pathway—is present in the human fetus from 20 weeks of gestation, but it does not become significantly active until about 34 to 36 weeks of gestation. This corresponds to the gestation at which the incidence of HMD falls, and increased amounts of lecithin—derived from pulmonary fluid—can be detected in the liquor amnii by amniocentesis (Gluck and Kulovich, 1973).

Asphyxia

At the moment of birth, some infants already have abnormal lung function (Hey and Hull, 1971). These infants have presumably already started to lose surfactant as a result of a period of intrauterine asphyxia. The development of HMD in such infants is inevitable.

Low birth weight infants frequently suffer intrapartum asphyxia, and as a result of this they become acidotic, hypoxic, hypercapnic and cold. Such infants are therefore at risk of HMD due to the sensitivity of surfactant synthesis to these adverse factors.

HMD may also develop in infants who have apparently normal lungs at birth and were not asphyxiated. If the immediate postnatal care of the infant is such that he develops the conditions known to inhibit surfactant synthesis, then surfactant, present at birth, will rapidly disappear, and HMD will develop within 3 to 4 h (Hey and Hull, 1971; Thibeault and Hobel, 1974).

Infants of diabetic mothers

Although some authorities disagree (Usher, Allen and McLean, 1971), these infants have an increased incidence of HMD (Pildes, 1973). This is the result of delayed activation of the dipalmitoyl lecithin synthetic pathway in infants of diabetic mothers (Whitfield, Sproule and Brudenell, 1973).

Caesarean section

Usher et al (1971) demonstrated that infants delivered by Caesarean section have an increased incidence of HMD. Although the reasons for this were not clear, possible factors included lack of placento-fetal transfusion, inhalation of amniotic fluid or blood, and absence of a compressing action of the vagina emptying fluid out of the infant's lungs. However, it has been suggested that the increased incidence of HMD following Caesarean section is related to the indication for section (Bevilacqua et al, 1973). These authors showed that infants born by elective section had a lower incidence of HMD than vaginally delivered infants of the same gestation, and Dunn (1973) has shown that the higher incidence of HMD in the infant born by Caesarean section can be abolished by ensuring an adequate placento-fetal transfusion.

Gabert, Bryson and Stenchever (1973) showed that the incidence of HMD is not increased in infants delivered by Caesarean section, provided there is evidence of normal surfactant production before delivery. The data of Fedrick and Butler (1972) supports the theory that pulmonary maturity is the major factor in deciding whether or not an infant delivered by Caesarean section develops HMD. They showed that there was a much higher incidence of HMD in infants delivered by Caesarean section before the onset of labour, compared with infants delivered by Caesarean section in labour. The former group is likely to include a number of infants whose lecithin synthesis had not matured.

Effect of drugs

Much of the recent research into HMD has been devoted to the effect of drugs on the synthesis and release of surfactant. It is now realised that many drugs can induce the choline incorporation pathway for surfactant (Farrell and Zachman, 1973). These include steroids (Liggins, 1969; Avery, 1975) and opiates (Taeusch et al, 1973a). Steroids have been used for this purpose in humans (Liggins and Howie, 1972), and infants born to heroin addicted mothers have a very low incidence of HMD (Glass, Rajegowda and Evans, 1971).

Drugs may also play a part in releasing surfactant from the granular pneumonocytes in which it is believed to be synthesised. Cholinergic (Goldenberg, Buckingham and Sommers, 1969), and adrenergic drugs (Wyszogrodski, Taeusch and Avery, 1975) may stimulate maximal release of surfactant in addition to the release of surfactant which takes place with the onset of breathing (Taeusch et al, 1974). This release of surfactant will only benefit the premature infant if other factors known to decrease the quantities of surfactant in the lung can be avoided in the immediate postnatal period.

Variation in the age at activation of the choline incorporation pathway

Certain conditions such as prolonged rupture of the membranes, fetal infection, or intrauterine growth retardation accelerate the activation of the choline incorporation pathway (Gluck and Kulovich, 1973; Bauer, Stern and Colle, 1974). Such infants will have adequate dipalmitoyl lecithin and are less likely to develop HMD even if delivered at short gestation. Other conditions, notably maternal diabetes and severe erythroblastosis are associated with delayed activation of the choline incorporation pathway and an increased risk of HMD postnatally (Whitfield et al, 1973).

Pathophysiology of HMD

Once the infant is depleted of surfactant he develops pulmonary oedema leading to desquamation of surfactant synthesising cells. Increased capillary permeability caused by hypoxia and acidaemia makes the oedema worse, and the full blown picture of atelectasis and hyaline membranes lining the alveolar ducts soon develops. The pulmonary artery pressure stays at systemic level (Chu et al, 1967) and the infant remains hypoxic and acidaemic. The hypoxaemia is largely due to intrapulmonary shunting (Prod'hom et al, 1965) but small right to left shunts occur at the level of the foramen ovale and the ductus arteriosus. The infant with established HMD has a very low pulmonary compliance, residual gas volume, and alveolar ventilation. The dead space is increased and the airways resistance is normal. These derangements of function and blood gases persist until surfactant reappears with the recovery of surfactant synthesis from about 36 h of age. Recovery is heralded by the appearance of surfactant and precursors in laryngeal aspirates (Gluck et al, 1972).

Prevention of RDS

The observation of Liggins (1969) that steroids infused into lambs resulted in accelerated pulmonary maturity, led to a plethora of experimental work on their use to accelerate lecithin biosynthesis in other animals and humans. Liggins's work has been confirmed in sheep and other species (Avery, 1975). However, it is important to realise that in animals the steroid has to be injected into the fetus; injection into the mother either has no effect, or results in fetal death (Motoyama et al, 1971). Furthermore, rabbit fetuses so treated have a decreased cell number in the 'treated' lungs (Carson, Taeusch and Avery, 1973), though catch-up growth occurs within one month postnatally (Kotas, Mims and Hart, 1974).

There is undoubtedly a species difference in the placental transfer of corticosteroids. In man steroids can cross the placenta in sufficient quantities to be physiologically active and even cause adrenal suppression, though cortisol may be metabolised to cortisone in the placenta (Murphy et al, 1974).

Liggins and Howie (1972) gave two injections of 6 mg of dexamethasone 12 h apart to women in premature labour. This resulted in a significant decrease in the incidence and mortality from HMD, though a surprisingly large number of infants died shortly after birth. In our experience death from HMD is unusual under 12 h of age except in infants below 1 kg birthweight. The beneficial effects of dexamethasone were only seen in women with spontaneous premature labour at less than 32 weeks gestation and in whom delivery could be postponed for at least 48 h after entering the trial. Treatment was of no benefit if delivery was postponed for more than seven days, or in women electively delivered at short gestation. The fact that therapy was successful in preventing RDS only in women with spontaneous onset of labour in whom delivery could be postponed for at least 48 h needs careful interpretation, since other factors which accelerate pulmonary maturity were not controlled in the study. Thus, prolonged membrane rupture, with or without ascending infection, is associated with a decreased incidence of HMD (Bauer et al, 1974), and beta-adrenergic drugs, used in some cases to delay delivery, release surfactant from the alveolar lining cells (Wyszogrodski et al, 1975). Although the dexamethasone was administered with the purpose of accelerating dipalmitoyl lecithin synthesis, there was no evidence in the Liggins and Howie study for a rise in liquor lecithin levels even in the cases in whom HMD was successfully prevented. Furthermore when Spellacy et al (1973) gave large doses of dexamethasone over a two week period to women between 28 and 32 weeks of gestation, they only produced small increases in the amount of lecithin present in the liquor. However, recent work has suggested that there can be a delay of up to a week between surfactant levels rising in the lung, and there being a detectable surge of lecithin in the liquor.

Since steroids may have a detrimental effect on the fetus when given prenatally, causing, for instance, intrapartum stillbirth (Liggins and Howie, 1972), adrenal suppression (Murphy et al, 1974) or decreased lung growth (Carson et al, 1973), further confirmatory controlled trials are required, such as that reported by Kennedy (1974), where attempts are made to control for other surfactant inducers, before recommending that steroids be routinely given to mothers in premature labour. Nevertheless it seems likely that it will prove possible within the next few years to administer some drug to accelerate the induction of the choline incorporation pathway in infants likely to be delivered prematurely. This should reduce the incidence of HMD.

Antenatal detection of surfactant production

When the choline incorporation pathway is activated at the thirty-fourth to thirty-sixth week of gestation, there is a rise in the amount of lecithin in

8

the amniotic fluid. This can be equated with lung maturity, and a decreased risk of HMD developing postnatally. The lecithin level in liquor has been assayed in four ways: by measuring the lecithin/sphingomyelin ratio (Gluck et al, 1971), by measuring the absolute amounts of lecithin (Bhagwanani, Fahmy and Turnbull, 1973), by measuring the concentration of palmitate (Warren, Holton and Allen, 1974), and by using a simple physical test on the liquor, such as the shake test (Clements et al, 1972). The simplicity of the shake test should make it a routine bedside investigation wherever induction of labour is contemplated and gestation is uncertain, provided the limitations of the test are recognised (Shephard, Buhi and Spellacy, 1974) and the hazards of amniocentesis are guarded against (Cook, Shott and Andrews, 1974). Some assay of fetal pulmonary lecithin levels is the best test of fetal maturity, because what matters to the infant is not that his lower femoral epiphysis is present (Murdoch and Cope, 1957), or that he has the right proportion of fat cells in the liquor (Brosens and Gordon, 1966) or his head is the right size (Campbell, 1969), but that his surfactant synthesising pathways are mature. Nevertheless, it is important to realise that HMD has been reported in infants with mature lecithin/sphingomyelin ratios (Zachman et al, 1973) and with good shake tests (Thibeault and Hobel, 1974).

Treatment

The management of HMD, which is a self-limiting disease lacking specific treatment, is to keep the infant alive until spontaneous recovery occurs.

It is important to stress that the classical teaching of 'minimal handling' of these sick infants is still true. Anything that disturbs the infant, such as a heel prick, or even physical examination, can cause deterioration. Major interference such as endotracheal tube suction and repeated arterial puncture, can cause irretrievable deterioration. For these reasons treatment is geared to monitoring and managing the infant with the minimum of physical interference once the initial procedures, such as arterial catheterisation and connection of monitors have been carried out. The adverse effects of overhandling the infant are particularly true for capillary blood gas analysis or percutaneous arterial sampling, which are traumatic and inaccurate at this age (Goddard et al, 1974). However, frequent blood gas analysis is mandatory, since reliable clinical assessment of the degree of oxygenation is virtually impossible in low birthweight infants (Goldman et al, 1973).

All infants with HMD requiring more than 40 per cent oxygen should have an indwelling arterial line, preferably in the umbilical artery, or alternatively a cut down into the radial or temporal artery. Although horrific complications following umbilical artery catheterisation have been reported—haemorrhage, paraplegia (Aziz and Robertson, 1973), massive aortic thrombosis (Neal et al, 1972) and bits left behind (Lackey and Taber, 1972), in our experience these complications are extremely rare. In 1968 we reported our initial experience with nearly 400 umbilical artery catheterisations (Gupta, Roberton and Wigglesworth, 1968). Only one surviving child had any long-term sequel—a missing tip to her toe. Since that time we have had no further long-term sequelae, and no mortality attributable directly to the catheters.

Umbilical catheters give easy access for blood gas analysis and biochemical monitoring without disturbing the baby. However, the amount of blood removed should always be carefully recorded and transfusions given as required to replace the blood loss and maintain the haematocrit.

The arterial catheter is also of use for continuous blood pressure monitoring. Great care has to be taken when connecting pressure transducers to the catheter, since they may work loose and massive haemorrhage result.

In addition to blood gas analyses and blood pressure recording, monitoring of respiration and heart rate should also be carried out. Apnoeic attacks are common in infants with HMD, and the quicker they can be detected and terminated the better. Heart rate must always be monitored, especially when some form of assisted ventilation is being used. Dead babies may be ventilated if the nursing staff mistake transmitted mechanical noises from the ventilator for the heart beat. Bearing these problems in mind, treatment can be considered under the following headings:

Temperature control.
Acid base homeostasis.
Oxygen therapy.
Metabolic, cardiovascular, and general support.
Feeding.

Each of these factors has not only to be controlled, but controlled as soon after birth as possible. Great attention to detail is required during the first few minutes and hours.

Temperature control

Hypothermia has deleterious effects at all ages. There are two specific problems in the premature newborn: the oxygen requirement of non-shivering thermogenesis (Scopes, 1966) and the sensitivity of surfactant synthesis to temperatures of less than 35°C (Gluck et al, 1972). Hey (1971) has defined the temperature at which naked and clothed infants should be nursed in an attempt to keep their oxygen consumption minimal—the so-called neutral temperature range. It is important to emphasise that naked infants less than 1500 g birthweight should be kept in an environmental temperature no more than 1 to 1.5°C lower than their rectal temperature. But as Hey (1975) has pointed out, the *optimal* temperature range may be even narrower than the neutral temperature range, since hyperthermia as well as hypothermia is harmful. Perlstein, Edwards and Sutherland (1970) showed that apnoeic attacks are more frequent with rising incubator temperature, and there may also be an increased mortality with comparatively high sustained environmental temperatures which are within the neutral temperature range of minimal oxygen consumption (Yashiro et al, 1973). The study of Aynsley-Green, Roberton and Rolfe (1975) has shown that some commercially available incubators provide an unstable thermal environment with large temperature swings to levels below those recommended (Hey, 1971) followed by rapid rises in temperature of the type which cause apnoea (Perlstein et al, 1970). Overhead radiant heaters also have disadvantages, since evaporative water loss in excess of 60 ml/kg/day may occur, especially in infants less than 30 weeks gestation who transude large amounts of fluid through the intact skin (Fanaroff et al, 1972). Not only is maintenance of environmental temperature of importance for survival, but the studies of Davies and Tizard (1975) have shown that cerebral palsy is significantly commoner among those low birthweight infants who had the lowest body temperature on the first day of life.

Acid base homeostasis

There is no doubt that a low pH should be corrected, not only because of the deleterious effects of acidaemia on the central nervous system (Dawes, Hibbard and Windle, 1964), cardiovascular function and cellular metabolism (Opie, 1965), but because of the pH sensitivity of surfactant synthesis. Which base to use, and at what rate to infuse it, remains undecided. Some advocate THAM (Gupta, Dahlenburg and Davis, 1967) though this may cause apnoea (Roberton, 1970) and its theoretical superiority over sodium bicarbonate is disputed (Heird et al, 1972). Sodium bicarbonate is also potentially dangerous when administered as a bolus of hypertonic solution even at the recommended rate of 1 ml/min (Baum and Roberton, 1975). In a trial comparing THAM with sodium bicarbonate in a group of very sick infants (van Vliet and Gupta, 1973), babies receiving THAM had a lower mortality. The amount of base they received was not stated and since the THAM was given as a more dilute solution yielding fewer bicarbonate molecules per millilitre than the bicarbonate solution used, the results could be interpreted as showing the deleterious effect of bicarbonate. Rapid infusion of base has been recommended since it may be followed by a rapid rise in arterial Po_2 (Gupta et al, 1967; Russell and Cotton, 1968). However, our own studies using either frequent sampling (Baum and Roberton, 1975) or an indwelling arterial oxygen electrode (Goddard et al, 1974) have not confirmed this except in rare cases. Such a rise probably occurs after less than 1 in 10 infusions of base.

Adequate oxygenation, blood volume maintenance, and ventilator therapy will minimise the need for base infusion. However, if base is required the following guidelines may be followed:

(a) There is probably little need to raise the pH above 7.25, the level below which surfactant synthesis decreases.

(b) In an emergency, such as cardiac arrest or extreme bradycardia, 5 to 10 ml of intravenous 8.4 per cent sodium bicarbonate should be given at 1 ml/min. In such a situation the importance of rapid pH correction for myocardial function outweighs the hazards of the rapid hypertonic infusion with its consequent fluid shift. The neonatal cardiovascular system is able to tolerate sudden increases in blood volume such as occur with placental transfusion at birth.

(c) In other circumstances the optimum rate of bicarbonate infusion is not known, but a rate of 1 mEq/min should not be exceeded.

(d) THAM (3.6 or 7 per cent) should only be given to infants who are being artificially ventilated. It may be given (at 1 ml/min) to mature infants with a severe acidaemia (e.g. following severe birth asphyxia) who are hyperventilating, when the more rapid correction of CSF pH with THAM (Holmdahl et al, 1961) may be preferable. I have never seen THAM cause apnoea in such cases.

Oxygen therapy

This is the most complicated and difficult part of therapy in HMD. The infant's arterial Po_2 should be kept within the normal range of 60 to 90 mmHg (Roberton et al, 1968), avoiding the risks of retrolental fibroplasia due to too high a Po_2 in the retinal arteries and without exposing the infant to a high inspired oxygen concentration with the hazard of pulmonary damage (Clark and Lambertsen, 1971).

RETROLENTAL FIBROPLASIA (RLF)

It must be emphasised that the environmental oxygen concentration is only of indirect relevance in the aetiology of RLF, which is caused by a toxic effect of high blood oxygen tensions on the pericytes of the developing retinal capillaries in the premature infant. The capillary endothelium dies and there is a reactive overgrowth of new vessels, with haemorrhage, scarring and distortion of the retina and macula resulting in either blindness or severe visual handicap. The dangers of retrolental fibroplasia are maximum in the infant with comparatively normal lungs of very low birthweight (less than 1250 g) (Alden et al, 1972), who is receiving oxygen at relatively low concentrations for the treatment of apnoeic attacks (Mushin, 1971). RLF is virtually unknown in infants weighing more than 2 kg at birth.

Although RLF has developed in infants who have received supplementary oxygen at low concentrations for considerable periods of time, and there are reports of infants in whom RLF has developed when no supplementary oxygen has been given (Zacharias, 1960), it is estimated that RLF is unlikely to develop if the retinal P_aO_2 remains less than 160 mmHg. (This is the P_aO_2 found in newborn infants breathing 40 per cent oxygen.) In the presence of a right to left shunt through a patent ductus arteriosus, the P_aO_2 of blood withdrawn from an umbilical artery should be kept less than 90 mmHg to prevent retinal P_aO_2 exceeding 160 mmHg (Roberton and Dahlenburg, 1969).

Clinical examination of the retina to detect arterial constriction as an early sign of excessive oxygen therapy with a risk of RLF is of no value (Baum and Bulpitt, 1970).

PULMONARY OXYGEN TOXICITY (BRONCHOPULMONARY DYSPLASIA)

There is no doubt that pure oxygen, especially at pressures greater than 1 bar, is rapidly toxic to mammalian pulmonary epithelium (Clark and Lambertsen, 1971). In the last seven years there have been many reports of infants with HMD dying with severely damaged lungs showing marked perialveolar fibrosis and bronchial wall damage. This condition, which is histologically different from the appearance of pulmonary oxygen toxicity in normal lungs even when they are artificially ventilated (de Lemos et al, 1969), has been called bronchopulmonary dysplasia. The most striking fact about the published cases of bronchopulmonary dysplasia is that not only were they receiving high concentrations of oxygen, but they initially had very abnormal lungs with severe HMD, and had been ventilated by a *positive* pressure ventilator (Northway, Rosan and Porter, 1967; Hawker, Reynolds and Taghizadeh, 1967; Pusey, MacPherson and Chernick, 1969; Barnes et al, 1969; Becker and Kopper, 1969; Banerjee, Girling and Wigglesworth, 1972; Bryan et al, 1973) at pressures in excess of 30 cmH$_2$O (Hawker et al, 1967; Becker and Koppe, 1969; Barnes et al, 1969). Fatal pulmonary disease of this type is very rare in infants breathing oxygen spontaneously, receiving continuous distending pressure, or receiving negative pressure ventilation (Stern et al, 1970), although some radiological change may occur in survivors of these types of therapy (Shepard et al, 1968). This suggests that it is the high positive inflating pressures applied to lungs already damaged by HMD which cause bronchopulmonary dysplasia. Furthermore, changing the technique of IPPV from a fast respiratory frequency at high pressures, to a slower frequency at lower pressures using positive end expiratory pressure (PEEP) (Herman and Reynolds, 1973) has virtually eliminated bronchopulmonary dysplasia even though high inspired oxygen concentrations are still used (Reynolds and Taghizadeh, 1974). Nevertheless, prolonged inhalation of greater than 60 per cent oxygen probably does cause some degree of histological change (Banerjee et al, 1972), and as such should be avoided as potentially harmful. Inhalation of pure oxygen is particularly inadvisable. Not only is oxygen toxicity more likely but it may also destroy surfactant (Clark and Lambertsen, 1971), and it promotes atelectasis, since all the gas is rapidly absorbed from alveoli which contain only oxygen and no nitrogen. Because of the potential hazards of inspired oxygen concentrations of greater than 60 per cent, they should be avoided if at all possible, *but never at the expense of an arterial Po$_2$ below 55 to 60 mmHg.*

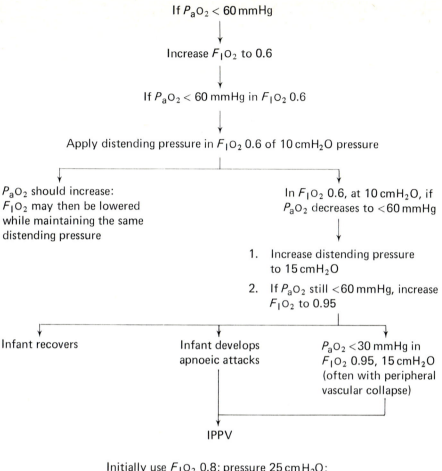

If $P_aO_2 < 60$ mmHg

↓

Increase F_IO_2 to 0.6

↓

If $P_aO_2 < 60$ mmHg in F_IO_2 0.6

↓

Apply distending pressure in F_IO_2 0.6 of 10 cmH$_2$O pressure

P_aO_2 should increase:
F_IO_2 may then be lowered
while maintaining the same
distending pressure

In F_IO_2 0.6, at 10 cmH$_2$O, if
P_aO_2 decreases to <60 mmHg

↓

1.   Increase distending pressure
     to 15 cmH$_2$O

2.   If P_aO_2 still <60 mmHg, increase
     F_IO_2 to 0.95

Infant recovers

Infant develops
apnoeic attacks

P_aO_2 <30 mmHg in
F_IO_2 0.95, 15 cmH$_2$O
(often with peripheral
vascular collapse)

IPPV

Initially use F_IO_2 0.8; pressure 25 cmH$_2$O;
PEEP 5 cmH$_2$O; rate 40/min; I : E ratio 2 : 1

(Avoid pressures > 30 cmH$_2$O if at all possible)

Figure 1   Management of oxygen therapy in an infant with HMD (F_{IO2} 0.6 or 0.95 = inspired O_2 concentrations of 60 or 95 per cent)

Management of oxygen therapy

The management of oxygen therapy is outlined in Fig. 1, and is based on having blood gas analyses at least four hourly. Sufficient oxygen is administered to keep the P_aO_2 in the range 60–90 mmHg. Once oxygen concentrations greater than 60 per cent are required, continuous distending pressure is used.

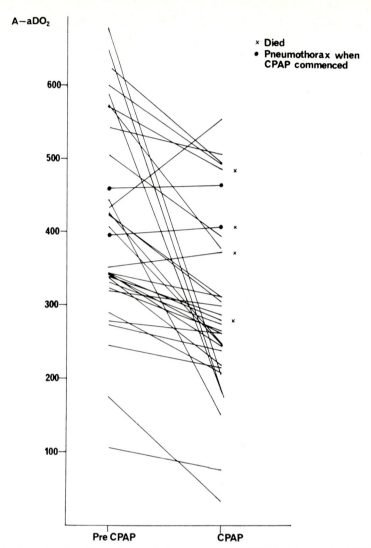

Figure 2   A−a Do_2 (mmHg) before and after commencing CDP in infants with RDS (from Baum and Roberton, 1974). A fall in the alveolar–arterial oxygen difference means improved oxygenation

(a) CONTINUOUS DISTENDING PRESSURE (CDP), CONTINUOUS POSITIVE AIRWAYS PRESSURE (CPAP)

The use of this technique, since it was first described by Gregory et al (1971), has been a major advance in the therapy of HMD. Many reports, including two controlled trials (Fanaroff et al, 1973; Rhodes and Hall, 1973) have shown that CDP improves arterial oxygenation in the vast majority of infants to whom it has been applied (Fig. 2). The technique has been fully reviewed recently (Chernick, 1973). The P_aO_2 improves immediately CDP is applied (Goddard et al, 1974) (Fig. 3), though the mechanism of this rise is not fully understood. Although there is an instantaneous improvement in the regularity of respiration (Speidel and Dunn, 1975) (Fig. 3), there is a deterioration in lung mechanics, with a fall in tidal volume, ventilation and compliance, and an increase in total resistance (airways plus CDP apparatus) and thus in the work of breathing. The functional residual capacity is usually

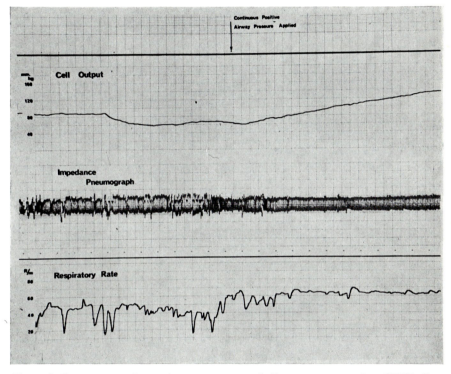

Figure 3 Improvement in respiratory pattern and P_aO_2 on commencing CPAP. P_aO_2 continuously recorded using an indwelling probe (Goddard et al, 1974). Time marked in minutes

increased (Gregory et al, 1971; Bancalari, Garcia and Jesse, 1973; Yu, Rolfe and Roberton, 1975). It seems likely that the improvement in P_aO_2 is due to this increase in functional residual capacity and a reduction in the right to left physiological shunt at pulmonary level (Chernick, 1973; Bancalari et al, 1973).

CDP can be applied in various ways: using a head box (Gregory et al, 1971; Dunn, 1974) or bag (Barrie, 1973), an endotracheal tube (Gregory et al, 1971), a negative pressure chamber (Fanaroff et al, 1973), a face mask (Rhodes and Hall, 1973), or nasal prongs (Kattwinkel et al, 1973). Pressures greater than 10 cmH₂O are rarely required, though levels up to 15 cmH₂O have been used successfully.

The systems listed all have individual problems of application. With the head box, access to the infant's head is impossible, oral feeding is unsafe and extraction of the baby for resuscitation can be difficult. Vert, Andre and Sibout (1973) have suggested that the tight neck seal may cause a raised intracranial venous pressure and thus intraventricular haemorrhage, though this has not been our experience (Baum and Roberton, 1974). Local injury from the neck seal may occur (Turner, Evans and Brown, 1975; Krauss and Marshall, 1975).

With the negative pressure chamber, the problems are the reverse. Access to the head is good, but access to the trunk for clinical or radiological assessment is impossible without discontinuing CDP.

The use of an endotracheal tube has recognised hazards, such as obstruction, infection and laryngeal damage, and should preferably be avoided except when distending pressure is needed to wean an infant off positive pressure ventilation, or when long-term distending pressure is used as in the treatment of pulmonary oedema (Roberton, 1974).

In a comparison of distending pressure given by tube, negative pressure box, or face mask, Olinsky, MacMurray and Swyer (1973) found no difference in survival between the three groups, though infants receiving distending pressure by endotracheal tube had the tube in situ and received therapy for a longer period than the other two groups.

Nasal prongs and face masks have the obvious advantage of allowing free access to all parts of the infant, without the hazards of endotracheal tubes. Initial experience with these techniques have been very encouraging and suggests that they may prove to be the optimal way of applying CDP.

There are few complications of CDP. Bronchopulmonary dysplasia does not occur (Baum and Roberton, 1974). Pneumothorax may occur in up to 24 per cent of cases (Chernick, 1973). This is higher than the incidence of pneumothorax in spontaneously breathing cases of HMD, but lower than that in infants being ventilated with the addition of PEEP (Berg et al, 1975). Cystic changes may occur in the lungs (Fig. 4); they resolve spontaneously. Applying distending pressure to the lungs could theoretically have two other effects. Firstly, it could result in CO_2 retention, but we did not find this. Secondly, it could impede venous return to the heart as does intermittent positive pressure ventilation (Morgan et al, 1966), and thus lower the cardiac output and blood pressure. What information there is on cardiovascular function during distending pressure (Gregory et al, 1971; Yu, Rolfe and Roberton, 1975) has not shown it to have any deleterious effect during the severe phase of the illness.

Hypoventilation and cardiovascular changes with distending pressure are probably minimised in HMD by the applied pressure being contained by the abnormal lungs (Chernick, 1973). However, if CDP is applied to the lungs of an infant with normal compliance, considerable hypoventilation and CO_2 retention can occur (Fig. 5).

When CDP is applied, the P_aO_2 rises (Fig. 2), and it is then usually possible to decrease the inspired oxygen concentration (Fig. 1). However, in many cases after an initial decrease in the inspired oxygen requirement, more oxygen is required as the disease progresses. The oxygen concentration is

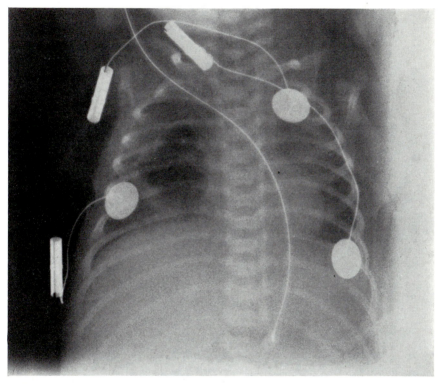

Figure 4 Cystic change in right lung of an infant receiving CDP. The cysts had cleared spontaneously within seven days

then increased to 90 per cent if necessary and pressures up to 15 cmH$_2$O used so long as the infant continues to breathe spontaneously. This appears to be less harmful to the infant, and in particular to his lungs, than intubating him and commencing IPPV. When discontinuing CDP, first the oxygen concentration is reduced to less than 60 per cent, and then the pressures are gradually reduced. These infants are remarkably sensitive to very low pressures, and discontinuing CDP from a level of 2 to 3 cmH$_2$O can cause considerable deterioration in oxygenation (Baum and Roberton, 1974) (Fig. 6).

(b) POSITIVE PRESSURE VENTILATION

The use of IPPV for treating HMD in low birthweight infants has become increasingly successful in recent years. In Oxford, 60 per cent of infants with HMD who require IPPV survive (Table 5). When using IPPV the infant is ventilated initially as recommended by Reynolds (1975). High concentrations of oxygen are administered at a respiratory frequency of 30 to 40/min, and an inflating pressure of 25 cmH$_2$O water with a positive and expiratory

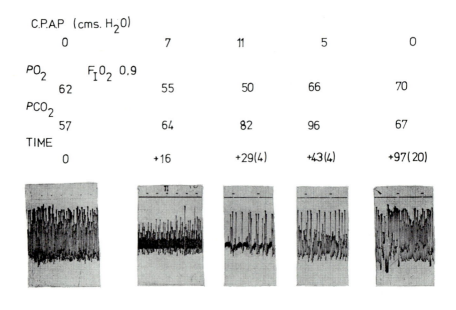

AH ♀ 702041

Figure 5 Effect of CDP on an infant with normally compliant lungs. Time in minutes: time 0, just before CDP applied, and 16, 29, 43 and 97 min later. Values in brackets are minutes elapsed since CDP pressure change. Blood gas measurements (mmHg) were taken at these times, and the respiratory patterns are shown in the tracings. As CPAP increases, Pco_2 increases and respiratory excursion decreases

pressure (PEEP) of 5 cmH$_2$O of water, and an inspiratory/expiratory (I/E) ratio of 2:1. Only ventilators which are capable of this degree of control of pressure, rate, PEEP and I/E ratio should be used for HMD. These initial settings are satisfactory for maintaining adequate oxygenation in most infants with HMD.

It is my practice to try to keep the ventilator pressure less than 30 cmH$_2$O and the oxygen concentration less than 60 per cent. However, if at these settings adequate P_aO_2 levels cannot be achieved by variation in PEEP or I/E ratio, the oxygen concentration may be increased up to 90 per cent, in preference to inflating pressures greater than 30 cmH$_2$O, since it is pressure more than oxygen which causes bronchopulmonary dysplasia (see above).

Infants with HMD do not suffer significant cardiovascular effects from these ventilator settings, apart from a slight lowering of blood pressure. However, it is important to maintain the infant's blood volume and haematocrit by transfusions whenever necessary. Naso-endotracheal tubes are used

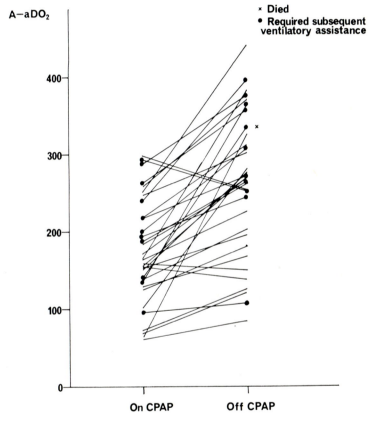

Figure 6   A$-$a Do$_2$ (mmHg) when CPAP discontinued in infants recovering from RDS. The increasing alveolar–arterial oxygen differences indicated deteriorating oxygenation

for long-term ventilation, but peroral tubes are adequate for 24 to 48 h of therapy. A snugly fitting endotracheal tube is important. I have seen infants receiving inflation pressures greater than 35 cmH$_2$O, remain inadequately ventilated due to a large leak round the tube. It is easier to ventilate infants when a larger endotracheal tube is used, such tubes are less likely to slip down into a mainstem bronchus, and lower pressures can be used. I try never to use an endotracheal tube smaller than 3 mm diameter or a French gauge 12, and prefer to use a 3.5 mm diameter or a French gauge 14 tube; these have not caused laryngeal or subglottic stenosis. Furthermore, large tubes make endotracheal suction easier. If the infants have retained secretions, suction may be required every 15 to 30 min, whereas in the early stages of HMD, when secretions are rarely a problem, four to six hourly suction is all that is required. Seriously ill infants deteriorate very rapidly during endotracheal suction and should always be connected to a heart rate monitor or a continuous P_aO_2 monitor during the procedure. If the heart rate drops by more than 25 per cent, or the P_aO_2 to below 40 mmHg, suction should be discontinued, and IPPV recommenced.

(c) INDICATIONS FOR VENTILATION

In the infant with HMD, the major indication for IPPV is apnoea. There is rarely any need to ventilate an infant because of deranged blood gas values;

Table 5   Ventilator survivors, United Oxford Hospitals, July 1972 to December 1973

Diagnosis	Ventilated	Survived	% Survival
RDS	39	23	58.9
Birth asphyxia	9	2	22.2
Extreme prematurity			
<1.0 kg	9	2	22.2
Infection[a]	8	2[b]	25
Malformation	7	—	—
Recurrent apnoea	2	2	100
Miscellanea[c]	3	—	—
Total	77	31	40.3

[a] 2 group B beta-haemolytic streptococci, 2 E. coli, 1 Proteus, 1 Pseudomonas, 1 H. influenzae, 1 negative culture.
[b] Proteus and H. influenzae.
[c] 1 pulmonary haemorrhage, 1 rhesus hydrops, 1 undiagnosed severe haemolytic anaemia.

many such infants survive without requiring IPPV, and CDP makes it possible to improve the oxygenation of infants with severe HMD, without resorting to IPPV. The concept of only ventilating for apnoea is not as drastic as it sounds; the infant maintains adequate blood gases until he suddenly deteriorates, often following some manipulation, and becomes apnoeic. Infants rarely deteriorate to a condition of unremitting cyanosis with irregular gasping respiration. If they do, they are ventilated.

(d) WEANING OFF IPPV

Infants should be ventilated for as short a time as possible. They should not be sedated to prevent them breathing out of phase with the ventilator unless they are so restless that gas exchange is being impeded. Once an infant starts to breathe spontaneously, an attempt is made to try to 'wean' him off IPPV. Should an infant show no signs of breathing spontaneously while on the ventilator at a time when recovery is anticipated, the pressure and rate are gradually lowered to encourage him to make respiratory efforts, until either the blood gases become unsatisfactory, or the infant starts to breathe.

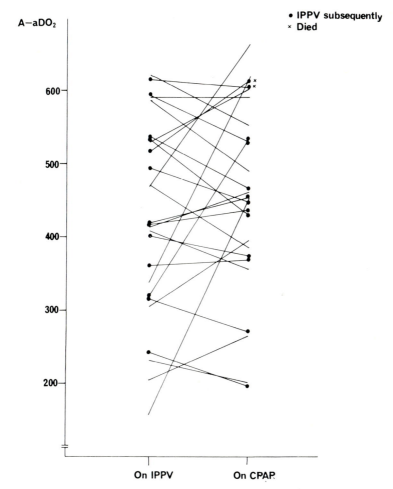

Figure 7 A−a D_{O_2} (mmHg) when changing from IPPV to CDP. In half the cases the A−a D_{O_2} fell indicating that oxygenation *improved*

The use of CDP through the endotracheal tube connected to the ventilator is invaluable in this situation (Baum and Roberton, 1974). Many spontaneously breathing infants cannot maintain an adequate P_aO_2 even in 90 per cent oxygen at atmospheric pressure when IPPV is discontinued, but will do so if CDP is applied. When changing from IPPV to CDP, the P_aO_2 is not only maintained, but in some cases it may rise (Fig. 7). Once the infant is breathing well on CDP and has a normal P_aO_2, the steps shown in Figure 1 are reversed. As always when weaning off CDP, the last few centimetres of pressure must be gradually and carefully discontinued.

(e) OTHER VENTILATOR PROBLEMS

Infection: the routine prophylactic use of antibiotics is unnecessary. Nevertheless, it is important to be constantly on the alert for signs of supervening bacterial infection when an endotracheal tube is in situ and secretions are a problem, or there is an otherwise unexplained clinical deterioration in the infant. In our unit, during 1972 and 1973, 71 per cent of infants with HMD who were ventilated for more than 12 h commenced antibiotics on the first day of IPPV. All infants who required more than three days of IPPV received antibiotics. Only three infants with HMD who were ventilated never received

Table 6   Incidence of suspected infection[a] in infants receiving IPPV for longer than 12 h (United Oxford Hospitals, 1972 to 1973)

	No.	% with +ve cultures
Infants already receiving antibiotics pre IPPV	13	69.2 (9)
Infants starting antibiotics within 12 h of starting IPPV	19	63.1 (12)
Infants starting antibiotics after 12 h IPPV (max. 84 h)	10	90 (9)
Infants not receiving antibiotics on IPPV	3	33 (1)
Total	45	68.9 (31)

[a] Infection is defined as a positive culture from either the tip of the endotracheal tube or from secretions aspirated up the tube.

any antibiotics, and all of these died within 36 h of being ventilated. One of these had a pneumococcal septicaemia (Table 6).

Pneumothorax: when IPPV and PEEP are used, up to 40 per cent of cases will develop an air leak (Berg et al, 1975). If an infant on IPPV deteriorates suddenly without obvious cause such as mechanical respirator failure or a blocked tube, the development of a pneumothorax should be assumed until proved otherwise by chest x-ray. Clinical signs of pneumothorax in this situation are rarely helpful.

General supportive measures

Blood pressure and blood volume: there is considerable evidence that the mortality rate from HMD is less in premature infants who have had delayed clamping of the umbilical cord and received a placental transfusion (Moss and Monset-Couchard, 1967; Usher et al, 1971), though not all authorities agree (Yao and Lind, 1974). There is, however, good evidence that critically ill neonates with systolic blood pressures of less than 40 mmHg have a bad prognosis (Hall and Oliver, 1971; Alden et al, 1972). A falling pressure during the course of the disease may also indicate hypoxia or a blood volume deficit, and carries a bad prognosis if untreated (Stahlman et al, 1972). I have a strong clinical impression that infants with HMD, especially if receiving CDP or IPPV, deteriorate if the haematocrit falls below 40 per cent. For these reasons, blood pressure is continuously monitored and frequent (four to six hourly) haematocrits are done on all sick infants, particularly those weighing less than 1500 g. Frequent transfusions are given to keep the haematocrit greater than 40 per cent and the systolic blood pressure greater than 40 mmHg. Abnormal haematocrit and blood pressure values are also corrected as quickly as possible in the first hour or two of life. Transfusion—by slow infusion of 5 to 10 ml of fresh blood—must be given at haematocrits of 40 per cent. At haematocrits less than this heart failure may be precipitated when a transfusion is given to an already stressed circulation; a single volume exchange transfusion of packed cells is a much safer way of raising the haematocrit if it has inadvertently fallen to values below 35 per cent. The work of

Table 7   Incidence of hypocalcaemia (<3.0 mEq/litre) in infants with pulmonary disease

	Hypocalcaemia <3.0	Ca >3.0
Severe pulmonary disease (requiring IPPV or CPAP)	41	35
Pulmonary disease RDS (without IPPV or CPAP)	10	46

$\chi^2 = 16.22$; $P > 0.001$.

Delivoria-Papadopoulos, Roncevic and Oski (1971) on the levels of 2,3-diphosphoglycerate in adult and fetal blood provides a further reason for giving frequent transfusions of adult cells, though we have not used exchange transfusion routinely in the management of low birthweight infants with HMD as they recommend.

Fluid and electrolyte balance: there is often a marked variability in plasma sodium (but not potassium) in infants receiving theoretically appropriate electrolyte supplements in oral feeding or intravenous infusions. For this reason electrolytes should be checked daily in all seriously ill infants with HMD, especially those on IPPV or receiving intravenous fluids.

Hypocalcaemia: first and second day hypocalcaemia is very common in infants with severe HMD. This may be related to infusions of base (Radde et al, 1972), asphyxia and hypoxia (Tsang and Oh, 1970) or even the calciuretic effect of frusemide or other diuretics used (Savage et al, 1975). Values below 3 mEq/litre are common in the sick infant (Roberton and Smith, 1975) (Table 7). Some infants are asymptomatic, but others are extremely irritable and 'jittery' and difficult to ventilate. Hypocalcaemia may also be of importance in causing recurrent apnoea (Gershanik, Levkoff and Duncan, 1972). We give calcium gluconate supplements to all such infants whose serum calcium falls to 3 mEq/litre. It is interesting to speculate whether such low calcium levels play a role in causing the ductus arteriosus to stay patent, since Kovalčik (1963) showed that the ability of the guinea-pig ductus arteriosus to constrict in response to oxygen was abolished in a calcium free medium.

Diuretics: there are theoretical grounds for using diuretics in HMD; there is marked pulmonary interstitial oedema and frusemide, as well as being diuretic, may improve pulmonary oedema by direct vascular effects (Dikshit et al, 1973). However, in a small study of its use in HMD, there was no improvement in blood gases in the first 24 h in infants who received the drug (Savage et al, 1975). It caused a marked diuresis of calcium and sodium, though the calcium excretion was insufficient to account for the degree of fall in serum calcium level in the first 48 h of life.

Steroids: there is no place for postnatal corticosteroid therapy as a surfactant inducer. This does not improve survival in HMD (Baden et al, 1972), and may increase the incidence of intraventricular haemorrhage (Taeusch et al, 1973b). Furthermore, infants with HMD have high circulating cortisol levels (Reynolds 1973).

Disorders of blood coagulation: it is now fashionable to implicate consumption coagulopathy (disseminated intravascular coagulation (DIC)) in many disease states. Although it has been suggested that DIC plays a part in the aetiology of HMD or its complications (Markarian et al, 1971a, b), other studies do not confirm this (Chessells and Wigglesworth, 1972). Infants who do show evidence of consumption coagulapathy have other aetiological factors such as hypothermia, asphyxia or hypoglycaemia (Ekelund and Finnstrom, 1972), or the coagulation abnormality is the result, and not the cause, of the haemorrhage.

Feeding

Infants suffering from HMD are usually premature. The importance of adequate early feeding in such infants at a time of maximum brain growth is increasingly recognised (Dobbing, 1974). Calories are required not only for this purpose, but also to minimise the risk of hypoglycaemia and jaundice in the first few days of life (Smallpeice and Davies, 1964). Cornblath (1969) showed an increased mortality associated with the use of gastrostomy feeding, and many infants with HMD tolerate hourly feeds of human breast milk through a fine indwelling nasogastric tube. However, gavage feeding is not without its hazards; there may be a fall in arterial P_aO_2 (Wilkinson and Yu, 1974) or an increased frequency of severe apnoeic attacks (Roberton, unpublished data). We have not tried naso-jejunal feeding, which also has its complications (Heird, 1974), and if gavage feeds are not tolerated we have found intragastric drip feeding of expressed breast milk to prove a satisfactory alternative in very low birthweight infants.

The more severely ill infants with HMD develop an ileus (Dunn, 1963), and oral feeding is not tolerated. When this occurs, intravenous fluids are required. In the short term 10 per cent dextrose with appropriate electrolyte supplements is adequate (Sinclair et al, 1970), but intravenous feeding regimens (Shaw, 1973) in sick infants are being increasingly used. However, these techniques have considerable attendant hazards, and require scrupulous attention to detail. When to use them to best advantage in infants with HMD is as yet unresolved. There is no place, at the moment at least, for their routine use, either to supplement or replace oral feeding.

Persistent Ductus Arteriosus

In the last five years a number of severely affected cases of HMD have been described, whose clinical condition and blood gases deteriorated further during the second week of their illness. They were usually receiving some form of intermittent positive pressure ventilation (Siassi et al, 1969; Kitterman et al, 1972). They developed cardiomegaly, clinical and radiological signs of pulmonary oedema, bounding pulses and a systolic murmur in the pulmonary area suggesting a widely patent ductus arteriosus. They probably represent the severest end of the spectrum of infants with patent ductus arteriosus described by Girling and Hallidie-Smith (1971), many of whom had not had HMD, and only five of whom required any therapy for heart failure. The high incidence of patent ductus arteriosus in the very sick premature infant is probably due to several factors: persisting elevation of the right heart pressure (Chu et al, 1967), inhibition of ductus-closure by hypoxia particularly in the premature (McMurphy et al, 1972) and perhaps even the presence of hypocalcaemia (Kovalčik, 1963).

Many such infants respond adequately to conventional therapy, including long-term continuous positive airways pressure (Roberton, 1974), plus digoxin and diuretics (Krovetz and Rowe, 1972). A more heroic surgical approach has been recommended for the seriously ill child (Kitterman et al, 1972). The operative mortality rate is high in severely affected infants, and many of the milder cases operated on would probably survive with conventional therapy for left ventricular failure, since even in the cases requiring long-term CDP, the prognosis for spontaneous closure of the ductus arteriosus is good. Although operative closure often results in a more rapid recovery, it is a matter of judgement in individual centres whether the risks of several weeks' CDP are greater than the risks of general anaesthesia and thoracotomy. The use of high oxygen tensions to close the ductus (Dunn and Speidel, 1973) must remain controversial, because of the high risk of retrolental fibroplasia in these very low birthweight infants.

RDS Variants

There have been attempts to separate off the mild, short duration respiratory illness seen usually in mature infants. (Transient tachypnoea of the newborn—Avery, Gatewood and Brumley, 1966; Type II RDS—Sundell et al, 1971; Benign respiratory distress—Taylor, Allen and Stinson, 1971). By definition the infants survive and there are no postmortem data. Laryngeal washings have a normal lecithin/sphingomyelin ratio (Barr, Jenkins and Baum, 1975). The x-ray findings are unremarkable, or suggest 'wet' lungs (Kuhn, Fletcher and De Lemos, 1969). Such infants are probably suffering from a mixture of birth asphyxia with metabolic acidaemia, non-meconium aspiration syndromes and delayed clearing of the intrapulmonary fluid. Clinically they merge into, and are impossible to differentiate from, the more typical forms of these diseases and from HMD.

Persistence of the transitional circulation

This undoubtedly seems to be a genuine variant, different from the entity of severe HMD in full-term infants (Roberton et al, 1967). In some cases it is contributed to by hyperviscosity (Fouron and Hébert, 1973), but in others it is idiopathic (Gersony, 1973). The infant is deeply cyanosed, with an arterial Po_2 less than 40 mmHg whilst breathing 100 per cent oxygen, even on IPPV (Brown and Pickering, 1974). Should he die the usual abnormality found is a widely patent ductus arteriosus and foramen ovale. The lungs usually look surprisingly normal on chest x-ray and at postmortem, though there may be small areas of haemorrhage and aspiration. The heart sounds are normal, murmurs are absent, and the pulses are unremarkable. The picture mimics cyanotic congenital heart disease, and these infants may be investigated by cardiac catheterisation and angiocardiography. At some stage during the first 24 h, they suddenly improve, become pink and remain normal thereafter. Occasionally, when they have not improved spontaneously in the first 24 h, exchange transfusions have been carried out using fresh adult blood in the hope that the higher P_{50} (Delivoria-Papadopoulos et al, 1971) will improve oxygenation of the ductus arteriosus to induce it to constrict (Brown and Pickering, 1974). Other than this form of treatment, expectant management in high oxygen concentrations is required. I know of no attempts to use hyperbaric oxygen in such infants.

Mortality Rate in HMD

An overall mortality rate of 25 to 30 per cent was usually quoted in the 1960s (Roberton et al, 1968). The recent advances in neonatal intensive care described here have undoubtedly resulted in a considerable reduction in the mortality from HMD, though it is difficult to identify which components of the treatment outlined above are responsible for this. Comparisons of mortality rates in hyaline membrane disease over different periods in time and between different units are of little value. Not only are there differences in the diagnostic criteria for HMD—particularly at the mild end of the spectrum —and variable exclusion of infants weighing less than 1 kg in the reported series, but neonatal units dealing with a large number of babies referred from other hospitals will always have a higher mortality rate from HMD than units dealing with 'inborn' babies only. Nevertheless, it is clear that the mortality rate has fallen. Our own figures for HMD are given in Tables 4 and 8. It can be seen that there is an overall mortality now of 10 per cent. If only infants who establish adequate spontaneous respiration at birth are considered, the mortality rate is approximately 5 per cent, and death is usually due to recognised complications of the disease (Table 8). However, infants in respiratory failure and requiring IPPV from the moment of birth have a 50 per cent mortality. Dunn (1974) has reported similar findings. Infants with hyaline membrane disease who breathe spontaneously but eventually deteriorate and require IPPV have a much better survival rate (Table 5).

It is therefore reasonable to give a mortality rate of about 5 per cent for hyaline membrane disease in low birthweight infants weighing more than 1000 g provided adequate respirations are established at birth. There is still

Table 8 Mortality rate from HMD (United Oxford Hospitals, 1972 to 1973)

	No.	Dead	% Deaths
HMD breathing spontaneously from birth	133	7[a]	5.3
HMD in respiratory failure from birth	16	8	50
Total HMD	149	15	10

[a] Additional cause of death

Pneumothorax	3
Intraventricular haemorrhage	2
H. influenzae septicaemia	1

a high mortality rate in those rare infants in respiratory failure from birth. This group provides a major challenge to further improvements in perinatal and neonatal care.

Sequelae of HMD

There are two potential sequelae for low birthweight infants surviving HMD. Firstly there is the risk of brain damage in low birthweight infants who suffered neonatal hypoxia and acidaemia. The more recent surveys of such infants (Davies and Stewart, 1975) show that they are surviving with a very low incidence of cerebral palsy and handicap, and an intelligence quotient compatible with their social background. Although most infants survive with normal lungs there is an increased risk of long-term pulmonary sequelae in infants who have been ventilated and have had severe bronchopulmonary dysplasia. This will be discussed fully in the section on chronic lung disease of prematurity.

ASPIRATION SYNDROMES

These develop after inhalation of amniotic fluid, particularly if it contains blood or meconium. Although the fetus makes regular respiratory movements in utero (Boddy and Dawes, 1975), these do not result in amniotic fluid being drawn into the lungs which are filled with a fluid actively secreted by the pulmonary alveolar epithelium, and having a totally different chemical composition from liquor amnii (Olver, Reynolds and Strang, 1972). However, if asphyxiated in utero the fetus may gasp and aspirate the amniotic fluid or its contents. If asphyxiated during delivery, the infant may also gasp and inhale either liquor or liquid contents of the birth canal such as antiseptic creams or maternal faeces.

Table 3 shows the incidence of aspiration syndromes in the United Oxford Hospitals in 1972 to 1973. They were responsible for 12 per cent of pulmonary disease in the unit, and occurred in 0.5 per cent of all births. Most cases were mild; in only eight instances were the infants sick enough for umbilical artery catheterisation to be indicated. No infant required IPPV, and none died. This disease seems to be more common in North America (Leake, Gunther and Sunshine, 1974; Gregory et al, 1974). Swyer (1969) was able to describe 95 cases over a 22 month period, of whom 28 required IPPV, and of these only six survived.

The illness which follows aspiration depends on the maturity of the infant and what is aspirated. In premature infants meconium aspiration is rare since the fetus rarely passes meconium in utero before 36 weeks (Desmond et al, 1957); asphyxia and aspiration result in HMD developing. In term infants, aspiration of substances other than meconium causes tachypnoea shortly after birth, with non-specific x-ray changes. It may be difficult to differentiate from mild HMD, and from infants hyperventilating with acidaemia due to asphyxia.

Meconium aspiration is the most severe type of aspiration syndrome, and the severity of the illness is related to the amount of meconium aspirated. The disease is most likely to develop when meconium is seen in the airway on direct laryngoscopy after delivery and is inhaled before it can be sucked out (Gregory et al, 1974). Of the 39 cases of aspiration syndrome in a two year period (Table 3) only 11 were due to meconium aspiration. The severe pulmonary illness is characterised by chemical pneumonitis and air trapping beyond the sticky meconium in the lower airways. The x-ray shows overdistended lungs, with areas of patchy atelectasis. Neither pneumomediastinum nor pneumothorax occurred in the infants referred to in Table 3, though these are frequent complications and facilities for urgent thoracentesis should always be available for an infant with meconium aspiration.

The incidence of aspiration syndromes can be minimised by careful clearing of foreign substances from the mouth and oropharynx of the infant immediately after delivery. In those cases where meconium is present, this is best done at direct laryngoscopy. If aspiration occurs, the infant is treated according to the routine supportive care outlined for HMD. When meconium was present in the oropharynx, antibiotics and perhaps steroids should be used. Bryan (1967) has shown that meconium enhances bacterial infection in rat lungs. Steroids have been suggested (Avery and Fletcher, 1974) on the grounds that meconium causes an irritant chemical pneumonitis, though there is no proof of their efficacy in this condition and I rarely use them.

PERIODIC BREATHING AND APNOEIC ATTACKS

This subject is of both practical and theoretical interest: practical because of the relationship between period breathing, apnoeic attacks and intra-ventricular haemorrhage—a major cause of death in low birthweight infants (Fedrick and Butler, 1970); theoretical, because of analogies between the patterns of fetal respiratory movements in utero, periodic breathing and apnoea postnatally, and the sudden infant death syndrome.

Pauses in respiration of varying duration are frequent in low birthweight infants. They may be very transient, lasting a few seconds only, and end spontaneously, or last for a minute or longer and end only after physical stimulation or IPPV. The pauses may be symptomatic of serious underlying disease, though they commonly develop in otherwise well, low birthweight infants from the fourth to the fifth day of life. It is a matter of definition when a short pause in respiration ceases to be part of the spectrum of periodic breathing, and becomes an apnoeic attack.

Periodic Breathing

Periodic breathing is usually defined as episodes of apnoea lasting more than 3 s, and less than 10 s (Rigatto and Brady, 1972a; Fenner et al, 1973), without cyanosis and with no or minimal alteration in the heart rate and blood pressure (Girling, 1972). It is a normal physiological variant found during rapid eye movement sleep in adults (Webb, 1974) and the newborn (Parmelee et al, 1967). It occurs most frequently in the very premature infant (Fenner et al, 1973), in whom it does not develop until 24 to 48 h of age (Chernick, Heldrich and Avery, 1964; Fenner et al, 1973), or later (Rigatto and Brady, 1972a).

The cause of periodic breathing is unknown. Chernick et al (1964) and Fenner et al (1973) documented hypocapnia, whereas Rigatto and Brady (1972a, b) found an increased $P\text{co}_2$, with a shift to the right in the CO_2 response curve. However, most authors agree that it is abolished by inhalation of carbon dioxide enriched gas (up to 4 per cent), or by increasing the inspired oxygen concentration (Wilson, Long and Howard, 1942; Chernick et al, 1964; Rigatto and Brady, 1972a, b; Fenner et al, 1973).

Periodic breathing probably represents 'hunting' by the immature nervous system in response to the general sensory and chemoreceptor input from arterial Po_2 and Pco_2. As a result the oscillatory control mechanisms of respiration in the infant becomes so pronounced that apnoea may result (Hathorn, 1972).

So long as periodic breathing does not develop into apnoeic attacks causing heart rate changes and cyanosis (Daily, Klaus and Meyer, 1969), it is harmless, and there is no need to treat it.

Apnoeic Attacks

These are defined as periods of respiratory arrest lasting longer than 30 s and usually associated with cyanosis and cardiovascular changes. Prolonged

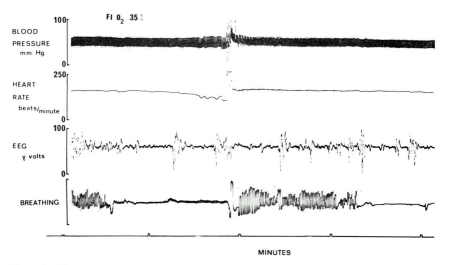

Figure 8 Two prolonged apnoeic attacks. In the first there is only a minor degree of brady-cardia after nearly 90 s and in the second respirations restarted at the end of the trace

apnoeic attacks develop in two distinct circumstances in premature infants. Firstly, well, premature infants who have usually been breathing periodically, develop longer and longer periods of apnoea, which may or may not be associated with their heart rate changes. Secondly, apnoeic episodes develop as an indication of serious underlying disease, such as HMD, hypoglycaemia, septicaemia or even minor seizures. Most commonly they are associated with HMD (Girling, 1972), when they have a grave prognosis often indicating an intracranial haemorrhage. This type of attack develops earlier in life than periodic breathing and may persist for at least two weeks (Daily et al, 1969). It is not known whether these two types of apnoeic attack have similar causes and mechanisms.

A wide variety of cardiovascular responses occur during the attacks. In otherwise healthy, small, preterm infants there may be no cardiovascular changes even during attacks lasting 30 to 40 s, or there may be a gradual fall in heart rate and a rise in blood pressure at the end of an attack, or even a rapidly developing reflex bradycardia and hypertension at the onset of apnoea (Figs. 8, 9). In contrast, more constant and more severe cardiovascular changes tend to occur during apnoeic attacks in infants with severe hyaline membrane disease. Girling (1972) observed three patterns: (a) no change in heart rate or blood pressure in 6 out of 47 attacks; (b) a falling heart rate and increasing blood pressure in 22 out of the 47 attacks; (c) a falling heart rate and falling blood pressure in 19 instances.

In infants with HMD, Daily et al (1969) described changes of type (b) with occasional transient increases in the heart rate at the start of an apnoeic attack.

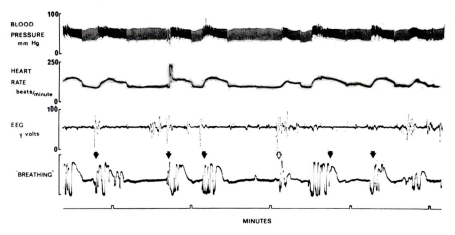

Figure 9 Frequent short apnoeic attacks with reflex bradycardia. Solid arrows indicate spontaneous end to an apnoeic attack, while the open arrows indicate its termination following peripheral stimulation

The prolonged apnoeic attacks in healthy infants can occur in either phase of sleep, and at normal blood gas tensions, but there are no comparable data available on the apnoeic attacks in serious illness described by Girling (1972). However, it is tempting to speculate that his group (a) were not hypoxic even during the attack, that group (b) were responding to asphyxia and hypoxia with hypertension and reflex bradycardia and group (c) were seriously ill infants with impending cardiovascular collapse. 'Healthy' pre-term infants having prolonged apnoeic attacks usually respond to gentle peripheral stimulation by starting to breathe, and are a group where a care-fully controlled increase of 2 to 4 per cent in the inspired oxygen concentra-tion is justified to decrease the number of prolonged attacks. The mechanism by which this works is not understood since severe apnoeic attacks may develop with normal arterial blood gas tensions (Roberton, 1974, unpublished observations). It is very important that these infants are not treated by high inspired oxygen concentrations during and after the apnoea. High $F_{I}O_2$ in infants with normal lungs results in very high P_aO_2 values and it is infants with recurrent apnoea, not those with severe HMD, who have recently been found to have developed retrolental fibroplasia (Mushin, 1971).

If the infant who has a prolonged apnoeic attack does not start to breathe after peripheral stimulation, the apnoeic attack should be terminated by inflating the lungs (using a bag and mask or endotracheal tube) with the gas mixture he was breathing before the apnoeic attack. Should the apnoeic attacks become so frequent that positive pressure ventilation is required, these infants' normal lungs can be ventilated easily, at low pressures and at low oxygen concentrations. Bronchopulmonary dysplasia does not develop, and the mortality rate is low (Reid and Mitchell, 1966).

Infants in whom apnoeic attacks develop as a symptom of serious illness, for instance HMD, as in Girling's groups (a) and (b), also respond initially to peripheral stimulation. However, Girling's group (c) infants needed active resuscitation (intubation and ventilation) in 7 out of 19 apnoeic attacks. If such infants do not establish spontaneous respiration after an apnoeic attack, IPPV is necessary and even when apnoea is due to deterioration in HMD the prognosis is reasonably good (Table 5).

Environmental temperature and apnoea

Perlstein and his co-workers (1970) showed that increasing the environmental temperature to greater than 36.6°C was associated with a raised body temperature and an increased incidence of apnoeic attacks. Also, apnoea occurred more often at 36.8°C compared with 36.0°C in the series described by Daily et al (1969). It may be that mild cooling is part of the sensory input required to maintain the respiratory drive in low birthweight infants, and that this is removed by increasing the environmental temperature.

Relationship of neonatal apnoea to fetal breathing

It is known that fetal respiratory movements occur during periods of rapid eye movements and EEG activity, and that fetal 'apnoea' occurs when there are no eye movements and comparative quiet on the EEG (Boddy and Dawes, 1975). During rapid eye movement (REM) sleep, the newborn behaves like the fetus, with irregular but persistent breathing of regular periodicity (Hathorn, 1972) and continuous EEG activity. In non-REM sleep the EEG is periodic in the human newborn, but respiration is very regular. However, should apnoea develop at such a time the infant tends to revert to the fetal pattern, and the apnoea may persist (Roberton, 1974, unpublished data).

Relationship of apnoeic attacks to intraventricular haemorrhage (IVH)

Very low birthweight infants who develop intraventricular haemorrhage usually present with a run of severe apnoeic attacks. It is not clear whether the intraventricular haemorrhage causes the apnoeic attacks or vice versa. However, during a prolonged apnoeic attack there is a rise in blood pressure and progressive acidaemia and hypoxia which increase the already marked capillary fragility in premature infants. The surge in blood pressure may be transmitted directly to the vascular zona germinativa over the basal ganglia, resulting in rupture of the arteries or capillaries and, aggravated by the haemorrhagic tendency produces a massive haemorrhage into the lateral ventricles (Hambleton and Wigglesworth, 1975). Such infants usually die, though a small number survive after IPPV, and develop post-haemorrhagic hydrocephalus (Larroche, 1972).

There is no specific treatment for IVH once it has occurred. However, by prevention of conditions known to cause apnoea, and careful monitoring to detect and rapidly terminate such attacks, the chain of events described in the last paragraph may be prevented.

Table 9 Histological diagnosis in cases of pneumonia 1958. Perinatal mortality survey

Pneumonia (total cases)	386
Haemorrhagic pneumonia	83 ⎫
HMD	65 ⎬ 201
IVH	35 ⎪
Extrapulmonary sepsis	18 ⎭

Data from Fedrick and Butler (1971a), *Biologia Neonatorum*, **17**, 458.

PNEUMONIA

Pneumonia in the newborn may be discussed under three headings: intrapartum pneumonia—pulmonary infection acquired in utero or during the infant's passage through the birth canal; postnatally acquired pneumonia presenting during the first week of life; pulmonary infection acquired during positive pressure ventilation using an endotracheal tube.

It is difficult to obtain a true incidence of neonatal pneumonia. Thus, in the 1958 perinatal mortality survey, only 25 per cent of the infants who were found histologically to have pneumonia had been registered as such at death (Federick and Butler, 1971a). The incidence of fatal neonatal pneumonia was 2.84 per 1000 live births. There were 386 cases; in 201 of these some other condition was found on histological examination of the lungs (Table 9).

In the 1970 Registrar General's annual report for England and Wales, 195 early neonatal deaths were attributed by certification to pneumonia (0.25/1000 live births). Even if one postulates that the accuracy of certification has not improved compared with the 25 per cent recognition rate of 1958, this still suggests that the incidence of fatal neonatal pneumonia has decreased during the last 12 years, despite the increased use of positive pressure ventilation. The frequency of primary pneumonia in the Oxford Unit is low (Table 3), though many infants who receive IPPV also develop pulmonary infection.

Intrapartum Pneumonia

It is important to distinguish patients in whom pulmonary infection developed during intra-uterine life, from those due to inhalation of infected material during passage through the birth canal. In the former the infant will be ill at birth, whereas in the latter symptoms may not develop for up to 48 h after birth.

True intrapartum pneumonia

These infants present at or soon after delivery with signs of respiratory distress. In many cases it is impossible to differentiate them clinically or radiologically from infants with HMD due to surfactant deficiency since both groups frequently suffer from intrapartum asphyxia. The differential diagnosis can only be surmised on the basis of a history suggestive of systemic or localised infection in the mother, such as a pyrexia of unknown origin, rigors, purulent vaginal discharge or premature rupture of the membranes. Infants with lung disease at birth will have leucocytes in the alveoli. In the majority of cases these do not represent endogenous polymorphs produced by the fetus, but direct invasion of the lung from the infected liquor amnii, or aspiration of this material should the infant have become asphyxiated in utero. This view of the sequence of events in congenital pneumonia is supported by clinical (Davies, 1971) and experimental studies (Lauweryns et al, 1973). In either case, the end result is the presence of infected material in the lungs of a highly susceptible infant who, if he is to survive, must mount his own polymorphonuclear leucocyte and antibody response.

It is much better to prevent this disease than to treat it. Since the likelihood of an infected birth canal and chorioamnionitis increase with the duration of membrane rupture (Federick and Butler, 1971b), the current policy of active management of labour now being pursued by many obstetricians should result in not only a shorter labour and shorter period of membrane rupture, but less chorioamnionitis, and fewer cases of congenital pneumonia. Prophylactic antibiotics are not given routinely to infants born after prolonged rupture of membranes, even when there is a suspicion of chorioamnionitis. Firstly, such a policy has never been shown to be beneficial, and it may even be harmful (Habel et al, 1972). Furthermore, it must be remembered that of the 386 cases of pneumonia dying during the first month of life in the perinatal mortality survey, only 51 had had membranes ruptured for more than 48 h, and 189 had had membranes ruptured for 6 h or less. Even if one only considers infants dying within 48 h of birth, when *congenital* pneumonia was the probable cause of death, 80 out of the 155 deaths had membranes ruptured for less than 6 h.

However, should an infant be born from a potentially infected birth canal, irrespective of the duration of membrane rupture, *and have respiratory difficulty*, then there is no way congenital infection can be excluded, and broad spectrum antibiotics should be given.

Infections caused by bacteria derived from birth canal

There has recently been a marked increase in serious infection due to group B beta-haemolytic streptococci (McCracken, 1973). This may be partially explained by the low level of natural immunity to the organism, plus ineffective phagocytosis of the coccus in many humans (Klesius et al, 1973). The organism is present in the vagina of 5 to 25 per cent of all parturient females. Most infants born to colonised mothers become colonised themselves, but some may acquire the organism from nursery personnel, who are frequently carriers. Most of the infants who become colonised remain asymptomatic, but the reported incidence of symptomatic infection in colonised infants ranges from 1.1 per cent (Baker and Barrett, 1973) to 16.7 per cent (Franciosi, Knostman and Zimmerman, 1973).

Should the infant be infected with group B beta-haemolytic streptococcus of serological subgroup Ia or III, it is most likely to present with an acute respiratory illness within 6 to 12 h of birth (Baker and Barrett, 1973). Alternatively the disease may develop at any time from the second day of life with signs of septicaemia, and the predominant pathological finding is a purulent meningitis (Barton, Feigin and Lins, 1973). The acute pulmonary form of the disease runs a fulminating course. Even if suspected and treated early with penicillin, virtually all infants with subgroup I infection die, but with other group B streptococci including the subgroup III, the mortality rate is lower (46 per cent in the Baker and Barrett series, 1973).

The emergence of this particular infection emphasises the importance of including penicillin G in the antibiotic treatment of all infants with infection in the first 48 h of life. Opinions vary as to treatment of the healthy newborn infant who is found to be colonised with the group B beta-haemolytic streptococcus. The majority of these children remain well, but for the present it is probably wise to give a five day course of oral penicillin.

Postnatally Acquired Pneumonia

An infant, irrespective of gestation, who develops signs of respiratory illness after the first 4 h of life should be regarded as having pneumonia until proved otherwise. It is usually possible to exclude pneumothorax, congenital heart disease, or other intrathoracic disease by clinical examination, chest x-ray and ECG. Infection due to Gram-positive organisms (with the recent exception of the group B beta-haemolytic streptococcus) has been largely eliminated from the newborn nursery by the prevention of umbilical cord sepsis (Gupta et al, 1968), and the use of hexachlorophene for washing the infant and his attendants (Simon, Yaffe and Gluck, 1961). The current pre-eminence of the Gram-negative organisms has been well reviewed by Gotoff and Behrman (1970). It is worth remembering that many infants with bacterial pneumonia may also have septicaemia, and may develop meningitis.

Treatment for postnatally acquired pneumonia should be with penicillin and kanamycin in the first place. Ampicillin has no therapeutic place with this group of infants, since many hospital acquired *E. coli* are now ampicillin resistant (Anderson, Datta and Shaw, 1972). The penicillin and kanamycin regimen would be modified in certain circumstances as follows: (a) cloxacillin in place of, or together with, penicillin if staphylococci are suspected or present, (b) gentamicin for kanamycin if the nursery flora is becoming kanamycin resistant (Anderson et al, 1972; Baker, Barrett and Clark, 1974), (c) gentamicin plus carbenicillin replacing kanamycin if *Pseudomonas aeruginosa* infection is suspected.

Unusual organisms are increasingly being recognised in the newborn nursery. *Haemophilus influenzae*, previously regarded as not a significant pathogen in the newborn, has been described as causing pneumonia (Ingman, 1970), and *Haemophilus parainfluenzae* has also been described (Zinner et al, 1972).

Infection in Association with Endotracheal Intubation and IPPV
(Table 6)

It is our general experience that most infants requiring long-term ventilation for hyaline membrane disease, at some period whilst on the ventilator will develop signs suggesting pulmonary infection, such as: aspiration of infected looking material up the endotracheal tube, and/or positive cultures of the aspirate; radiological changes of collapse/consolidation in which infection cannot be excluded; non-specific signs of infection in the infant, irrespective of his pulmonary symptoms.

In infants who already have severe pulmonary disease due to HMD, it is very important not to overlook coexisting pneumonia. Such infants should receive broad spectrum antibiotics whenever there is a suspicion of infection. Most such infants do indeed have positive bacterial cultures of the aspirates from their endotracheal tubes (Table 6). We use the antibiotics indicated above, and usually give a 10 days' course unless there is a rapid improvement in the infant's condition and the cultures are sterile. At the end of the 10-day course, even though cultures continue to be positive, if the baby is well, the drugs may be discontinued. With an endotracheal tube in situ, Gram-negative organisms including *Pseudomonas* will persist as 'commensals' and do not need to be treated.

Despite the management outlined above, there are still some infants who die on the ventilator and who show evidence at postmortem of serious lung infection.

MASSIVE PULMONARY HAEMORRHAGE (HAEMORRHAGIC PULMONARY OEDEMA)

Many conditions may be associated with small amounts of interstitial pulmonary haemorrhage—such as HMD, pneumonia and pulmonary oxygen toxicity. However, massive pulmonary haemorrhage is a distinct clinical entity in which the infant collapses with blood flowing up his trachea and out of his mouth and nose. Histologically there is massive intra-alveolar haemorrhage. It has been estimated that about one in 1000 liveborn infants die of this condition (Fedrick and Butler, 1971c). Its aetiology is probably multifactorial, being related to severe birth asphyxia (Rowe and Avery, 1966), cold (Mann and Elliot, 1957), rhesus haemolytic disease (Chessells and Wigglesworth, 1971), congenital heart disease (Esterly and Oppenheimer, 1966) and small for dates infants (Fedrick and Butler, 1971b). Many of these babies also have haemostatic failure (Chessells and Wigglesworth, 1971). Cole et al (1973) have postulated that this condition is haemorrhagic pulmonary oedema. The fluid which exudes up the trachea is a mixture of whole blood and a plasma ultrafiltrate, and only rarely has a haematocrit greater than 10 per cent. The normally small pores in fetal lung capillary epithelium are presumably distended for blood to pass through them. Cole et al (1973) postulate that the distension is due to left heart failure and venous congestion. Infants who develop massive pulmonary haemorrhage are often seriously ill, and are likely to have a lowered cardiac output with a raised left atrial pressure causing pulmonary capillary distension and haemorrhage.

Although the condition carries a high mortality (Cole et al, 1973) the concept of haemorrhagic pulmonary oedema encourages approaches similar to those used in pulmonary oedema of other types—particularly the use of positive pressure ventilation (Robin, Cross and Zelis, 1973). Using IPPV, six cases of massive pulmonary haemorrhage have been treated by us in the last year and four have survived (Trompeter et al, 1975).

PNEUMOTHORAX AND PNEUMOMEDIASTINUM

Incidence

These conditions are not rare, but the incidence is difficult to obtain since many infants probably have a pneumothorax which is not detected clinically (Chernick and Reed, 1970). However, an overall incidence for pneumothorax of 1 to 2 per cent has been given (Steele et al, 1971). Perhaps less than 10 per cent of pneumothoraces which are radiologically present cause symptoms, since the incidence of clinically apparent pneumothorax is reported as less than 0.1 per cent (Howie and Weed, 1957). Pneumomediastinum probably occurs more frequently than pneumothorax (Steele et al, 1971), though if it develops in isolation it is probably symptomatic in less than 10 per cent of cases (Morrow, Hope and Boggs, 1967). About 25 per cent of cases of pneumothorax have a coexisting pneumomediastinum (Chernick and Reed, 1970). In addition to such large extrapulmonary collections of air as pneumothorax and pneumomediastinum, it is increasingly recognised that interstitial pulmonary emphysema may occur simultaneously and often precedes the development of these lesions, particularly in cases of HMD (Thibeault et al, 1973). In the United Oxford Hospitals in the last two years there was an incidence of 3.5 pneumothoraces and allied conditions per 1000 live births (Table 10).

Pathology

In the neonatal period many cases of pneumomediastinum and pneumothorax are due to air leaking along the bronchovascular bundles into the mediastinum, and finally rupturing into the pleural cavity (Macklin, 1939).

Table 10   Incidence of symptomatic pneumothorax and pneumomediastinum (United Oxford Hospitals, 1972 to 1973)

Total cases:			
Pneumothorax		25	
Solo pneumomediastinum		4	
Pulmonary cysts		2	
		0.35% of all live births	

	Cases of pneumothorax	Drained	Survived
RDS breathing spontaneously	3	3	2
RDS + CDP/IPPV[a]	8	6	5
Terminal in very low birth weight	2	—	—
Associated with congenital malformation	2	—	—
Solo pneumothorax[a]	10	3	10
Total	25	12	17

[a] One infant in each of these two groups was born outside the United Oxford Hospitals.

The recent work of Stahlman, Cheatham and Gray (1973) showing that interstitial emphysema, particularly in infants receiving high pressure IPPV, is due to rupture into the lymphatic system, is consistent with Macklin's hypothesis. In other cases, rupture of lung subpleurally must also take place (Chernick and Avery, 1963). This is probably more likely to happen in the newborn premature infant who has fewer interalveolar connections through the pores of Kohn (Chernick and Reed, 1970). The pressures required to cause alveolar rupture in the normal neonatal lung are probably in the range of 50 cmH$_2$O or higher (Rosen and Laurence, 1965).

Aetiology

These conditions used to be diagnosed most commonly in the first few hours of life, mainly in infants who presented with respiratory difficulty in the delivery room, or who had the meconium aspiration syndrome (Howie and Weed, 1957; Chernick and Avery, 1963). This group now accounts for only 40 per cent of the pneumothoraces in Oxford (Table 10). The normal infant can generate sufficiently high pressures during spontaneous respiration to cause alveolar rupture (Karlberg et al, 1962), and over-vigorous positive pressure resuscitation of the apnoeic newborn may cause pneumothoraces to develop (Chernick and Avery, 1963; Chernick and Reed, 1970). Hey and Lenney (1973) have shown that many commonly used resuscitation devices give much higher pressures than is indicated on the control. In this way pressures in excess of 50 cmH$_2$O may frequently be delivered.

With the increasing use of positive pressure ventilation as well as CDP in infants with HMD, the incidence of pneumothorax has increased considerably and this may occur at any time during IPPV. As many as 40 per cent of infants on positive pressure ventilation plus PEEP develop signs of an air leak (Berg et al, 1975). There is a lower incidence with CDP alone. In our experience (Baum and Roberton, 1974) 12.1 per cent of infants with HMD receiving CDP develop pneumothoraces. In addition to rupture into the lungs, the air may track into the pericardium or the abdominal cavity (Aranda, Stern and Dunbar, 1972; Singh, Wigglesworth and Stern, 1972).

Signs, Symptoms and Diagnosis

With a pneumomediastinum alone, or a small non-tension pneumothorax, the signs may be minimal or absent (Morrow et al, 1967; Chernick and Reed, 1970). With a pneumothorax it is sometimes possible to detect mediastinal shift or poor air entry to the affected side of the chest and the heart sounds may be muffled with a pneumomediastinum. Infants with a large tension pneumothorax not only show signs of severe respiratory difficulty due to pulmonary collapse, but since the mediastinum is displaced and compressed, the venous return is impaired, cardiac output falls, and the baby becomes cyanosed and hypotensive. Even then it may be difficult clinically to ascribe the collapsed state of the infant to a pneumothorax. A most useful sign in this condition is abdominal distension and rigidity. This does not mean a pneumo-peritoneum; it is due to the pneumothorax pushing down the diaphragm and compressing the intra-abdominal contents. The development of a pneumo-thorax must always be considered in the differential diagnosis of sudden deterioration of an infant receiving IPPV.

The only satisfactory way to diagnose this condition is by x-ray. Since pneumomediastina are often missed on anteroposterior views, any infant with respiratory distress must have a lateral as well as an anteroposterior chest radiograph. It is important to realise that the clinical deterioration, when a pneumothorax develops in an infant with HMD, may appear disproportionate to the initial radiographic abnormality in the AP projection. However, not only does a small quantity of air in the pleural cavity seriously compromise gas exchange in an infant who already has severe pulmonary disease, but a

9

horizontal beam lateral chest x-ray will show that the lungs have collapsed on to the posterior thoracic wall, and that the volume of air in the pleural cavity is quite large (MacEwan et al, 1971).

Treatment

Pneumothorax

If a baby with a pneumothorax is deteriorating rapidly, the chest should be aspirated using a number one needle attached via a three-way tap to a 20 ml syringe. Having thus aspirated the pneumothorax, one must be prepared to insert a chest drain as soon as possible, especially if the condition occurred during IPPV therapy.

In other infants with HMD who develop a pneumothorax, the blood gases deteriorate and even if the infant does not collapse, the pneumothorax should be drained as quickly as possible after radiological confirmation. When a drain is inserted into such a patient it should not only be attached to an underwater seal, but also to 3 to 5 cmH$_2$O negative pressure to keep the lung expanded (Chernick and Reed, 1970).

A pneumothorax may be treated conservatively when an infant does not have deteriorating blood gas values and the pneumothorax is genuinely small on x-ray. This is often the case when the lesion develops in conditions other than HMD (Table 10). After the insertion of an umbilical catheter to monitor blood gases, the infant is kept in as high an oxygen concentration as is felt to be safe in terms of lung and retinal toxicity, in an attempt to speed up the absorption of the pneumothorax by washing out nitrogen (Chernick and Avery, 1963).

Pneumomediastinum

The use of high inspired oxygen concentrations to accelerate nitrogen washout from the interstitial sacs of air is the only possible therapy for pneumomediastina which are usually multilocular in the connective tissue of the mediastinum. Surgical drainage would not be feasible.

Pneumopericardium

This develops when air which has tracked into the mediastinum also ruptures into the pericardial cavity and is trapped there. The air is under pressure and causes cardiac tamponade, with hypotension and a decreased cardiac output. The chest radiograph shows a striking appearance with a ring of air obviously contained within the pericardium and surrounding a cardiac shadow which is normal or even decreased in size. The condition is easily treated by needle aspiration of the pericardial cavity, performed conventionally through the xiphoid route. This usually produces dramatic relief (Singh et al, 1972).

CHRONIC LUNG DISEASE OF PREMATURITY

It is recognised that signs of pulmonary disease may persist in low birth-weight infants who survive serious respiratory illness in the neonatal period. There are three major manifestations of this.

Pulmonary infection

Several studies have shown that infants who survive HMD not only have more frequent chest infections during the first year of life, but when they occur they are more severe and often require assisted ventilation (Shepard et al, 1968). This usually takes the form of severe bronchiolitis with positive cultures for respiratory syncytial virus. The reason for this increased susceptibility to pulmonary disease is not clear, but the likelihood of serious infection decreases with increasing age (Stahlman et al, 1973).

Persisting dyspnoea and pulmonary dysfunction

Many infants who have had classical respiratory distress syndrome have signs of persisting pulmonary disease for several weeks after recovery. In the milder form of the disease infants breathe at 50 to 70/min and have a moderate degree of intercostal recession. A few fine high-pitched crepitations are heard in the lungs. Radiologically various minor changes are seen, including small areas of atelectasis and small fluffy opacities suggesting pulmonary oedema. The most severe pulmonary sequelae are seen in infants surviving IPPV who have the condition of bronchopulmonary dysplasia. Westgate et al (1969) have shown that infants with the milder sequelae have slight hypoxaemia with increased $A - a$ Do_2 during the first year of life which they believe is due to ventilation perfusion imbalance in the injured lung. This had resolved by the age of 12 months.

In the recent survey of Bryan et al (1973) survivors of HMD were divided into three groups: (a) infants recovering from HMD; (b) infants recovering from HMD and IPPV; (c) group (b) infants with bronchopulmonary dysplasia. All groups had a decreased functional residual capacity (FRC) and dynamic compliance at one month, and groups (b) and (c) still had abnormal compliance at the age of two to four months. By six to twelve months only those with bronchopulmonary dysplasia had a reduced compliance, and by then they had developed signs of air trapping with the increased FRC. All survivors aged one month had a raised $P_a co_2$ and low $P_a o_2$ compared with controls. The $P_a co_2$ remained high only in infants with bronchopulmonary dysplasia, though the $P_a o_2$ was low to the age of 12 months in all ventilated infants, particularly those with bronchopulmonary dysplasia. Thus, serious pulmonary physiological impairment was common.

Late onset of respiratory disease (Wilson–Mikity syndrome)

This usually occurs in very low birthweight infants and presents with gradually increasing respiratory difficulty from the age of one to two weeks, usually *without* preceding HMD or IPPV. The disease may remain very mild with little more than a slight increase in respiratory rate and a few non-specific x-ray changes. However, in a small percentage of cases the disease becomes very much more severe.

This severe form of chronic chest disease has a mortality of up to 25 per cent (Hodgman et al, 1969), and has the marked radiological changes initially described by Wilson and Mikity (1960). The infant is severely dyspnoeic, and the x-ray of the chest shows multiple cystic honeycomb lesions bilaterally. The infant becomes progressively hypoxaemic and develops CO_2 retention, and eventually dies aged three to four months in respiratory failure with overdistended lungs, and in some cases cor pulmonale. At postmortem the histology of the lungs is quite distinct from that in bronchopulmonary dysplasia (Hodgman et al, 1969).

Aetiology

There are six potential contributory factors in the aetiology of the lung complications listed above:

Residual effects of HMD
Infection
Pulmonary oedema with a patent ductus arteriosus
Pulmonary immaturity
Oxygen toxicity
Ventilator therapy at high pressures

Residual effects of HMD
There is no doubt that this disease causes widespread damage and destruction of the pulmonary alveolar epithelium. Although bronchopulmonary dysplasia cannot be the result of inadequately healed HMD, many of the milder sequelae may represent delayed healing of the damaged alveolar lining.

Infection
Many infants, particularly those with endotracheal tubes in situ on the ventilator, have recurrent infection. There is no doubt that infection damages the lungs at all ages, and in the premature infant with HMD it may contribute to delayed healing of the alveolar epithelium and the long-term sequelae.

Pulmonary oedema with a patent ductus arteriosus
Infants with severe HMD and particularly those with bronchopulmonary dysplasia, and also infants with the Wilson–Mikity syndrome often have a patent ductus arteriosus (Kitterman et al, 1972), a raised right heart pressure, and radiological and clinical signs of pulmonary oedema. Although the patent

ductus and the pulmonary oedema may contribute to the problems of the infant during the acute phase of his illness, the histology of established bronchopulmonary dysplasia or Wilson–Mikity syndrome is quite different from that of chronic pulmonary oedema in children and adults. However, the neonatal lung may react differently to the presence of chronic interstitial oedema, especially if complicated by interstitial haemorrhage as a result of HMD, pulmonary oxygen toxicity, or positive pressure ventilation.

Pulmonary immaturity

Burnard et al (1965) showed that the airways of the immature lung are abnormally compliant, and tend to collapse very readily during expiration. This results in air trapping, and emphysematous change distally in the lung. They postulated that when mild, this caused the mild end of the spectrum of late onset respiratory difficulty, and when severe was responsible for the Wilson–Mikity syndrome. They, and others (Swyer et al, 1965) have documented such changes, with an increased airways resistance in infants with the Wilson–Mikity syndrome.

Oxygen toxicity

The role of this in chronic pulmonary disease is difficult to assess. There is no doubt that many very low birthweight infants have survived prolonged exposure to oxygen concentrations greater than 60 per cent without any obvious serious lung disease. Except in infants who have been ventilated, lung function studies on survivors of HMD are usually normal or only transiently abnormal (Stahlman et al, 1973; Bryan et al, 1973). Many of these infants have had prolonged high oxygen therapy. A few survivors have symptoms and signs of airways obstruction, but these infants have a strong family history of atopy and do not seem to have had a more prolonged exposure to oxygen in the neonatal period. Nevertheless, oxygen toxicity may contribute to some of the minor sequelae reported by Westgate et al (1969), Stahlman et al (1973) and Bryan et al (1973). It is, however, very unlikely to be the cause of the Wilson–Mikity syndrome, which usually develops in infants who did not have HMD and were not exposed to concentrations of oxygen greater than 30 to 40 per cent. In summary, there is as yet no evidence that oxygen on its own causes any significant long-term pulmonary sequelae.

Ventilator therapy

It is clear that virtually all infants with bronchopulmonary dysplasia have a specific disease which is causally related to high pressure intermittent positive pressure ventilation. The mechanism of the disease is not understood, but it is probably partially due to simple physical distortion and destruction of the lungs by high inflation pressures and fast inspiratory flow rates. Interstitial emphysema of the lung (Stahlman et al, 1973; Thibeault et al, 1973), and the disruption of the pulmonary parenchyma which this causes, may also aggravate any fibrosing reaction. It is in this group of infants that there are persisting severe abnormalities in pulmonary function and blood gas status (Bryan et al, 1973). Occasional cases have also occurred following the use of negative pressure ventilation (Shepard et al, 1968). Infants with bronchopulmonary dysplasia also have a further increased susceptibility to serious respiratory infection compared with non-ventilated cases of HMD (Bryan et al, 1973; Stahlman et al, 1973).

Although ventilator therapy at high pressure may be the single most important factor in the aetiology of bronchopulmonary dysplasia, it has no role in the aetiology of Wilson–Mikity syndrome, which develops in infants who have not been ventilated.

Conclusions

It is thus apparent that more than one factor must be involved in most cases of chronic pulmonary disease. It is difficult to say what causes the increased incidence of respiratory infection in survivors with no radiological or clinical abnormality. This could simply be the aftermath of the mild changes outlined above. At the other end of the scale, premature infants who survive after prolonged IPPV at high pressure suffer several or all of the six factors listed above—epithelial damage, infection, pulmonary oedema, the collapsing airways of prematurity, oxygen toxicity and the disruptive forces of IPPV, of which the latter is perhaps the single most significant factor. Children with Wilson–Mikity syndrome probably represent a specific entity due to airways obstruction caused by the collapsing airways of the premature lung, perhaps aggravated by pulmonary oedema.

II. DISEASES OF INFANCY

BRONCHIOLITIS

This is a disease of infancy. Ninety per cent of cases occur before the age of 12 months (Miller, 1973). The maximum incidence is between two and six months of age. It is characterised by signs of severe respiratory distress with fewer x-ray changes and signs on auscultation of the chest than might be expected from the clinical severity of the illness. It accounts for 20 per cent of the total admissions to hospital with respiratory tract infections under 12 months of age (Miller, 1973) and has a mortality in a recent series of 0.7 per cent (Court, 1973b).

Signs and Symptoms

The clinical manifestations of the disease can be divided into two stages; mild upper respiratory signs in the early catarrhal stage of the disease, progressing to the second stage when the signs are due to the marked narrowing and obstruction of the terminal airways causing severe dyspnoea and cyanosis. The signs of the disease have recently been well reviewed by Court (1973a).

The infant is often dehydrated due to fever, inadequate fluid intake and increased insensible water loss with tachypnoea. Restlessness is common; this is a characteristic feature of a hypoxic *infant* in marked contradistinction to the hypoxic neonate who lies very still. Although cyanosis was only detected in a quarter of Court's series (1973a), many infants will have low P_aO_2 values even though these may be above the level at which cyanosis appears.

On auscultation of the chest a few fine crepitations may be heard, but more characteristically in over two-thirds of cases there are inspiratory and expiratory rhonchi in all lung fields.

The disease persists for four to five days, by which time the chest signs start to improve, and by seven to ten days after the bronchiolitis became apparent the children are clinically and radiologically back to normal.

Aetiology

In 1957, Chanock and his co-workers demonstrated that what had hitherto been known as chimpanzee-coryza agent could be a cause of respiratory illness in children (Chanock, Roizman and Myers, 1957). Further studies by Chanock et al (1961) showed that this agent, now renamed respiratory syncytial virus (RSV), could be cultured from throat swabs of seriously ill infants with bronchiolitis and pneumonia. Although other viruses can be cultured from a small percentage of cases of bronchiolitis (Poole and Tobin, 1973), nearly 80 per cent of such cases in epidemic years are positive for RSV (Gardner, 1973).

The major aetiological mystery is why RSV infection causes the illness of bronchiolitis in infancy with signs of severe airways obstruction, since at other ages the spectrum of disease caused by the virus is different. Outbreaks of neonatal RSV infection (Neligan et al, 1970) are associated with upper respiratory tract infection and only mild pulmonary signs and symptoms, and in older children and adults RSV infection is again associated with a mild respiratory infection (Poole and Tobin, 1973).

There is evidence that there may be an abnormal immune response when an infant is infected with this virus. This concept developed following the trial of a killed parenterally injected RSV vaccine used in the United States (Kapikian et al, 1969). Infants immunised with this vaccine developed an unusually severe respiratory disease when exposed to a wild RSV epidemic even if they were more than 12 months old—an age at which severe bronchiolitis is comparatively unusual. This led to the suggestion that bronchiolitis due to natural RSV infection may also be the result of an abnormal immune response. Chanock et al (1970) suggested that this could be a type III reaction between the virus and neutralising IgG maternal antibodies still circulating in the infant, at a time when the antibody levels were low and local levels of IgA in the infant's respiratory mucosa had not yet risen to protective levels. This is analogous to infants immunised parenterally with killed vaccine, who have neutralising serum IgG antibodies but no mucosal IgA antibodies.

Gardner, McQuillin and Court (1970) postulated that bronchiolitis is the result of a type I hypersensitivity reaction. In the rare case of pneumonia due to RSV, the lungs are full of RSV at postmortem, whereas in fatal bronchiolitis very little RSV can be identified in the lungs which do, however, contain IgG antibodies. But the amount of antibody detected by immunofluorescent techniques, appeared to be insufficient to account for a type III reaction. Gardner, therefore, rejected the Chanock hypothesis of a type III reaction and suggested that bronchiolitis represented a second exposure to RSV, the first (?neonatal) exposure having caused only IgE antibodies to appear in the lung.

The presence or absence of mucosal IgA is probably one of the major determinants of whether bronchiolitis develops when infection with RSV occurs. Kim et al (1969) has shown that RSV specific IgA does appear in nasal secretions of infants recovering from RSV positive bronchiolitis. Chanock et al (1970) have shown that possession of such an antibody during RSV infection does not necessarily prevent local upper respiratory tract disease, but does prevent the development of serum antibodies of the sort that might precipitate a type III reaction and bronchiolitis. The Scottish study by Ross, Pinkerton and Assaad (1971) showed that bronchiolitis developed in infants who were immunologically immature and produced IgA and IgG slowly and in inadequate amounts when exposed to RSV. They did not regard maternal antibody levels, or abnormal reactions between antibody and the RSV, as being of importance in the aetiology of bronchiolitis, which they suggested was the response of the immunologically immature lung to RSV infection.

The most recent publication from the Chanock group (Parrott et al, 1973) supports the concept of Ross et al (1971). Parrott et al (1973) have shown that children may develop severe bronchiolitis without levels of maternal antibody that would cause a type III reaction, and they agree there is an immature immune response since many infants with bronchiolitis have no anti-RSV IgA and IgG.

These views are not incompatible with the hypothesis of Gardner et al (1970). Mild neonatal infection (Neligan et al, 1970) might have sensitised the respiratory epithelium whilst leaving it unprotected by IgA or IgG, as shown by Ross et al (1971) and Parrott et al (1973). Vaccinated children would also have no IgA, but they would have high levels of IgG. In such circumstances a type III response could well occur, and it may be noted that although these infants developed an illness similar to bronchiolitis, it had some unusual features such as age distribution, and the severity of the pulmonary signs and radiological changes.

Epidemiology

Outbreaks of bronchiolitis occur usually at two-yearly intervals, in the months November to March (Glezen and Denny, 1973; Miller, 1973), though there may be annual epidemics (Mufson et al, 1973). The disease is spread by droplet and is highly infectious with an incubation period of five to eight days (Ditchburn et al, 1971). There is a high incidence of nosocomial infections in hospital in-patients (Ditchburn et al, 1971).

Five groups of children have an increased susceptibility to RSV infection:

Low socio-economic status

There is a much higher incidence of RSV infection in children from the low socio-economic groups. The reason for this is multifactorial, including such things as overcrowding and family size (Gardner, 1968).

Obesity

The study of Tracey, De and Harper (1971) demonstrated that fat children had an increased incidence and severity of bronchiolitis. This was independent of social class. The mechanism remains obscure, though an increased liability to impaired alveolar hypoventilation due to obesity has been implicated.

Survivors of severe neonatal pulmonary disease

It is now recognised that infants who survive HMD, particularly those who were ventilated (Stahlman et al, 1973), not only have an increased incidence if bronchiolitis, but develop it in a more severe form often requiring IPPV.

Children with some predisposing abnormalities

Certain underlying conditions, such as those associated with mental subnormality (e.g. Down's syndrome, spina bifida and hydrocephalus) or congenital heart disease are associated with an increased incidence and severity of serious respiratory illness in childhood (Court, 1973b).

Family history of atopy

It has long been recognised that many children who have infantile bronchiolitis later develop asthma, and that there is a higher incidence of atopic disease in their first degree relatives (Simon and Jordan, 1967). It has been suggested that children with bronchiolitis from which RSV is not isolated are also more likely to develop asthma subsequently (Simon and Jordan, 1967). Consistent with this possibility are the observations of higher IgE levels in infants with RSV-negative bronchiolitis (Polmar, Robinson and Minnefor, 1972) and the higher incidence of subsequent asthma in cases of wheezy bronchitis with raised IgE levels (Foucard, 1974).

Diagnosis

The clinical picture of bronchiolitis in an infant is characteristic. However, it is important to establish whether the illness is due to RSV or bacterial infection. RSV infection can be confirmed either by direct culture or by using the technique of immunofluorescence. Using this latter technique, diagnosis is possible within 24 h of the infant's admission to hospital (Gardner and McQuillin, 1968). Laryngeal or nasopharyngeal aspirates are treated with rabbit anti-RSV antibody followed by a fluorescein-conjugated antirabbit globulin, and the preparation is then examined under dark ground illumination using blue light from a mercury vapour lamp. Cells which have RSV absorbed on to their surface can then be easily identified by their fluorescence. During the first 24 h, bacterial infection cannot be excluded.

In bronchiolitis the chest x-ray shows overdistended lungs. The presence of significant consolidation, together with a polymorphonuclear leucocytosis, suggests that any pulmonary disease is due to bacterial infection.

Treatment

Since this disease is usually viral, there is no specific therapy, and treatment is directed to intensive supportive care of the seriously ill child. This has recently been well reviewed by Phelan and Stocks (1974).

Hydration

Most of these infants are dehydrated. Furthermore they are too dyspnoeic to bottle feed and, except in mild and convalescent cases, the presence of an indwelling nasogastric tube will further aggravate the compromised respiratory function by increasing nasal airway resistance. Intravenous fluid should therefore be administered using dextrose saline with potassium supplements.

Oxygen and acid-base status

The most serious abnormality in such infants is hypoxaemia (Simpson and Flenley, 1967), a low P_aO_2 being almost universally present on admission. For this reason blood gas analysis should be routine in these patients. The hypoxaemia may be one of the causes of the infants' restlessness which often improves when sufficient oxygen is administered to maintain the arterial P_aO_2 in the normal range. Intermittent arterial puncture is probably as bad for the very sick infant with bronchiolitis as it is for the premature infant with HMD, and the use of an indwelling arterial cannula should then be considered.

Oxygen administration is advised in all cases. There is no risk of depression of ventilation at this time of life, since these infants will always be CO_2 responsive. They do not, however, tolerate face masks, and since oxygen tents are notoriously poor providers of a high oxygen concentration, the oxygen level within the tent should be checked frequently with a paramagnetic oxygen analyser, to ensure that levels of at least 40 per cent are being given. The oxygen flow into the tent in litres per minute is a valueless measurement. Small infants can, of course, be successfully nursed in a conventional incubator.

Acidaemia rarely needs correction since rehydration and oxygenation in an infant with normal kidneys results in a rapid spontaneous correction of the base deficit. Furthermore, bolus injection of sodium bicarbonate has its hazards, and should only be used in the presence of peripheral vascular collapse and impending or actual cardiac arrest. Arterial Pco_2 values which are rising are an indication of worsening respiratory failure, but I would agree with Phelan and Stocks (1974) that the decision to intubate and ventilate such infants should only be taken after consideration of the infant's overall condition, and not on the basis of arterial Pco_2 values alone.

Hypotension

At the risk of being repetitious, the blood pressure should always be recorded. If there is evidence of shock or hypotension, acidaemia should first be corrected and blood transfusion given if necessary. Any infant with a haemoglobin concentration below 9 g/100 ml should be transfused, with diuretic cover is required.

Heart failure

If this is present, with tachycardia or signs of fluid retention, standard therapy with digoxin and diuretics should be instituted. It is important to remember that infants can be both dehydrated *and* in heart failure.

Antibiotics

If there is any doubt that the illness is not due to RSV infection, antibiotic cover should be given until microbiological diagnosis is confirmed by immuno-fluorescence. The Newcastle group recommended penicillin and cloxacillin (Gardner, 1968). However, since the bacteria which kill at this age are rarely penicillin sensitive, and may be Gram-negative, the recommendation of Phelan and Stocks (1974) to give methicillin and gentamicin is to be preferred. It is interesting to note that in a report of respiratory deaths under two years of age, of the seven 'normal' infants who died, that is, infants with no pre-disposing abnormality, two had virus infections (one RSV and one para-influenza III), and five *Staphylococcus aureus*. Only one of the five with staphylococcal infection had received a penicillinase resistant penicillin (Court, 1973b).

Bronchodilators

There is no place for the use of β-adrenergic drugs or the methyl-xanthines in infants with bronchiolitis. They are ineffective at producing bronchodilatation, possibly because of the relative paucity of bronchiolar musculature at this age.

Steroids

The use of steroids remains more controversial. Controlled trials have shown no significant benefit of therapy with various steroids in bronchiolitis (Leer et al, 1969). The American Academy of Pediatrics (1970) has actively discouraged their use in this disease. Nevertheless, in an infant who is in extremis, no harm comes from giving 100 to 200 mg of intravenous hydrocortisone, and clinical impression suggests that some of these infants do improve in the hour after such an injection.

Outcome

Infants who are not shocked or in respiratory failure when they arrive in hospital should survive, even though they may require a period of positive pressure ventilation. Recovery is complete, although these children do have recurrent chest disease, and there is an increased incidence of asthma and allied diseases on long-term follow-up.

Prevention

The mortality rate from both bronchiolitis and other RSV infections is such that a vaccine is being sought. The killed virus vaccine referred to above was clearly unsatisfactory, but there is hope that the newer temperature sensitive mutants of RSV instilled intranasally will confer effective mucosal (IgA) immunity (Kim et al, 1973).

SUDDEN INFANT DEATH SYNDROME—SIDS
(cot deaths, sudden unexpected death)

It has been recognised since the time of Solomon (1 Kings iii. 16–19) that a percentage of infants die suddenly and unexpectedly. In the majority of these cases no obvious cause of death is found at postmortem examination.

In the United Kingdom—as in the United States—SIDS has only recently become a registrable cause of death. For this reason many such cases have previously been registered as respiratory or other infections, and it is difficult to obtain an estimate of the true incidence of the condition. In an attempt to do this for the United Kingdom, Carpenter and Shaddick (1965) estimated that 70 per cent of respiratory deaths in infancy reported to coroners were cases of SIDS. Seven years earlier Banks (1958) in a survey commissioned by the Minister of Health had estimated that there were 1432 cot deaths in the United Kingdom a year. In published series the average incidence of SIDS is 2.2 to 2.3/1000 live births (Fitzgibbons et al, 1969; Valdes-Dapena, 1970; Froggatt, Lynas and MacKenzie, 1971). This represents about one-third of the infant deaths between one month and 12 months (Richards and McIntosh, 1972; Bergman et al, 1972). Thus, the annual mortality from SIDS in the United Kingdom is approximately 1500 to 1700. SIDS is probably the largest single cause of infant mortality, and in the Washington study was the second major cause of death between the first week of life and 14 years of age, only accidental deaths occurring in greater numbers (Bergman et al, 1972).

Epidemiology

The work of Valdes-Dapena (1967), Froggatt et al (1971), and Bergman et al (1972) among others has established the pattern of occurrence of SIDS. The dead infants are usually discovered between midnight and 08.00 hours, most commonly in the winter months, and infants between two and six months

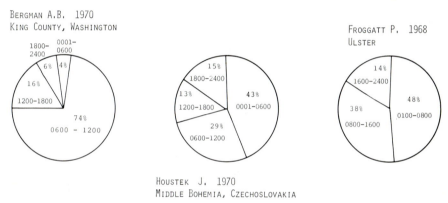

Figure 10 Time of day at which deaths have been discovered, as reported by three different studies

of age are particularly afflicted. There is a preponderance of males (Figs. 10 to 12). Lower social class, paternal unemployment, illegitimacy, over-crowding, poor obstetric factors, decreased maternal age and increased maternal parity, large family size and failure to attend well-baby clinics, all increase the likelihood of SIDS (Valdes-Dapena, 1967; Froggatt et al, 1971; Bergman et al, 1972; Richards and McIntosh, 1972; Protestos et al, 1973). There is also an increased incidence of SIDS in infants born prematurely (Table 11; Bergman, 1970), twins (Carpenter, 1972) and infants with a sibling who suffered SIDS (Valdes-Dapena, 1967). Comprehensive though the literature is on the conditions under which SIDS occurs, it has unfortunately provided little information which has helped to elucidate their cause.

Pathology

Before discussing the pathology of sudden infant death syndrome, it is important to realise that between 15 to 20 per cent of babies who are found dead in their bed have some major abnormality detectable at postmortem.

The diseases which were implicated in Beckwith's study (1970) are listed in Table 12. There are also small numbers of infants in whom it is difficult to be certain whether the degree of histological change in the lungs indicates *fatal* pulmonary infection, or whether it is more compatible with the degree of infiltration and bronchial wall desquamation found in SIDS (Beckwith, 1970). It should be remembered that cot deaths may be infanticide, and in

Table 11   Gestational age of infants with sudden infant death syndrome (Washington, USA, 1965 to 1967)

Gestational age in weeks	SIDS rate/1000 live births
< 34	7.34
34	27.5
35	3.2
36	2.2
37	2.3
38	2.5
39	1.0
> 40	1.9

Data from Bergman (1970).

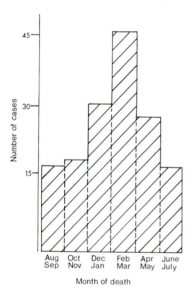

Figure 11   Bimonthly incidence of cot deaths (Froggatt et al, 1971)

the published series there are usually several infants in whom a subdural haemorrhage, hanging, or 'suffocation' are the cause of death (Beckwith, 1970; Richards and McIntosh, 1972). There is marked similarity in the social background of infants who are battered, and those who are the victims of SIDS. Nevertheless, the vast majority of cases of SIDS are accidental, and there is no suspicion of criminal assault.

The morbid anatomical findings of SIDS have been reviewed by Beck-

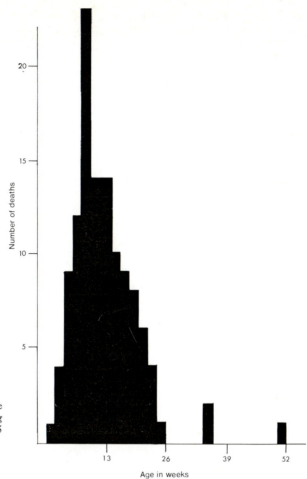

Figure 12 Age incidence of cot deaths in King County, Washington, 1965 to 1967 (Bergman, 1970)

Table 12 Identifiable cause of death in infants found dead

206 cases of sudden infant death		
SIDS	149	
Doubtful	19	
Bronchitis		13
? Violent		6
Explained	38	
Septicaemia (9 meningococci)		12
Pulmonary infection		9
Cardiac (4 carditis, 2 CHD)		6
Congenital malformations		3
Gastroenteritis		3
? Violent		5

Data from Beckwith (1970).

with (1970). The characteristic finding is the presence of petechiae on the intrathoracic structures together with a small amount of pulmonary oedema, alveolar haemorrhage, and minimal inflammatory exudate in the bronchi.

Aetiology

A large number of theories have been advanced to explain SIDS (Valdes-Dapena, 1967). Table 13 lists some of the more unlikely ones. I have included suffocation by pillows in this list as unlikely to cause sudden death because most investigators feel that the normal infant is capable of turning his head to one side when lying prone. Moreover, in 95 per cent of American cases of SIDS, the infants were sleeping without a pillow in the cot (Bergman et al,

Table 13   Sudden infant death syndrome: aetiologies which have been postulated but appear highly unlikely

Status thymolymphaticus
Cardiac arrhythmia
Laryngospasm
Abnormality of calcium metabolism and parathyroids
Cortisol deficiency
Electrolyte imbalance
Acidaemia
Inborn error of protein metabolism
Hypothermia
Hyperthermia
Deficiencies of vitamins C, D and E
Selenium deficiency
Dislocation of atlanto-axial joint
Extradural haemorrhage
Suffocation—pillows
Diving reflex

1972). Cardiac arrhythmia may be responsible in a small number of infants who die in their cots. However, it is not a feature of the usual type of SIDS.

Other theories of SIDS which have been postulated require further discussion:

Immunoglobulin deficiency

The maximum incidence of SIDS between two and six months is difficult to explain. The trough of IgG levels in the human newborn following the postnatal fall in transplacentally acquired maternal IgG is concurrent with the peak incidence of SIDS. It was, therefore, postulated that an immune mechanism may be at the basis of SIDS. However, careful studies have shown no difference in immunoglobulin levels between cases of SIDS and matched controls (Valdes-Dapena, 1970).

Infection

The age distribution of cases of SIDS is very similar to the age of distribution of infantile deaths with lower respiratory tract disease (Carpenter, 1972). Also, cot deaths and lower respiratory tract infection are more common in the winter months and in the poorer socio-economic groups (Gardner, 1968), and a small number of cases of infants found dead undoubtedly have an overwhelming pulmonary infection. Furthermore, many cot death children, while not seriously ill when last seen alive, did have a minor degree of upper respiratory tract infection, or were 'off-colour' (Carpenter, 1972; Richards and McIntosh, 1972). However, there is a vast difference in the reported incidence of positive cultures for viruses or bacteria in cases of SIDS. For viruses it ranges from 0 to 100 per cent, and for bacteria from 2 to 41 per cent. The subject has been well reviewed by Valdes-Dapena (1967, 1970). There seems little to support the theory that infection plays a major role in SIDS.

Milk allergy

Although occasional cases of cot deaths have been described in infants who have been exclusively breast fed (Bergman et al, 1972), there is no doubt at all that the syndrome is very much more common in infants who have been exposed to cows' milk protein from an early age. It has been suggested that these infants are hypersensitised to this protein, and if cows' milk is inhaled during sleep a lethal anaphylactic reaction results. Cases of SIDS may have higher levels of antibodies to cows' milk protein in their plasma than controls, and their sera are capable of producing passive cutaneous anaphylaxis to cows' milk protein (Coombs, 1965). Other work (Peterson and Good, 1963) has, however, failed to show any significant difference between cases of SIDS and control subjects in the level of antimilk antibodies in the serum, or the amount of antibody detectable by immunofluorescent techniques in different parts of the respiratory tract (Valdes-Dapena and Felipe, 1971).

When milk was instilled into the upper respiratory tract of guinea-pigs sensitised to cows' milk, a severe anaphylactic reaction developed and they died. These animals had the histological changes in their lungs of anaphylaxis. However, if the sensitised guinea-pig was lightly anaesthetised to mimic sleep, it became apnoeic and died without a struggle when milk was introduced into the larynx (Parish et al, 1960), and the histological changes in the lungs was similar to those seen in the SIDS. Unsensitised guinea-pigs continued to breathe satisfactorily.

Despite the fact that an immunological cause for the increased incidence of SIDS in bottle-fed infants does not seem to have been substantiated, the epidemiological association between SIDS and bottle feeding remains to be explained.

Reflex apnoea as a cause of sudden infant death syndrome

Most of the recent research on SIDS has led to the conclusion that there is a group of infants who are prone to develop apnoea, during which they make no spontaneous effort to restart breathing and may die during the attack.

Research has been directed towards identifying such infants, and delineating those factors which could provoke an apnoeic attack.

It is well known that periodic breathing, including transient apnoea, is seen in the rapid eye movement phase of sleep in newborn infants (Parmelee et al, 1967) as well as in adults. Steinschneider (1972) in a study of five infants in whom there was a strong family history of SIDS, was able to show that the infants had an increased incidence of apnoeic attacks during sleep, and some of these lasted longer than 15 s. Furthermore, two of the infants studied subsequently died of SIDS. Prolonged reflex apnoea which persists in the face of progressive hypoxia, acidaemia and bradycardia, up to the point of the EEG becoming isoelectric, is also seen in the newborn premature infant, as shown earlier.

The fact that some infants may just become apnoeic and die could explain why many cases of SIDS occur without the parents sleeping in the same bedroom being wakened, or without disturbing the clothes in the cot. However, it seems that not only do cases of SIDS have an increased liability to recurrent apnoea of this type, but some further factor is required to trigger the apnoea.

One of these factors may be upper respiratory tract obstruction. Shaw (1970) suggested that nasal obstruction was the sole cause of SIDS. Cross and Lewis (1971) described an infant whom they studied in a body plethysmograph; when the sealing cuff round the infant's face was deflated, progressive apnoea occurred without any sort of struggle. They postulated that this was due to a misplaced cuff occluding the infant's airway by pushing the tongue back into the pharynx. What was striking about this infant was that it tolerated this obstruction and became apnoeic without any sort of struggle. The analogy with SIDS is obvious. Also, Anderson and Rosenblith (1971) found an increased incidence of SIDS in infants who scored badly on their tactile adaptive scores. This tests the response of infants to nasal obstruction. Further studies on rabbits (Wealthall, 1973) and on human infants (Swift and Emery, 1973) have shown that some newborn make no attempt to withdraw from bilateral nasal occlusion, and certain animals may become progressively apnoeic and die. That infants with SIDS may have been having frequent apnoeic attacks, is also suggested by the data of Naeye (1973) who found that these infants have hypertrophy of the muscle in the small pulmonary arterioles compatible with recurrent episodes of hypoxia. Many cases of SIDS have had mild upper respiratory tract infections, and nasal obstruction during sleep in such an infant might trigger a severe apnoeic attack in a susceptible infant and cause death. The infants studied by Steinschneider (1972) certainly showed an increased incidence of prolonged apnoeic attacks (greater than 15 s) when they had an upper respiratory tract infection, and the cases of SIDS with infections, described by Stevens (1965), developed apnoeic attacks and bradycardia from which they could not be resuscitated.

The role of cows' milk in SIDS may be explained by the data of Johnson, Robinson and Salisbury (1973). They have shown that the introduction of heterologous milk into the larynx is one of the stimuli which will initiate reflex apnoea. Introduction of some physiological solution, such as liquor amnii or normal saline, did not interfere with respiration, nor did the introduction of autologous milk (e.g. sheep's milk into lambs). Their data also showed that although apnoea was more difficult to induce in older animals, when it did occur serious cardiorespiratory collapse ensued, corresponding to the increased risk of SIDS in humans beyond the neonatal period, and the considerable difficulty often encountered in trying to resuscitate 'near-miss' cases of SIDS (Stevens, 1965). The studies of Salisbury (personal communication) have shown that a newborn infant has much more irregular respiration and a tendency to periods of apnoea when receiving a cows' milk feed than when receiving a feed of expressed breast milk.

Conclusion

A working hypothesis for the aetiology of SIDS is that some infants are prone to develop reflex apnoea progressing to cardiac arrest and death during the first six months of life. These infants are a small percentage of the whole, but are those specifically at risk from sudden infant death syndrome. Events which may trigger one of these episodes of apnoea include the introduction of heterologous milk into the pharynx, or the presence of upper respiratory tract obstruction such as might be caused by an intercurrent upper respiratory infection. This theory explains two of the major epidemiological correlates of cot death: the mild respiratory illness preceding death, and the sparing of breast-fed infants. The other epidemiological findings may merely be selecting out infants born into households where lower and upper respiratory tract infection with obstruction are more common, together with a lower incidence of breast feeding.

ACKNOWLEDGEMENTS

The author wishes to acknowledge the help of Professor J. P. M. Tizard and Dr J. D. Baum in the preparation of this chapter.

REFERENCES

Alden, E. R., Mandelkorn, T., Woodrum, D. E., Wennberg, R. P., Parks, C. R. & Hodson, W. A. (1972) Morbidity and mortality of infants weighing less than 1000 grams in an intensive care nursery. *Pediatrics*, **50**, 40–49.

American Academy of Pediatrics, Committee on Drugs (1970) Should steroids be used in treating bronchiolitis? *Pediatrics*, **46**, 640–642.

Anderson, F. M., Datta, N. & Shaw, E. J. (1972) R factors in hospital infection. *British Medical Journal*, **3**, 82–85.

Anderson, R. B. & Rosenblith, J. F. (1971) Sudden unexpected death syndrome. *Biology of the Neonate*, **18**, 395–406.

Aranda, J. V., Stern, L. & Dunbar, J. S. (1972) Pneumothorax with pneumoperitoneum in a newborn infant. *American Journal of Diseases of Children*, **123**, 163–166.

Avery, M. E. & Fletcher, B. D. (1974) *The Lung and its Disorders in the Newborn Infant*, 3rd edn, p. 238. Philadelphia and London: Saunders.

Avery, M. E. (1975) Pharmacological approaches to acceleration of fetal lung maturation. *British Medical Bulletin*, **31**, 13–17.

Avery, M. E., Gatewood, O. B. & Brumley, G. (1966) Transient tachypnea of the newborn. *American Journal of Diseases of Children*, **111**, 380–385.

Aynsley-Green, A., Roberton, N. R. C. & Rolfe, P. (1975) Air temperature recordings in infant incubators. *Archives of Disease in Childhood*, **50**, 215–219.

Aziz, E. M. & Robertson, A. F. (1973) Paraplegia. A complication of umbilical artery catherisation. *Journal of Pediatrics*, **82**, 1051–1052.

Baden, M., Bauer, C. R., Colle, E., Klein, G., Taeusch, H. W. Jr & Stern, L. (1972) A controlled trial of hydrocortisone therapy in infants with respiratory distress syndrome. *Pediatrics*, **50**, 526–534.

Baker, C. J. & Barrett, F. F. (1973) Transmission of group B streptococci among parturient women and their neonates. *Journal of Pediatrics*, **83**, 919–925.

Baker, C. J., Barrett, F. F. & Clark, D. J. (1974) Incidence of kanamycin resistance among *E. coli* isolates from neonates. *Journal of Pediatrics*, **84**, 126–130.

Bancalari, E., Garcia, O. L. & Jesse, M. J. (1973) Effects of continuous negative pressure on lung mechanics in idiopathic respiratory distress syndrome. *Pediatrics*, **51**, 485–493.

Banerjee, C. K., Girling, D. J. & Wigglesworth, J. S. (1972) Pulmonary fibroplasia in newborn babies treated with oxygen and artificial ventilation. *Archives of Disease in Childhood*, **47**, 509–518.

Banks, A. L. (1958) An enquiry into sudden death in infancy. *Monthly Bulletin*, Ministry of Health, London, **17**, 182–191.

Barnes, N. D., Glover, W. J., Hull, D. & Milner, A. D. (1969) Effects of prolonged positive-pressure ventilation in infancy. *Lancet*, **2**, 1096–1099.

Barr, P. A., Jenkins, P. A. & Baum, J. D. (1975) Lecithin/sphingomyelin ratio in the hypopharyngeal aspirate of newborn infants. Paper presented to the Paediatric Research Society, Bristol. March 1975.

Barrie, H. (1973) Continuous positive airway pressure for respiratory distress syndrome. *Lancet*, **2**, 851

Barton, L. L., Feigin, R. D. & Lins, R. (1973) Group B beta hemolytic streptococcal meningitis in infants. *Journal of Pediatrics*, **82**, 719–723.

Bauer, C. R., Stern, L. & Colle, E. (1974) Prolonged rupture of membranes associated with a decreased incidence of respiratory distress syndrome. *Pediatrics*, **53**, 7–12.

Baum, J. D. & Bulpitt, C. J. (1970) Retinal vasoconstriction in premature infants with increased arterial oxygen tensions. *Archives of Disease in Childhood*, **45**, 350–353.

Baum, J. D. & Roberton, N. R. C. (1975) Immediate effects of alkali infusion in infants with respiratory distress syndrome. *Journal of Pediatrics*, **87**, 255–261.

Baum, J. D. & Roberton, N. R. C. (1974) Experience with the use of distending pressure in infants with respiratory distress syndrome. *Archives of Disease in Childhood*, **49**, 771–781.

Becker, M. J. & Koppe, J. G. (1969) Pulmonary structural changes in neonatal hyaline membrane disease treated with high pressure artificial respiration. *Thorax*, **24**, 689–694.

Beckwith, J. B. (1970) Observations on the pathological anatomy of the sudden infant death syndrome. In *Sudden Infant Death Syndrome*, ed. Bergman, A. B., Beckwith, J. B. & Ray, C. G., pp. 83–107. Seattle: University of Washington Press.

Berg, T. J., Pagtakhan, R. D., Reed, M. H., Langston, C. & Chernick, V. (1975) Bronchopulmonary dysplasia and lung rupture in hyaline membrane disease. *Pediatrics*, **55**, 51–54.

Bergman, A. B. (1970) Sudden infant death syndrome in King County, Washington: epidemiologic aspects. In *Sudden Infant Death Syndrome*, ed. Bergman, A. B., Beckwith, J. B. & Ray, C. G., pp. 47–54. Seattle and London: University of Washington Press.

Bergman, A. B., Ray, C. G., Pomeroy, M. A., Wahl, P. W. & Beckwith, J. B. (1972) Studies of the sudden infant death syndrome in King County, Washington. III. Epidemiology. *Pediatrics*, **49**, 860–870.

Bevilacqua, G., Baroni, M., Cavatorta, E., Mansani, F. E., Maretti, M. & Ottaviani, A. (1973) Risk to the newborn from Caesarean section. In *Perinatal Medicine*. Proceedings of the Third European Congress of Perinatal Medicine, ed. Bossart, H., Cruz, J. M., Huber, A., Prod'hom L. S. & Sistek, L., pp. 149–158. Bern, Stuttgart, Vienna: Hans Huber.

Bhagwanani, S. G., Fahmy, D. & Turnbull, A. C. (1973) Bubble stability test compared with lecithin assay in prediction of respiratory distress syndrome. *British Medical Journal*, **1**, 697–700.

Boddy, K. & Dawes, G. S. (1975) Fetal breathing. *British Medical Bulletin*, **31**, 3–7.

Brosens, I. & Gordon, H. (1966) The estimation of maturity by cytological examination of the liquor amnii. *Journal of Obstetrics and Gynaecology of the British Commonwealth*, **73**, 88–90.

Brown, R. & Pickering, D. (1974) Persisting transitional circulation. *Archives of Disease in Childhood*, **49**, 883–885.

Bryan, C. S. (1967) Enhancement of bacterial infection by meconium. *Johns Hopkins Medical Journal*, **121**, 9–13.

Bryan, M. H., Hardie, M. J., Reilly, B. J. & Swyer, P. R. (1973) Pulmonary function studies during the first year of life in infants recovering from the respiratory distress syndrome. *Pediatrics*, **52**, 169–178.

Burnard, E. D., Grattan-Smith, P., Picton-Warlow, C. G. & Grauaug, A. (1965) Pulmonary insufficiency in prematurity. *Australian Paediatric Journal*, **1**, 12–24.

Campbell, S. (1969) The prediction of fetal maturity by ultrasonic measurement of the biparietal diameter. *Journal of Obstetrics and Gynaecology of the British Commonwealth*, **76**, 603–609.

Carpenter, R. G. (1972) Epidemiology. In *Sudden and Unexpected Deaths in Infancy (cot deaths)*, ed. Camps, F. E. & Carpenter, R. G., pp. 7–14. Bristol: John Wright and Sons Ltd.

Carpenter, R. G. & Shaddick, C. W. (1965) Role of infection, suffocation and bottle-feeding in cot death; an analysis of some factors in the histories of 110 cases and their controls. *British Journal of Preventive and Social Medicine*, **19**, 1–7.

Carson, S. H., Taeusch, H. W. Jr & Avery, M. E. (1973) Inhibition of lung cell division after hydrocortisone injection into fetal rabbits. *Journal of Applied Physiology*, **34**, 660–663.

Chanock, R. M., Roizman, B. & Myers, R. (1957) Recovery from infants with respiratory illness of a virus related to chimpanzee coryza agent (CCA). I. Isolation properties and characterization. *American Journal of Hygiene*, **66**, 281–290.

Chanock, R. M., Kim, H. W., Vargosko, A. J., Deleva, A., Johnson, K. M., Cumming, C. & Parrott, R. H. (1961) Respiratory syncytial virus I. Virus recovery and other observations during 1960 outbreak of bronchiolitis, pneumonia and minor respiratory diseases in children. *Journal of the American Medical Association*, **176**, 647–653.

Chanock, R. M., Kapikian, A. Z., Mills, J., Kim, H. W. & Parrott, R. H. (1970) Influence of immunological factors in respiratory syncytial virus disease of the lower respiratory tract. *Archives of Environmental Health*, **21**, 347–355.

Chernick, V. (1973) Continuous negative chest wall pressure therapy for hyaline membrane disease. *Pediatric Clinics of North America*, **20**, 407–417.

Chernick, V. & Avery, M. E. (1963) Spontaneous alveolar rupture at birth. *Pediatrics*, **32**, 816–824.

Chernick, V. & Reed, M. H. (1970) Pneumothorax and chylothorax in the neonatal period. *Journal of Pediatrics*, **76**, 624–632.

Chernick, V., Heldrich, F. & Avery, M. E. (1964) Periodic breathing of premature infants. *Journal of Pediatrics*, **64**, 330–340.

Chessells, J. M. & Wigglesworth, J. S. (1971) Haemostatic failure in babies with rhesus isoimmunisation. *Archives of Disease in Childhood*, **46**, 38–45.

Chessells, J. M. & Wigglesworth, J. S. (1972) Coagulation studies in preterm infants with respiratory distress and intracranial haemorrhage. *Archives of Disease in Childhood*, **47**, 564–570.

Chu, J., Clements, J. A., Cotton, E. K., Klaus, M. H., Sweet, A. Y. & Tooley, W. H. (1967) Neonatal pulmonary ischemia. I. Clinical and physiological studies. *Pediatrics*, **40**, 709–782.

Clark, J. M. & Lambertsen, C. J. (1971) Pulmonary oxygen toxicity—a review. *Pharmacological Reviews*, **23**, 37–133.

Clements, J. A., Platzker, A. C. G., Tierney, D. F., Hobel, C. J., Creasy, R. K., Margolis, A. J., Thibeault, D. W., Tooley, W. H. & Oh, W. (1972) Assessment of the risk of the respiratory-distress syndrome by a rapid test for surfactant in amniotic fluid. *New England Journal of Medicine*, **286**, 1077–1081.

Cole, V. A., Normand, I. C. S., Reynolds, E. O. R. & Rivers, R. P. A. (1973) Pathogenesis of hemorrhagic pulmonary edema and massive pulmonary hemorrhage in the newborn. *Pediatrics*, **51**, 175–187.

Cook, L. N., Shott, R. J. & Andrews, B. F. (1974) Fetal complications of diagnostic amniocentesis: a review, and report of a case with pneumothorax. *Pediatrics*, **53**, 421–424.

Coombs, R. R. A. (1965) An experimental model for cot deaths. In *Sudden Death in Infants*, ed. Wedgewood, R. J. & Benditt, E. P., pp. 55–72. US Department of Health, Education and Welfare.

Cornblath, M. (1969) What place does gastrostomy feeding have in the care of sick premature infants? *Proceedings of 59th Ross Conference on Paediatric Research*, Ross Laboratories, Columbus, Ohio, pp. 53–56.

Court, S. D. M. (1973a) The definition of acute respiratory illness in children. *Postgraduate Medical Journal*, **49**, 771–776.

Court, S. D. M. (1973b) The management and outcome of children admitted to hospital. *Postgraduate Medical Journal*, **49**, 812–817.

Cross, K. W. & Lewis, S. R. (1971) Upper respiratory obstruction and cot death. *Archives of Disease in Childhood*, **46**, 211–213.

Daily, W. J. R., Klaus, M. & Meyer, H. B. P. (1969) Apnea in premature infants: monitoring, incidence, heart rate changes and an effect of environmental temperature. *Pediatrics*, **43**, 510–518.

Davies, P. A. (1971) Bacterial infection in the fetus and newborn. *Archives of Disease in Childhood*, **46**, 1–27.

Davies, P. A. & Stewart, A. L. (1975) Low birth weight infants: neurological sequelae. *British Medical Bulletin*, **31**, 85–91.

Davies, P. A. & Tizard, J. P. M. (1975) Very low birth weight, and subsequent neurological defect. *Developmental Medicine and Child Neurology*, **17**, 3–17.

Dawes, G. S., Hibbard, E. & Windle, W. F. (1964) The effect of alkali and glucose infusion on permanent brain damage in rhesus monkeys asphyxiated at birth. *Journal of Pediatrics*, **65**, 801–806.

de Lemos, R., Wolfsdorf, J., Nachman, R., Block, A. J., Leiby, G., Wilkinson, H. A., Allen, T, Haller, J. A., Morgan, W. & Avery, M. E. (1969) Lung injury from oxygen in lambs: the role of artificial ventilation. *Anesthesiology*, **30**, 609–618.

Delivoria-Papadopoulos, M., Roncevic, N. P. & Oski, F. A. (1971) Postnatal changes in oxygen transport of term, premature and sick infants; the role of red cell 2:3-diphosphoglycerate and adult haemoglobin. *Pediatric Research*, **5**, 235–245.

Desmond, M. M., Moore, J., Lindley, J. E. & Brown, C. A. (1957) Meconium staining of the amniotic fluid. *Obstetrics and Gynecology*, **9**, 91–103.

Dewhurst, C. J., Dunham, A. M., Harvey, D. R. & Parkinson, C. E. (1973) Prediction of respiratory-distress syndrome by estimation of surfactant in the amniotic fluid. *Lancet*, **1**, 1475–1477.

Dikshit, K., Vyden, J. K., Forrester, J. S., Chatterjee, K., Prakash, R. & Swan, H. J. C. (1973) Renal and extrarenal hemodynamic effects of furosemide in congestive heart failure after acute myocardial infarction. *New England Journal of Medicine*, **288**, 1087–1090.

Ditchburn, R. K., McQuillin, J., Gardner, P. S. & Court, S. D. M. (1971) Respiratory syncytial virus in hospital cross infection. *British Medical Journal*, **3**, 671–673.

Dobbing, J. (1974) The later growth of the brain and its vulnerability. *Pediatrics*, **53**, 2–6.

Donald, I. & Steiner, R. E. (1953) Radiography in the diagnosis of hyaline membrane disease. *Lancet*, **2**, 846–849.

Dunn, P. M. (1963) Intestinal obstruction in the newborn with special reference to transient functional ileus associated with respiratory distress syndrome. *Archives of Disease in Childhood*, **38**, 459–467.

Dunn, P. M. (1973) Caesarean section and the prevention of respiratory distress syndrome of the newborn. In *Perinatal Medicine*, Proceedings of the Third European Congress of Perinatal Medicine, ed. Bassart, H., Cruz, J. M., Huber, A., Prod'hom, L. S. & Sistek, L. pp. 138–145. Bern, Stuttgart, Vienna: Hans Huber.

Dunn, P. M. (1974) Continuous positive airway pressure (CPAP) using the Gregory box. *Proceedings of the Royal Society of Medicine*, **67**, 245–247.

Dunn, P. M. & Speidel, B. D. (1973) The use of oxygen to close patent ductus arteriosus in preterm infants. *Lancet*, **2**, 333–334.

Ekelund, H. & Finnström, O. (1972) Fibrin degradation products and plasminogen in newborn infants with respiratory disturbances and postnatal asphyxia. *Acta Pediatrica Scandinavica*, **61**, 661–669.

Esterly, J. R. & Oppenheimer, E. H. (1966) Massive pulmonary hemorrhage in the newborn. I. Pathologic considerations. *Journal of Pediatrics*, **69**, 3–11.

Fanaroff, A. A., Wald, M., Gruber, H. S. & Klaus, M. H. (1972) Insensible water loss in low birth weight infants. *Pediatrics*, **50**, 236–245.

Fanaroff, A. A., Cha, C. C., Sosa, R., Crumrine, R. S. & Klaus, M. H. (1973) Controlled trial of continuous negative external pressure in the treatment of severe respiratory distress syndrome. *Journal of Pediatrics*, **82**, 921–928.

Farrell, P. M. & Zachman, R. D. (1973) Induction of choline phosphotransferase and lecithin synthesis in the fetal lung by corticosteroids. *Science*, **179**, 297–298.

Fedrick, J. & Butler, N. R. (1970) Certain causes of neonatal death. II. Intraventricular haemorrhage. *Biology of the Neonate*, **15**, 257–290.

Fedrick, J. & Butler, N. R. (1971a) Certain causes of neonatal death. III. Pulmonary infection (a) clinical factors. *Biology of the Neonate*, **17**, 458–471.

Fedrick, J. & Butler, N. R. (1971b) Certain causes of neonatal death. III. Pulmonary infection (b) Pregnancy and delivery. *Biology of the Neonate*, **18**, 45–57.

Federick, J. & Butler, N. R. (1971c) Certain causes of neonatal death. IV. Massive pulmonary haemorrhage. *Biology of the Neonate*, **18**, 243–262.

Fedrick, J. & Butler, N. R. (1972) Hyaline-membrane disease. *Lancet*, **2**, 768–769.

Fenner, A., Schalk, U., Hoenicke, H., Wendenburg, A. & Roehling, T. (1973) Periodic breathing in premature and neonatal babies: incidence, breathing pattern, respiratory gas tensions, response to changes in the composition of ambient air. *Pediatric Research*, **7**, 174–183.

Fitzgibbons, J. P. Jr, Nobrega, F. T., Ludwig, J., Kurland, L. T. & Harris, L. E. (1969) Sudden, unexpected, and unexplained death in infants. *Pediatrics*, **43**, 980–988.

Foucard, T. (1974) A follow-up study of children with asthmatoid bronchitis. *Acta Paediatrica Scandinavica*, **63**, 129–139.

Fouron, J. C. & Hébert, F. (1973) The circulatory effects of hematocrit variations in normovolemic newborn lambs. *Journal of Pediatrics*, **82**, 995–1003.

Franciosi, R. A., Knostman, J. D. & Zimmerman, R. A. (1973) Group B streptococcal neonatal and infant infections. *Journal of Pediatrics*, **82**, 707–718.

Froggatt, P., Lynas, M. A. & MacKenzie, G. (1971) Epidemiology of sudden unexpected death in infants ('cot death') in Northern Ireland. *British Journal of Preventive and Social Medicine*, **25**, 119–134.

Gabert, H. A., Bryson, M. J. & Stenchever, M. A. (1973) The effect of cesarean section on respiratory distress in the presence of a mature lecithin sphingomyelin ratio. *American Journal of Obstetrics and Gynecology*, **116**, 366–368.

Gardner, P. S. (1968) Virus infections and respiratory disease of childhood. *Archives of Disease in Childhood*, **43**, 629–645.

Gardner, P. S. (1973) Respiratory syncytial virus infection. *Postgraduate Medical Journal*, **49**, 788–791.

Gardner, P. S. & McQuillin, J. (1968) Application of immunofluorescent antibody technique in rapid diagnosis of respiratory syncytial virus infection. *British Medical Journal*, **3**, 340–343.

Gardner, P. S., McQuillin, J. & Court, S. D. M. (1970) Speculation on pathogenesis in death from respiratory syncytial virus infection. *British Medical Journal*, **1**, 327–330.

Gershanik, J. J., Levkoff, A. H. & Duncan, R. (1972) The association of hypocalcaemia and recurrent apnoea in premature infants. *American Journal of Obstetrics, and Gynecology*, **113**, 646–652.

Gersony, W. M. (1973) Persistence of the fetal circulation: a commentary. *Journal of Pediatrics*, **82**, 1103–1106.

Girling, D. J. (1972) Changes in heart rate, blood pressure and pulse pressure during apnoeic attacks in newborn babies. *Archives of Disease in Childhood*, **47**, 405–410.

Girling, D. J. & Hallide-Smith, K. A. (1971) Persistent ductus arteriosus in ill and premature babies. *Archives of Disease in Childhood*, **46**, 177–181.

Glass, L., Rajegowda, B. K. & Evans, H. E. (1971) Absence of respiratory distress syndrome in premature infants of heroin addicted mothers. *Lancet*, **2**, 685–686.

Glezen, W. P. & Denny, F. W. (1973) Epidemiology of acute lower respiratory disease in children. *New England Journal of Medicine*, **288**, 498–505.

Gluck, L. & Kulovich, M. V. (1973) Lecithin/sphingomyelin ratios in amniotic fluid in normal and abnormal pregnancy. *American Journal of Obstetrics and Gynecology*, **115**, 539–546.

Gluck, L., Kulovich, M. V., Borer, R. C. Jr, Brenner, P. H., Anderson, G. G. & Spellacy, W. N. (1971) Diagnosis of the respiratory distress syndrome by amniocentesis. *American Journal of Obstetrics and Gynecology*, **109**, 440–445.

Gluck, L., Kulovich, N. V., Eidelman, A. I., Cordero, L. & Khazin, A. F. (1972) Biochemical development of surface activity in mammalian lung. IV. Pulmonary lecithin synthesis in the human fetus and newborn and etiology of the respiratory distress syndrome. *Pediatric Research*, **6**, 81–99.

Goddard, P., Keith, I., Marcovitch, H., Roberton, N. R. C., Rolfe, P. & Scopes, J. W. (1974) The use of a continuously recording intravascular oxygen electrode in the newborn. *Archives of Disease in Childhood*, **49**, 853–860.

Goldenberg, V. E., Buckingham, S. & Sommers, S. C. (1969) Pilocarpine stimulation of granular pneumocyte secretion. *Laboratory Investigation*, **20**, 147–158.

Goldman, H. I., Maralit, A., Sun, S. & Lanzkowsky, P. (1973) Neonatal cyanosis and arterial oxygen saturation. *Journal of Pediatrics*, **82**, 319–324.

Gotoff, S. P. & Behrman, R. E. (1970) Neonatal septicemia. *Journal of Pediatrics*, **76**, 142–153.

Gregory, G. A., Gooding, C. A., Phibbs, R. H. & Tooley, W. H. (1974) Meconium aspiration in infants—a prospective study. *Journal of Pediatrics*, **85**, 848–852.

Gregory, G. A., Kitterman, J. A., Phibbs, R. H., Tooley, W. H. & Hamilton, W. K. (1971) Treatment of the idiopathic respiratory distress syndrome with continuous positive airway pressure. *New England Journal of Medicine*, **284**, 1333–1340.

Gupta, J. M., Dahlenburg, G. W. & Davis, J. A. (1967) Changes in blood gas tensions following administration of amine buffer THAM to infants with respiratory distress syndrome. *Archives of Disease in Childhood*, **42**, 416–427.

Gupta, J. M., Roberton, N. R. C. & Wigglesworth, J. S. (1968) Umbilical artery catheterisation in the newborn. *Archives of Disease in Childhood*, **43**, 382–387.

Habel, A. H., Sandor, G. S., Conn, N. C. & McCrae, W. M. (1972) Premature rupture of membranes and effects of prophylactic antibiotics. *Archives of Disease in Childhood*, **47**, 401–404.

Hall, R. T. & Oliver, T. K. Jr (1971) Aortic blood pressure in infants admitted to a neonatal intensive care unit. *American Journal of Diseases of Children*, **121**, 145–147.

Hambleton, G. & Wigglesworth, J. S. (1975) Vascular studies on premature brain. *Archives of Disease in Childhood*, **50**, 744 (abstract).

Hathorn, M. K. S. (1972) Ventilation in newborn infants in different sleep states. In *Foetal and Neonatal Physiology*, ed. Comline, R. S., Cross, K. W., Dawes, G. S. & Nathanielsz, P. W., pp. 67–70. Cambridge: University Press.

Hawker, J. M., Reynolds, E. O. R. & Taghizadeh, A. (1967) Pulmonary surface tension and pathological changes in infants dying after respiratory treatment for severe hyaline membrane disease. *Lancet*, **2**, 75–77.

Heird, W. C. (1974) Nasojejunal feeding. *Journal of Pediatrics*, **85**, 111–113.

Heird, W. C., Dell, R. B., Price, T. & Winters, R. W. (1972) Osmotic effects of infusion of THAM. *Pediatric Research*, **6**, 495–503.

Herman, S. & Reynolds, E. O. R. (1973) Methods for improving oxygenation in infants mechanically ventilated for severe hyaline membrane disease. *Archives of Disease in Childhood*, **48**, 612–617.

Hey, E. N. (1971) The care of babies in incubators. In *Recent Advances in Paediatrics*, ed. Gairdner, D. M. T. & Hull, D., pp. 171–216. London: Churchill.

Hey, E. N. (1975) The thermal environment of the newborn. *British Medical Bulletin*, **31**, 69–74.

Hey, E. N. & Hull, D. (1971) Lung function at birth in babies developing respiratory distress. *Journal of Obstetrics and Gynaecology of the British Commonwealth*, **78**, 1137–1146.

Hey, E. N. & Lenney, W. (1973) Safe resuscitation at birth. *Lancet*, **2**, 103–104.

Hodgman, J. E., Mikity, V. G., Tatter, D. & Cleland, R. S. (1969) Chronic respiratory distress in the premature infant. Wilson–Mikity syndrome. *Pediatrics*, **44**, 179–195.

Holmdahl, M. H., Nahas, C. G., Hassam, D. & Verosky, M. (1961) Acid-base changes in the cerebrospinal fluid following rapid changes in the bicarbonate-carbonic acid ratio in the blood. *Annals of the New York Academy of Science*, **92**, 520–527.

Houstek, J. (1970) Sudden infant death syndrome in Czechoslovakia: epidemiologic aspects. In *Sudden Infant Death Syndrome*, ed. Bergman, A. B., Beckwith, J. B. & Ray, C. G., pp. 55–63. University of Washington Press.

Howie, V. M. & Weed, A. S. (1957) Spontaneous pneumothorax in the first 10 days of life. *Journal of Pediatrics*, **50**, 6–15.

Ingman, M. J. (1970) Neonatal *Hemophilus influenzae* septicemia, originating from maternal amnionitis. *American Journal of Diseases of Children*, **119**, 66–67.

Johnson, P., Robinson, J. S. & Salisbury, D. (1973) The onset and control of breathing after birth. In *Foetal and Neonatal Physiology*, ed. Comline, R. S., Cross, K. W., Dawes, G. S. & Nathanielsz, P. W., pp. 217–221. Cambridge: University Press.

Kapikian, A. Z., Mitchell, R. H., Chanock, R. M., Shvedoff, R. A. & Stewart, R. A. (1969) An epidemiologic study of altered clinical reactivity to respiratory syncytial (RS) virus infection in children previously vaccinated with an inactivated RS virus vaccine. *American Journal of Epidemiology*, **89**, 405–421.

Karlberg, P., Cherry, R. B., Escardo, F. E. & Koch, G. (1962) Respiratory studies in newborn infants. II. Pulmonary ventilation and mechanics of breathing in the first minutes of life, including the onset of respiration. *Acta Paediatrica Scandinavica*, **51**, 121–136.

Kattwinkel, J., Fleming, D., Cha, C. C., Fanaroff, A. A. & Klaus, M. H. (1973) A device for administration of continuous positive airway pressure by the nasal route. *Pediatrics*, **52**, 131–134.

Kennedy, J. L. Jr (1974) Antepartum betamethasone in the prevention of respiratory distress syndrome (abstract). *Pediatric Research*, **8**, 447.

Kim, H. W., Canchola, J. G., Brandt, C. D. M., Pyles, G., Chanock, R. M., Jensen, K. & Parrott, R. H. (1969) Respiratory syncytial virus disease in infants despite prior administration of antigenic inactivated virus. *American Journal of Epidemiology*, **89**, 422–434.

Kim, H. W., Arrobio, J. O., Brandt, C. D., Wright, P., Hodes, D., Chanock, R. M. & Parrott, R. H. (1973) Safety and antigenicity of temperature sensitive (TS) mutant respiratory syncytial virus (RSV) in infants and children. *Pediatrics*, **52**, 56–63.

Kitterman, J. A., Edmunds, L. H. Jr, Gregory, G. A., Heymann, M. A., Tooley, W. H. & Rudolph, A. M. (1972) Patent ductus arteriosus in premature infants. *New England Journal of Medicine*, **287**, 473–477.

Klesius, P. H., Zimmerman, R. A., Mathews, J. H. & Krushak, D. H. (1973) Cellular and humoral immune response to group B streptococci. *Journal of Pediatrics*, **83**, 926–932.

Kotas, R. V., Mims, L. C. & Hart, L. K. (1974) Reversible inhibition of lung cell number after glucocorticoid injection into fetal rabbits to enhance surfactant appearance. *Pediatrics*, **53**, 358–361.

Kovalčik, V. (1963) The response of the isolated ductus arteriosus to oxygen and anoxia. *Journal of Physiology*, **169**, 185–197.

Krauss, D. R. & Marshall, R. E. (1975) Severe neck ulceration from CPAP head box. *Journal of Pediatrics*, **86**, 286–287.

Krovetz, L. J. & Rowe, R. D. (1972) Patent ductus, prematurity and pulmonary disease. *New England Journal of Medicine*, **287**, 513–514.

Kuhn, J. P., Fletcher, B. D. & De Lemos, R. A. (1969) Roentgen findings in transient tachypnea of the newborn. *Radiology*, **92**, 751–757.

Lackey, D. A. & Taber, P. (1972) An unusual complication of umbilical artery catheterisation *Pediatrics*, **49**, 281–283.

Larroche, J. C. (1972) Post-haemorrhagic hydrocephalus in infancy. Anatomical study. *Biology of the Neonate*, **20**, 287–299.

Lauweryns, J., Bernat, R., Lerut, A. & Detournay, G. (1973) Intrauterine pneumonia, an experimental study. *Biology of the Neonate*, **22**, 301–318.

Leake, R. D., Gunther, R. & Sunshine, P. (1974) Perinatal aspiration syndrome: its association with intrapartum events and anesthesia. *American Journal of Obstetrics and Gynecology*, **118**, 271–275.

Leer, J. A. Jr, Green, J. L., Heimlich, E. M., Hyde, J. S., Moffet, H. L., Young, G. A. & Barron, B. A. (1969) Corticosteroid treatment in bronchiolitis. A controlled collaborative study in 297 infants and children. *American Journal of Diseases of Children*, **117**, 495–503.

Liggins, G. C. (1969) Premature delivery of foetal lambs infused with glucocorticoids. *Journal of Endocrinology*, **45**, 515–523.

Liggins, G. C. & Howie, R. N. (1972) A controlled trial of antepartum glucocorticoid treatment for prevention of the respiratory distress syndrome in premature infants. *Pediatrics*, **50**, 515–525.

McCracken, G. H. Jr (1973) Group B streptococci: the new challenge in neonatal infections. *Journal of Pediatrics*, **82**, 703–706.

MacEwan, D. W., Dunbar, J. S., Smith, R. D. & Brown, B. St. J. (1971) Pneumothorax in young infants—recognition and evaluation. *Journal of the Canadian Association of Radiologists*, **22**, 264–269.

Macklin, C. C. (1939) Transport of air along sheaths of pulmonic blood vessels from alveoli to mediastinum; clinical implications. *Archives of Internal Medicine*, **64**, 913–926.

McMurphy, D. M., Heymann, M. A., Rudolph, A. M. & Melmon, K. L. (1972) Developmental changes in constriction of the ductus arteriosus. Responses to oxygen and vasoactive agents in the isolated ductus arteriosus of the fetal lamb. *Pediatric Research*, **6**, 231–238.

Mann, T. P. & Elliot, R. I. K. (1957) Neonatal cold injury due to accidental exposure to cold. *Lancet*, **1**, 229–234.

Markarian, M., Githens, J. H., Rosenblut, E., Fernandez, F., Jackson, J. J., Bannon, A. E., Lindley, A., Lubchenco, L. O. & Martorell, R. (1971a) Hypercoagulatability in premature infants with special reference to the respiratory distress syndrome. I. Coagulation studies. *Biology of the Neonate*, **17**, 84–97.

Markarian, M., Lubchenco, L. O., Rosenblut, E., Fernandez, F., Lang, D., Jackson, J. J., Bannon, A. E., Lindley, A., Githens, J. H. & Martorell, R. (1971b) Hypercoagulatability in premature infants with special reference to the respiratory distress syndrome and hemorrhage. II. The effect of heparin. *Biology of the Neonate*, **17**, 98–111.

Miller, D. L. (1973) Collaborative studies of acute respiratory disease in patients seen in general practice and in children admitted to hospital. Aims, field methods and morbidity rates. *Postgraduate Medical Journal*, **49**, 749–761.

Morgan, B. C., Martin, W. E., Hornbein, T. F., Crawford, E. W. & Guntheroth, W. G. (1966) Hemodynamic effects of intermittent positive pressure respiration. *Anesthesiology*, **27**, 584–590.

Morrow, G., Hope, J. W. & Boggs, T. R. Jr (1967) Pneumomediastinum—a silent lesion in the newborn. *Journal of Pediatrics*, **70**, 554–560.

Moss, A. J. & Monset-Couchard, M. (1967) Placental transfusion. Early versus late clamping of the umbilical cord. *Pediatrics*, **40**, 109–126.

Motoyama, E. K., Orzalesi, M. M., Kikkawa, Y., Kaibara, M., Wu, B., Zigas, C. J. & Cook, C. D. (1971) Effect of cortisol on the maturation of fetal rabbit lungs. *Pediatrics*, **48**, 547–555.

Mufson, M. A., Levine, H. D., Wasil, R. E., Mocega-Gonzalez, J. E. & Krause, H. E. (1973) Epidemiology of respiratory syncytial virus infection among infants and children in Chicago. *American Journal of Epidemiology*, **98**, 88–95.

Murdoch, D. & Cope, I. (1957) Ossification centres as evidence of foetal maturity. *Journal of Obstetrics and Gynaecology of the British Commonwealth*, **64**, 382–384.

Murphy, B. E. P., Clark, S. J., Donald, I. R., Pinsky, M. & Vedady, D. (1974) Conversion of maternal cortisol to cortisone during placental transfer to the human fetus. *American Journal of Obstetrics and Gynecology*, **118**, 538–541.

Mushin, A. (1971) Ocular changes in premature babies receiving controlled oxygen therapy in the neonatal period. *Proceedings of the Royal Society of Medicine*, **64**, 779–780.

Naeye, R. L. (1973) Pulmonary arterial abnormalities in the sudden-infant-death syndrome. *New England Journal of Medicine*, **289**, 1167–1170.

Neal, W. A., Reynolds, J. W., Jarvis, C. W. & Williams, H. J. (1972) Umbilical artery catheterisation. Demonstration of arterial thrombosis by aortography. *Pediatrics*, **50**, 6–13.

Neligan, G. A., Steiner, H., Gardner, P. S. & McQuillin, J. (1970) Respiratory syncytial virus infection of the newborn. *British Medical Journal*, **3**, 146–147.

Northway, W. H. Jr, Rosan, R. C. & Porter, D. Y. (1967) Pulmonary disease following respirator therapy of hyaline-membrane disease. *New England Journal of Medicine*, **276**, 357–368.

Olinsky, A., MacMurray, S. B. & Swyer, P. R. (1973) Continus pressure breathing in RDS: comparative trial of three methods: Paper presented at the International Conference on Intensive Care of the Newborn, Banff, Canada.

Olver, R. E., Reynolds, E. O. R. & Strang, L. B. (1972) Foetal lung liquid. In *Foetal and Neonatal Physiology*, ed. Comline, R. S., Cross, K. W., Dawes, G. S. & Nathanielsz, P. W., pp. 186–207. Cambridge University Press.

Opie, L. H. (1965) Cardiac metabolism. The effect of some physiologic, pharmacologic and pathologic influences. *American Heart Journal*, **69**, 401–409.

Parish, W. E., Barrett, A. M., Coombs, R. R. A., Gunther, M. & Camps, F. E. (1960) Hypersensitivity to milk and sudden death in infancy. *Lancet*, **2**, 1106–1110.

Parmelee, A. H. Jr, Wenner, W. H., Akiyama, Y., Shultz, M. & Stern, E. (1967) Sleep states in premature infants. *Developmental Medicine and Child Neurology*, **9**, 70–77.

Parrott, R. H., Kim, H. W., Arrobio, J. O., Hodes, D. S., Murphy, B. R., Brandt, C. D., Camargo, E. & Chanock, R. M. (1973) Epidemiology of respiratory syncytial virus in Washington, DC. II. Infection and disease with respect to age, immunologic status, race and sex. *American Journal of Epidemiology*, **98**, 289–300.

Perlstein, P. H., Edwards, N. K. & Sutherland, J. M. (1970) Apnea in premature infants and incubator-air-temperature changes. *New England Journal of Medicine*, **282**, 461–466.

Peterson, R. D. A. & Good, R. A. (1963) Antibodies to cow's milk protein—their presence and significance. *Pediatrics*, **31**, 209–221.

Phelan, P. D. & Stocks, J. G. (1974) Management of severe viral bronchiolitis and severe acute asthma. *Archives of Disease in Childhood*, **49**, 143–148.

Pildes, R. S. (1973) Infants of diabetic mothers. *New England Journal of Medicine*, **289**, 902–904.

Polmar, S. H., Robinson, L. D. & Minnefor, A. B. (1972) Immunoglobulin E in bronchiolitis. *Pediatrics*, **50**, 279–284.

Poole, P. M. & Tobin, J. O'H. (1973) Viral and epidemiological findings in MRC/PHLS survey of respiratory disease in hospital and general practice. *Postgraduate Medical Journal*, **49**, 778–787.

Prod'hom, L. S., Levison, H., Cherry, R. B. & Smith, C. A. (1965) Adjustment of ventilation, intrapulmonary gas exchange and acid-base balance during the first day of life. *Pediatrics*, **35**, 662–676.

Protestos, C. D., Carpenter, R. G., McWeeny, P. M. & Emery, J. L. (1973) Obstetric and perinatal histories of children who died unexpectedly (cot death). *Archives of Disease in Childhood*, **48**, 835–841.

Pusey, V. A., MacPherson, R. I. & Chernick, V. (1969) Pulmonary fibroplasia following prolonged artificial ventilation of newborn infants. *Canadian Medical Association Journal*, **100**, 451–457.

Radde, I. C., Parkinson, D. K., Höffken, B., Appiah, K. E. & Hanley, W. B. (1972) Calcium ion activity in the sick neonate. Effect of bicarbonate administration and exchange transfusion. *Pediatric Research*, **6**, 43–49.

Reid, D. H. S. & Mitchell, R. G. (1966) Recurrent neonatal apnoea. *Lancet*, **1**, 786–788.

Reynolds, E. O. R. (1975) Management of hyaline membrane disease. *British Medical Bulletin*, **31**, 18–24.

Reynolds, E. O. R. & Taghizadeh, A. (1974) Improved prognosis of infants mechanically ventilated for hyaline membrane disease. *Archives of Disease in Childhood*, **49**, 505–515.

Reynolds, E. O. R., Roberton, N. R. C. & Wigglesworth, J. S. (1968) Hyaline membrane disease, respiratory distress and surfactant deficiency. *Pediatrics*, **42**, 758–768.

Reynolds, J. W. (1973) Serum total corticoid and cortisol levels in premature infants with respiratory distress syndrome. *Pediatrics*, **51**, 884–890.

Rhodes, P. G. & Hall, R. T. (1973) Continuous positive airway pressure delivered by face mask in infants with the idiopathic respiratory distress syndrome: a controlled study. *Pediatrics*, **52**, 1–5.

Richards, I. D. G. & McIntosh, H. T. (1972) Confidential enquiry into 226 consecutive infant deaths. *Archives of Disease in Childhood*, **47**, 697–706.

Rigatto, H. & Brady, J. P. (1972a) Periodic breathing and apnoea in preterm infants. I. Evidence for hypoventilation possibly due to central respiratory depression. *Pediatrics*, **50**, 202–218.

Rigatto, H. & Brady, J. P. (1972b) Periodic breathing and apnoea in preterm infants. II. Hypoxia as a primary event. *Pediatrics*, **50**, 219–228.

Roberton, N. R. C. (1970) Apnoea after THAM administration in the newborn. *Archives of Disease in Childhood*, **45**, 206–214.

Roberton, N. R. C. (1974) Prolonged CPAP for pulmonary oedema due to a patent ductus arteriosus in the newborn. *Archives of Disease in Childhood*, **49**, 585–587.

Roberton, N. R. C. & Dahlenburg, G. W. (1969) Ductus arteriosus shunts in the respiratory distress syndrome. *Pediatric Research*, **3**, 149–159.

Roberton, N. R. C., Gupta, J. M., Dahlenburg, G. W. & Tizard, J. P. M. (1968) Oxygen therapy in the newborn. *Lancet*, **1**, 1323–1329.

Roberton, N. R. C., Hallidie-Smith, K. A. & Davis, J. A. (1967) Severe respiratory distress syndrome mimicking cyanotic heart-disease in term babies. *Lancet*, **2**, 1108–1110.

Roberton, N. R. C. & Smith, A. (1975) Early neonatal hypocalcaemia. *Archives of Disease in Childhood*, **50**, 604–609.

Robin, E. D., Cross, C. E. & Zelis, R. (1973) Pulmonary edema. *New England Journal of Medicine*, **288**, 292–304.

Rosen, M. & Laurence, K. M. (1965) Expansion pressures and rupture pressures in the newborn lung. *Lancet*, **2**, 721–722.

Ross, C. A. C., Pinkerton, I. W. & Assaad, F. A. (1971) Pathogenesis of respiratory syncytial virus diseases in infancy. *Archives of Disease in Childhood*, **46**, 702–704.

Rowe, S. & Avery, M. E. (1966) Massive pulmonary hemorrhage in the newborn. *Journal of Pediatrics*, **69**, 12–20.

Russell, G. & Cotton, E. K. (1968) Effects of sodium bicarbonate by rapid injection and of oxygen in high concentration in respiratory distress syndrome of the newborn. *Pediatrics*, **41**, 1063–1073.

Savage, M. O., Wilkinson, A. R., Baum, J. D. & Roberton, N. R. C. (1975) Frusemide in respiratory distress syndrome. *Archives of Disease in Childhood*, **50**, 709–713.

Schlesinger, E. R. (1973) Neonatal intensive care: planning for services and outcomes following care. *Journal of Pediatrics*, **82**, 916–920.

Scopes, J. W. (1966) Metabolic rate and temperature control in the human baby. *British Medical Bulletin*, **22**, 88–91.

Shaw, E. B. (1970) Sudden unexpected death in infancy syndrome. *American Journal of Diseases of Children*, **119**, 416–418.

Shaw, J. C. L. (1973) Parenteral nutrition in the management of sick low birthweight infants. *Pediatric Clinics of North America*, **20**, 333–358.

Shepard, F. M., Johnston, R. B. Jr, Klatte, E. C., Burko, H. & Stahlman, M. (1968) Residual pulmonary findings in clinical hyaline-membrane disease. *New England Journal of Medicine*, **279**, 1063–1071.

Shephard, B., Buhi, W. & Spellacy, W. (1974) Critical analysis of the amniotic fluid shake test. *Obstetrics and Gynecology*, **43**, 558–562.

Siassi, B., Emmanouilides, G. C., Cleveland, R. J. & Hirose, F. (1969) Patent ductus arteriosus complicating prolonged assisted ventilation in respiratory distress syndrome. *Journal of Pediatrics*, **74**, 11–19.

Simon, G. & Jordan, W. S. Jr (1967) Infectious and allergic aspects of bronchiolitis. *Journal of Pediatrics*, **70**, 533–538.

Simon, H. J., Yaffe, S. J. & Gluck, L. (1961) Effective control of staphylococci in a nursery. *New England Journal of Medicine*, **265**, 1171–1176.

Simpson, H. & Flenley, D. C. (1967) Arterial blood-gas tensions and pH in acute lower-respiratory-tract infections in infancy and childhood. *Lancet*, **1**, 7–12.

Sinclair, J. C., Driscoll, J. M. Jr, Heird, W. C. & Winters, R. W. (1970) Supportive management of the sick neonate. Parenteral calories, water and electrolytes. *Pediatric Clinics of North America*, **17**, 863–893.

Singh, K. R., Wigglesworth, F. W. & Stern, L. (1972) Pneumopericardium in the newborn— a complication of respirator management *Canadian Medical Association Journal*, **106**, 1195–1196.

Smallpeice, V. & Davies, P. A. (1964) Immediate feeding of premature infants with undiluted breast-milk. *Lancet*, **2**, 1349–1352.

Spellacy, W. N., Buhi, W. C., Riggall, F. C. & Holsinger, K. L. (1973) Human amniotic fluid lecithin/sphingomyelin ratio changes with estrogen or glucocorticoid treatment. *American Journal of Obstetrics and Gynecology*, **115**, 216–218.

Speidel, B. D. & Dunn, P. M. (1975) Effect of continuous positive airway pressure on breathing pattern in infants with respiratory distress syndrome. *Lancet*, **1**, 302–304.

Stahlman, M., Blankenship, W. J., Shepard, F. M., Gray, J., Young, W. C. & Malan, A. F. (1972) Circulatory studies in clinical hyaline membrane disease. *Biology of the Neonate*, **20**, 300–320.

Stahlman, M., Cheatham, W. & Gray, M. E. (1973) Interstitial emphysema and chronic lung disease in post-respiratory hyaline membrane disease. Paper presented at the International Conference on Intensive Care of the Newborn, Banff, Canada.

Stahlman, M., Hedvall, G., Dolanski, E., Faxelius, G., Burko, H. & Kirk, V. (1973) A six-year follow-up of clinical hyaline membrane disease. *Pediatric Clinics of North America*, **20**, 433–446.

Steele, R. W., Metz, J. R., Bass, J. W. & Dubois, J. J. (1971) Pneumothorax and pneumo-mediastinum in the newborn. *Radiology*, **98**, 629–632.

Steinschneider, A. (1972) Prolonged apnoea and sudden infant death syndrome. *Pediatrics*, **50**, 646–654.

Stern, L., Ramos, A. D., Outerbridge, E. W. & Beaudry, P. H. (1970) Negative pressure artificial respiration: use in treatment of respiratory failure of the newborn. *Canadian Medical Association Journal*, **102**, 595–601.

Stevens, L. H. (1965) Sudden unexplained death in infancy. Observations on a natural mechanism of adoption of the face down position. *American Journal of Diseases of Children*, **110**, 243–247.

Sundell, H., Garrott, J., Blankenship, W. J., Shepard, F. M. & Stahlman, M. J. (1971) Studies on infants with type II respiratory distress syndrome. *Journal of Pediatrics*, **78**, 754–764.

Swift, P. G. F. & Emery, J. L. (1973) Clinical observations on response to nasal occlusion in infancy. *Archives of Disease in Childhood*, **48**, 947–951.

Swyer, P. R. (1969) An assessment of artificial respiration in the newborn. *Proceedings of 59th Ross Conference on Pediatric Research, Columbus, Ohio*, pp. 25–35.

Swyer, P. R., Delivoria-Papadopoulos, M., Levison, H., Reilly, B. J. & Balis, J. U. (1965) The pulmonary syndrome of Wilson and Mikity. *Pediatrics*, **36**, 374–384.

Taeusch, H. W. Jr, Carson, S. H., Wang, N. S. & Avery, M. E. (1973a) Heroin induction of lung maturation and growth retardation in fetal rabbits. *Journal of Pediatrics*, **82**, 869–875.

Taeusch, H. W. Jr, Wang, N. S., Baden, M., Bauer, C. R. & Stern, L. (1973b) A controlled trial of hydrocortisone therapy in infants with respiratory distress syndrome. II. Pathology. *Pediatrics*, **52**, 850–854.

Taeusch, H. W., Wyszogrodski, I., Wang, N. S. & Avery, M. E. (1974) Pulmonary pressure volume relationships in premature fetal and newborn rabbits. *Journal of Applied Physiology*, **37**, 809–813.

Taylor, P. M., Allen, A. C. & Stinson, D. A. (1971) Benign unexplained respiratory distress of the newborn infant. *Pediatric Clinics of North America*, **18**, 975–1004.

Thibeault, D. W. & Hobel, C. J. (1974) The interrelationship of the foam stability test, immaturity and intrapartum complications in the respiratory distress syndrome. *American Journal of Obstetrics and Gynecology*, **118**, 56–61.

Thibeault, D. W., Lachman, R. S., Laul, V. R. & Kwong, M. S. (1973) Pulmonary interstitial emphysema, pneumomediastinum and pneumothorax. *American Journal of Diseases of Children*, **126**, 611–614.

Tracey, V. V., De, N. C. & Harper, J. R. (1971) Obesity and respiratory infection in infants and young children. *British Medical Journal*, **1**, 16–18.

Trompeter, R., Yu, V. Y. H., Aynsley-Green, A. & Roberton, N. R. C. (1975) Massive pulmonary haemorrhage in the newborn infant. *Archives of Disease in Childhood*, **50**, 123–127.

Tsang, R. C. & Oh, W. (1970) Neonatal hypocalcaemia in low birth weight infants. *Pediatrics*, **45**, 773–781.

Turner, T., Evans, J. & Brown, J. K. (1975) Monoparesis: complication of constant positive airways pressure. *Archives of Disease in Childhood*, **50**, 128–129.

Usher, R. H., Allen, A. C. & McLean, F. H. (1971) Risk of respiratory distress syndrome related to gestational age, route of delivery and maternal diabetes. *American Journal of Obstetrics and Gynecology*, **111**, 826–832.

Usher, R., Saigal, S., O'Neill, A., Chua, L. & Surainder, Y. (1971) Red cell volume in respiratory distress syndrome (abstract). *Pediatric Research*, **5**, 415.

Valdes-Dapena, M. A. (1967) Sudden and unexpected death in infancy: a review of the world literature 1954–1966. *Pediatrics*, **39**, 123–138.

Valdes-Dapena, M. (1970) Progress in sudden infant death research 1963–1969. In *Sudden Infant Death Syndrome*. ed. Bergman, A. B., Beckwith, J. B. & Ray, C. G., pp. 3–13. Seattle and London: University of Washington Press.

Valdes-Dapena, M. A. & Felipe, R. P. (1971) Immunofluorescent studies in crib deaths: absence of evidence of hypersensitivity to cow's milk. *American Journal of Clinical Pathology*, **56**, 412–415.

Van Vliet, P. K. J. & Gupta, J. M. (1973) THAM v. sodium bicarbonate in idiopathic respiratory distress syndrome. *Archives of Disease in Childhood*, **48**, 249–255.

Vert, P., Andre, M. & Sibout, M. (1973) Continuous positive airway pressure and hydrocephalus. *Lancet*, **2**, 319.

Warren, C., Holton, J. B. & Allen, J. T. (1974) Assessment of fetal lung maturity by estimation of amniotic fluid palmitic acid. *British Medical Journal*, **1**, 94–96.

Wealthall, S. (1973) An animal model for cot death. Paper presented to Neonatal Society, Manchester.

Webb, P. (1974) Periodic breathing during sleep. *Journal of Applied Physiology*, **37**, 899–903.

Westgate, H. D., Fisch, R. O., Langer, L. O. Jr & Staub, H. P. (1969) Pulmonary and respiratory function changes in survivors of hyaline-membrane disease. *Diseases of the Chest*, **56**, 465–470.

Whitfield, C. R., Sproule, W. B. & Brudenell, M. (1973) The amniotic fluid lecithin/sphingomyelin area ratio (LSAR) in pregnancies complicated by diabetes. *Journal of Obstetrics and Gynaecology of the British Commonwealth*, **80**, 918–922.

Wilkinson, A. R. & Yu, V. Y. H. (1974) Immediate effects of feeding on blood gases and some cardiorespiratory functions in ill newborn infants. *Lancet*, **1**, 1083–1085.

Wilson, J. L., Long, S. B. & Howard, P. J. (1942) Respiration of premature infants. *American Journal of Diseases of Children*, **63**, 1080–1085.

Wilson, M. G. & Mikity, V. G. (1960) A new form of respiratory disease in premature infants. *American Journal of Diseases of Children*, **99**, 489–499.

Wyszogrodski, I., Taeusch, H. W. & Avery, M. E. (1975) Isoxuprine induced alterations of pulmonary pressure volume relationships in premature rabbits. *American Journal of Obstetrics and Gynecology*, (in press).

Yao, A. C. & Lind, J. (1974) Placental transfusion. *American Journal of Diseases of Children*, **127**, 128–141.

Yashiro, K., Adams, F. H., Emmanouilides, G. C. & Mickey, M. R. (1973) Preliminary studies on the thermal environment of low birthweight infants. *Journal of Pediatrics*, **82**, 991–994.

Yu, V. Y. H., Rolfe, P. & Roberton, N. R. C. (1975) Cardiorespiratory responses to continuous positive airways pressure in respiratory distress syndrome (submitted for publication).

Zacharias, L. (1960) Incidence of retrolental fibroplasia. *Pediatrics*, **25**, 726–727.

Zachman, R. D., Olson, E. B., Frantz, T. A., Bergseth, M. E. & Graven, S. N. (1973) Respiratory distress syndrome with amniotic fluid lecithin/sphingomyelin ratios greater than two. *Pediatric Research*, **7**, 395.

Zinner, S. H., McCormack, W. M., Lee, Y.-H., Zuckerstatter, M. H. & Daly, A. K. (1972) Puerperal bacteremia and neonatal sepsis due to hemophilus parainfluenzae: report of a case with antibody titers. *Pediatrics*, **49**, 612–614.

9
MISCELLANEOUS PROBLEMS

A. L. Muir   T. B. Stretton

In this chapter we first describe recent developments in bronchoscopy and then discuss pulmonary oedema, the lungs in renal disease, and shock lung.

BRONCHOSCOPY

In recent years there have been two significant advances in this long-established procedure. The first was the introduction by Sanders in 1967 of an attachment for the rigid bronchoscope to facilitate ventilation of the anaesthetised patient during bronchoscopy. The second was the development of a flexible fibreoptic instrument (Ikeda, Yanai and Ishikawa, 1968). More recently Ikeda has published his *Atlas of Flexible Bronchofiberscopy* (1974).

Whilst bronchoscopy under local anaesthesia may be safer than under a general anaesthetic, it is certainly more unpleasant for the subject when a rigid bronchoscope is being used. Given the choice, most patients elect to have a general anaesthetic for the procedure. Although 'ventilating broncho-scopes' have been described, and some operators have used cuirass ventilators to maintain breathing throughout the examination, it has been common anaesthetic practice to rely on apnoeic oxygenation ('diffusion respiration') when the bronchoscope is inserted into the patient's trachea. However, with the kind of device invented by Sanders (1967) the maintenance of breathing is made simple and effective. Utilising the Venturi principle, a high-pressure jet of oxygen, directed by means of an injection device into the proximal end of the bronchoscope, entrains room air down the tube, and the oxygen–air mixture issuing from the distal end of the instrument inflates the patient's lungs. The high-pressure jet of oxygen is delivered intermittently by a simple hand-operated on–off switch, oxygen being taken directly from a standard pipeline source at a pressure of approximately 4.0 bar. The Venturi injection device is simplicity itself. It consists essentially of a 16 to 19 gauge needle which is clamped to the proximal end of the bronchoscope with the needle-shaft lying adjacent to the wall of the 'scope and directed down its lumen. The high-pressure oxygen delivery tube is locked on to the luer hub of the needle which is bent outwards at a right angle to receive this.

Using apparatus of this type, with minor modifications or variation in design, ventilation and oxygenation of the anaesthetised and relaxed patient are both readily and efficiently maintained. The anaesthetist simply opens and closes the switch on the oxygen delivery tubing to inflate the lungs by intermittent positive pressure at a suitable frequency. The adequacy of ventilation is judged by inspection of the patient's chest movements.

With this technique the gas pressure and oxygen concentration issuing from the distal end of the bronchoscope are influenced by the pressure of the oxygen source, the dimensions of the Venturi injector and the size of the bronchoscope. Using a 16 s.w.g. Venturi attachment in combination with three sizes of Negus bronchoscopes ('adult', 'small adult' and 'adolescent'), Ball, Dundee and Stevenson (1973) recorded oxygen concentrations of 40 to 46 per cent and inflation pressures of 22 to 29 cmH_2O, the highest values being found with the narrowest bronchoscope. Insertion of a suction tube or telescope through the bronchoscope produced higher values for oxygen and inflation pressure by reducing the cross-sectional area of the tube and hence increasing resistance to the inflow of room air. Arterial pH, Pco_2 and Po_2 values in eight patients studied by Ball et al (1973) during bronchoscopic ventilation were 7.36 to 7.46, 28 to 43 and 85 to 200 mmHg, respectively.

There can be little doubt that this technique is both safe and satisfactory, and will be accepted as standard practice during bronchoscopy of the anaesthetised subject. The only objections likely to be raised by the bronchoscopist are to the noise from the Venturi and the degree of blow-back which is usually slight but can on occasion be somewhat excessive.

The second development, that of the flexible bronchoscope, is arguably of even greater importance. This instrument in no way replaces the rigid tube and may be regarded as either complementary or supplementary to the latter. Indeed, expertise with a rigid bronchoscope continues to be as necessary as ever. But the fibreoptic instrument has certain definite advantages for diagnostic bronchoscopy. With it, the procedure can be performed in the conscious subject, with a minimum of discomfort, using topical anaesthesia. The narrow diameter (4–6 mm) and flexibility of the tube permits greater penetration into and inspection of the bronchial tree. In particular, upper lobe examination is greatly facilitated. Subsegmental bronchi (the fourth division down) are readily accessible to the fibreoptic bronchoscope and with smaller diameter instruments this range will increase further. Small biospy samples may be taken from visible lesions, bronchial brushings can be obtained, and samples of secretion may be aspirated. The aspirate may be taken directly through the bronchoscope or through a fine polyethylene catheter inserted through the bronchoscope into more peripheral airways.

The entire procedure can be observed by an assistant using a secondary fibreoptic light pathway attached to the eyepiece of the bronchoscope. This kind of device, or 'lecturescope', is of obvious educational value. It also allows a trainee bronchoscopist to acquire the necessary manipulative skills with the bronchoscope whilst the teacher watches proceedings through the lecturescope. The major constraints in this educational relationship are that it can be lengthy and the conscious patient can also listen to any discussion that takes place.

Photographs may readily be taken through the bronchoscope though the image size is small and the fibreoptic bundles impose limitations in the quality of the end result. Nevertheless, this is a potentially valuable resource and has research as well as clinical applications (Sackner, 1975). Regional sampling and analysis of gas from the lungs can assist in the localisation of disordered lung function (Hugh Jones, 1967) and may be performed through a fibreoptic bronchoscope. These and other applications have been well reviewed by Sackner (1975).

There is some controversy, particularly in Britain, about the place of fibreoptic bronchoscopy in medical practice. The equipment is more expensive and more delicate than the traditional bronchoscope. It is also more difficult to sterilise. The required manipulative skills are different and are not always acquired readily, even by those who are skilled and experienced with rigid instruments. Moreover, it is possible to learn how to pass a fibreoptic bronchoscope into the bronchial tree without necessarily being able to intubate in the conventional way. This is potentially hazardous and it is most important to be able to insert an endotracheal tube before learning to manipulate a fibreoptic bronchoscope.

There are several ways of passing the fibreoptic instrument: through the nose or the mouth, either alone or through an endotracheal tube or rigid bronchoscope, and it can also be inserted through a tracheostomy tube. With the fibreoptic bronchoscope (fibrescope) in position, ventilation takes place through the space in the air passages alongside the instrument, and there must be adequate room for this to occur. When the fibrescope is used on its own, the operator has no control over the patient's airway throughout the entire procedure. While problems may never arise, the development of severe laryngospasm in such circumstances, or sudden cardiorespiratory arrest, would necessitate urgent endotracheal intubation. Hence the need for prior skill with this procedure.

Some operators prefer to carry out bronchoscopy in the traditional manner under general anaesthesia using a rigid bronchoscope, and pass the fibreoptic instrument through this for more extensive visualisation of the bronchial tree. Others prefer to insert an endotracheal tube and use this as an airway and a pathway for the fibrescope. Although this may be performed under local anaesthesia, a general anaesthetic seems kinder to the patient. Ventilatory assistance can then be given through the side arm of a T tube connected to the endotracheal tube. The fibrescope is inserted through a small hole in a rubber membrane or diaphragm which is tied over the end of the T tube, to prevent air leaking back past the fibrescope. The same effect can be achieved using a detachable cuff which is slipped over the fibrescope and inflated so as to occlude the proximal opening of the T tube (Reichert, Hall and Hyde, 1974).

Many bronchoscopists prefer to pass the fibrescope under local anaesthesia,

10

without using an airway, through either the nose or the mouth. The pernasal pathway is very satisfactory indeed, providing the dimensions of the nasal cavity are adequate to accommodate the tube, and this is the most frequently chosen route by bronchoscopists in the USA, (Credle, Smiddy and Elliott, 1974). The patient is able to remain semirecumbent or even sitting throughout the examination and there is no need for special positioning of the head. If the oral route is used and the patient is not edentulous, care must be taken to ensure that he does not bite the instrument.

Local anaesthesia is best achieved by the topical application of lignocaine in either 4 or 2 per cent concentration. The patient is premedicated $\frac{1}{2}$ to 1 h before the procedure with atropine, usually combined with a sedative. There is a wide choice of drugs suitable for sedation, though diazepam, which is justifiably popular in many other circumstances, appears less satisfactory in this context because the cough reflex remains brisk.

Anxiety has been expressed because the arterial Po_2 may fall during the procedure (*British Medical Journal*, 1974). In our experience the fall in Po_2 is modest and is of little consequence in patients with an initially normal Po_2. It is a simple matter to anticipate any aggravation of hypoxia in patients with pre-existing hypoxaemia by administering oxygen throughout the examination. This can be done by means of an appropriate mask designed to give a controlled increase in inspired oxygen. The fibrescope is then passed through a hole in the facepiece.

Major complications are rare. Thus, in the survey by Credle et al (1974), 193 American bronchoscopists recorded a total of some 24 500 examinations, with major complications in 22 patients and three deaths. Half of the major complications and one of the deaths were related to premedication or topical anaesthesia and of those attributed to the procedure itself, the most common problem was severe laryngospasm. With careful premedication, avoidance of excessive local anaesthesia and anticipation of undue hypoxaemia, the major complications should be significantly reduced, thereby making fibreoptic bronchoscopy an even safer procedure.

It is in the diagnostic (and research) field that this instrument has its place. Therapeutic procedures such as the removal of a foreign body or control of bleeding demand the use of a rigid, tubular bronchoscope, though on occasion the fibrescope has been satisfactorily utilised to clear bronchial secretions in the seriously ill patient.

Facilities for fibreoptic bronchoscopy will undoubtedly expand, though their provision will be limited in certain areas by financial considerations. There is concern that those receiving training in the technique should first master the use of the traditional bronchoscope, though it seems improbable that this policy will be universally accepted. But we repeat that it is most important for the bronchoscopist to be able to insert an endotracheal tube swiftly should the need arise, and adequate provision must be made for dealing with other respiratory or cardiac emergencies.

PULMONARY OEDEMA

Physicians commonly encounter the problem of pulmonary oedema and usually associate it with a raised hydrostatic pressure at the venous end of the pulmonary capillaries, but in recent years other mechanisms have attracted increasing attention. Pulmonary oedema may be most conveniently defined as a pathological state in which there is an increase in the extravascular liquid within the lung, though Staub (1974) has suggested that the concept of pulmonary oedema deserves to be extended to include changes in the rate of fluid and protein flow through the interstitium as well as in its liquid and protein content. The extra volume of liquid may be contained either in the interstitial compartment of the lung or in the alveolar gas space.

The interstitial space of the lung has two compartments: that between the alveolar epithelium and the capillary endothelium of the alveolar walls, the alveolar interstitial space; and the loose connective tissue of the interlobular septa and around the blood vessels and airways. The earliest manifestation of pulmonary oedema on light-microscopy is the accumulation of fluid in the loose interstitial perivascular and peribronchial spaces. This can be quite marked without any apparent change in alveolar wall interstitium or in the alveolar gas space (Staub, Nagano and Pearce, 1967). Only at a late stage in the development of the oedema is there leakage of fluid into the alveoli, first into the corners of the alveolar sacs and finally filling the alveoli with loss of alveolar volume. Even at the stage of alveolar oedema, the process is a patchy one, and does not involve the whole lung; an apparently normal alveolus may be adjacent to a fluid-filled alveolus. The preferential accumulation of fluid in the perivascular and peribronchial spaces suggests that there is a subatmospheric pressure in this loose interstitial space whilst the alveolar wall interstitium is subject to alveolar and therefore atmospheric pressure.

At first, analysis of the forces governing the passage of fluid from the capillaries assumed that these capillary walls were inert (Starling, 1896), but recently the importance of the permeability characteristics of the alveolar and capillary membranes has been stressed (Robin, Cross and Zelis, 1973). Pulmonary capillary membranes appear to have a higher permeability than alveolar membranes although the permeability of the latter may increase when alveoli are filled with liquid. Taylor and Gaar (1970) have estimated a pore radius of 6 to 10 Å for the pulmonary alveolar membrane and one of 40 to 50 Å for the capillary membrane. Permeability may be increased by haemodynamic factors. Thus, Pietra et al (1969), using stroma-free haemoglobin (approximately 60 Å) as an electron-dense marker, showed that high pulmonary capillary pressures seemed to widen the interendothelial cell-junctions and allow the passage of haemoglobin into the alveolar interstitial space.

The physicochemical forces governing transcapillary filtration of fluid (FF) can be expressed by the equation:

$$FF = k\left[(P_{cap} - P_{is}) - (\pi_{cap} - \pi_{is})\right]$$

where k is the water filtration coefficient and contains an expression of the surface area and the permeability characteristics of the pulmonary capillary membrane; P_{cap} is the pulmonary capillary hydrostatic pressure (normally about 10 mmHg); P_{is} is the interstitial fluid hydrostatic pressure; π_{cap} is the plasma colloid osmotic pressure (normally about 25 mmHg); π_{is} represents the interstitial fluid colloid osmotic pressure.

Approximate normal values for the two intracapillary pressures are indicated, though pulmonary capillary hydrostatic pressure will vary according to gravitational forces. The magnitude of the interstitial pressures is more difficult to establish. Meyer, Meyer and Guyton (1968) have presented evidence to show that the interstitial hydrostatic pressure is negative, whilst Staub (1971) has estimated that the interstitial colloid osmotic pressure is sufficiently high for liquid movement to occur even in the absence of a negative interstitial hydrostatic pressure. In addition to the physicochemical forces in the interstitial space, the movement of fluid is probably also influenced by surface tension forces at the air–liquid interface of alveolar–capillary units. These forces tend to draw liquid from the vascular bed into the alveolar space (Pattle, 1965). However, the effect of these forces, directed towards the alveoli, may be partly offset by alveolar pressure, which is approximately atmospheric. It thus seems likely that the net vectorial forces are such that fluid tends to accumulate within the interstitial space and normal lymph flow is essential to maintain a steady state in the water balance (Fig. 1). Certainly, an elevation of pulmonary venous pressure produces a prompt increase in pulmonary lymphatic flow (Földi, 1969). Although the amount of water in the lung increases when pulmonary venous pressure is increased or plasma proteins are decreased (Guyton and Lindsey, 1959) it is possible that fluid begins to accumulate only when the lymphatic drainage capacity is exceeded.

Abnormalities in any of the physicochemical forces or in membrane permeability can lead to the accumulation of an abnormal amount of fluid in the lung. The clinician most commonly encounters pulmonary oedema attributable to an increased pulmonary capillary pressure in left ventricular failure complicating ischaemic, hypertensive or valvular heart disease. The pulmonary capillary pressure is also increased in mitral stenosis and in pulmonary veno-occlusive disease. Overtransfusion may increase pulmonary capillary pressures and produce pulmonary oedema, and if non-colloid fluids have been used a low oncotic pressure may be implicated in the pathogenesis of the oedema. Decreased plasma oncotic pressure may well be important in the pulmonary oedema of hepatic disease and possibly also in a few patients with renal disease. However, there is good reason to believe that altered pulmonary capillary permeability is important in many patients with pulmonary oedema complicating renal failure (Merrill and Hampers, 1970;

Crosbie, Snowden and Parsons, 1972; Robin et al, 1973). Changes in alveolar and capillary permeability are also important in the production of oedema due to the inhalation of toxic gases such as nitrogen dioxide or due to circulating endotoxins. Experimentally, alloxan-induced pulmonary oedema is of this type. Cottrell and colleagues (1967) compared the electron microscopic appearances of haemodynamic and alloxan-induced pulmonary oedema. In the haemodynamic form the endothelium, the epithelium and their respective basement membranes appeared unaffected whilst in the alloxan form there

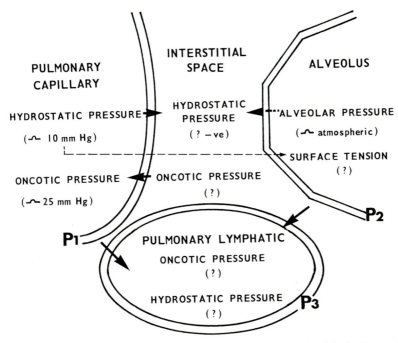

Figure 1 Diagrammatic representation of some of the forces involved in fluid transfer in the lung, where P_1, P_2 and P_3 represent the respective permeabilities of the capillary, alveolar and lymphatic membranes

was degeneration of both epithelium and endothelium. Effects due to the liberation of vasoactive substances have also been implicated in pulmonary oedema formation, and it has been shown in animal experiments that histamine can produce increased permeability of bronchial venules (Pietra et al, 1971). Such an effect could clearly be of importance in the genesis of interstitial oedema. A mechanical factor that may occasionally be responsible for the development of pulmonary oedema is the creation of an abnormally negative pressure in the interstitial space. This may be due to rapid re-expansion of the lung following hasty aspiration of a large pleural effusion or the application of excessive negative intrapleural pressure in the treatment of spontaneous pneumothorax (Ziskind, Weill and George, 1965).

Radiological Features of Pulmonary Oedema

When alveolar oedema develops there is filling of the gas space with fluid and there is loss of total alveolar volume. The radiographic appearance is due to the presence of the 'acinar shadow' which is the result of opacification of the air spaces supplied by one terminal bronchiole (Fraser and Paré, 1970). The shadows are often confluent and may be scattered throughout the lung fields though in many patients the distribution of the gas space oedema is around the hilum of the lung, producing the characteristic 'bat-wing' appearance; the reason for this particular anatomical distribution remains obscure.

Although the radiological diagnosis of gas space oedema is relatively easy, the recognition of the earlier interstitial oedema is more difficult, and it is far from certain how well the radiological features correlate with increased extravascular lung water. The important features are loss of normal sharp definition of pulmonary vascular markings and loss of demarcation of hilar shadows, later accompanied by thickening of the interlobular septa (B lines of Kerley). An increase in upper lobe vein size indicates pulmonary venous hypertension.

Haemodynamic correlations have been made by McHugh et al (1972) who found that, in patients with acute myocardial infarction, dilatation of upper lobe vessels occurred when pulmonary capillary pressure (i.e. 'wedge' pressure) was over 18 mmHg, whereas perihilar haze and diminished clarity of medium sized lung vessels were seen when this pressure lay between 18 and 22 mmHg. However, in 10 per cent of their cases there was a serious discrepancy in the correlation between the level of pulmonary capillary pressure and the radiological findings. In particular there was a group of patients with high pulmonary capillary pressures but without any radiological abnormality at the time of study, though positive x-ray findings developed subsequently.

Measurement of Pulmonary Oedema

Definite radiological features indicate quite marked pulmonary oedema and the clinical features of dyspnoea, orthopnoea and crepitations on auscultation also signify an advanced stage. Precise quantification of oedema is difficult. The most certain method is at autopsy, using the ratio of wet weight to dry weight of lung tissue, after correcting for the trapped blood volume, though even then other pathologies and postmortem changes influence the results. Even histological identification of oedema is not easy as it is only possible to stain the proteinaceous material left behind after the fixing process.

Double indicator dilution methods have been proposed to measure the amount of liquid in the lungs (Chinard and Enns, 1954; Levine, Mellins and Fishman, 1965; Goresky, Cronin and Wangel, 1969). The two indicators are injected simultaneously into the pulmonary artery and sampled 'downstream' in the aorta, in a way analogous to the derivation of dye-dilution curves for the measurement of cardiac output. One indicator (tritiated water) is freely diffusible whilst the other (radio-iodine labelled human serum albumin) remains in the vascular compartment. The difference in their mean transit times across the pulmonary vascular bed gives a measure of the water content of the lungs. Thermal and conductivity dilution curves have also been used, as heat is more diffusible than tritium (Noble and Severinghaus, 1972). But all these methods are critically dependent on the area of lung to which the indicators are delivered; water in unperfused areas cannot be measured. Other investigators have used changes in pulmonary impedance as a measure of the water content of the lungs (Van de Water, Miller and Milne, 1970; Severinghaus, 1971) but more information is required about its accuracy and reproducibility.

Lung Function in Pulmonary Oedema

When alveolar oedema occurs there is a marked reduction in vital capacity and in lung compliance in the tidal volume range. However, when oedematous lungs are forcibly inflated beyond the tidal range the succeeding deflation pressure–volume curve is similar to that of normal lungs (Cook et al, 1959; Levine et al, 1965) suggesting that the abnormal mechanical behaviour is better explained by altered 'surface phenomena' rather than by any intrinsic tissue change. The formation of alveolar oedema probably washes out the normal surfactant layer of the alveolar membrane and thus alters the normal pressure–volume relationships of the lung. Changes in pulmonary compliance in the early stages of interstitial oedema may be due to a decrease in lung volume and to an increase in pulmonary blood volume (Bø, Hauge and Waaler, 1973). In addition, a consistent increase in total airway resistance only occurs when alveolar oedema is grossly evident (Sharp et al, 1958, 1961). In earlier stages of pulmonary oedema changes in airway resistance are small and inconsistent.

Hypoxaemia and hypocapnia with respiratory alkalosis are the characteristic blood gas findings in pulmonary oedema, though carbon dioxide retention and respiratory acidosis may complicate the advanced stages. In addition, a metabolic acidosis develops as tissue perfusion becomes inadequate (Anthonisen and Smith, 1965; Avery, Samet and Sackner, 1970). The arterial hypoxia of clinical pulmonary oedema has been shown to be due to shunting of blood past unventilated alveoli (Pain, Stannard and Sloman, 1967), and in general the degree of hypoxia correlates with the degree of pulmonary oedema. Figure 2 shows the arterial blood gas tensions and mean pulmonary arterial pressures in patients with acute myocardial infarction. The patients, all without hypercapnia (Muir, 1970) were divided into two groups, those with an apparently uncomplicated myocardial infarction and those with clinical and radiological evidence of left ventricular failure. Patients with left ventricular failure all had low arterial oxygen tensions, but in addition some patients with neither clinical nor radiological features of pulmonary oedema also had low arterial oxygen tensions with increased venous admixture. However, mean pulmonary arterial pressures were raised in these latter patients, possibly due to otherwise undetected pulmonary oedema. These findings emphasise the difficulty in diagnosing early pulmonary oedema. They also suggest that, in man, arterial hypoxaemia due to ventilation–perfusion abnormalities is a relatively early feature of pulmonary oedema. This

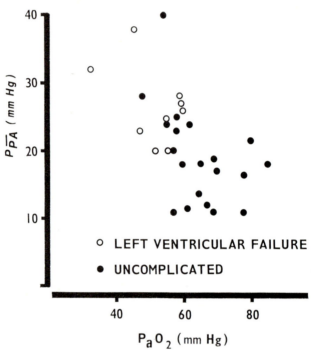

Figure 2   The relationship of mean pulmonary arterial pressure to arterial oxygen tensions in patients with myocardial infarction with (○) or without (●) left ventricular failure

is in contrast to the situation in experimental animal studies where pulmonary oedema has to be very marked before hypoxaemia becomes apparent (Said et al, 1964; Muir et al, 1972).

Changes in the distribution of pulmonary blood flow

West, Dollery and Heard (1965) noted that although pulmonary blood flow normally increased towards the base of the vertically suspended isolated lung, there was sometimes a reduction of blood flow to the base of the lung; this they ascribed to a cuff of perivascular oedema fluid accumulating around small extra-alveolar vessels. Thus, a reduction in blood flow to the base of the lungs might be expected in early interstitial pulmonary oedema. However, other investigators using intact animals were only able to demonstrate a reduction in blood flow when the oedema had become very marked (Naimark, Kirk and Chernecki, 1971; Muir et al, 1972). Moreover, within any one horizontal section of lung the reduction in blood flow was closely related to areas of alveolar oedema. In subsequent studies the mechanical factors that could cause a reduction in blood flow in alveolar oedema were examined separately. Neither a loss of regional lung volume nor filling of the alveoli with fluid, both prominent features of alveolar oedema, caused a reduction of blood flow. However, when hypo-osmotic plasma was instilled into the alveoli rather than iso-osmotic plasma there was a reduction in blood flow. It was reasoned that hypo-osmotic plasma was more likely than iso-osmotic plasma to cross the alveolar epithelial lining and cause a state resembling alveolar interstitial oedema, and perhaps the main mechanical factor causing a reduction in blood flow in alveolar oedema was interstitial fluid compressing the pulmonary capillaries (Muir, Hall and Hogg, 1972). These experimental studies suggest that a reduction in blood flow to the oedematous area is a relatively late feature in dogs. At this stage there is also likely to be a reduction of ventilation to the same area and this would tend to preserve normal arterial oxygen saturation rather than cause hypoxaemia; this was indeed the case in both these studies and in those of Said and colleagues (1964).

Distribution of ventilation

Less is known about the distribution of ventilation in pulmonary oedema. Once alveolar (gas space) oedema occurs, ventilation distribution must be considerably altered. Iliff, Greene and Hughes (1972) studied the distribution of ventilation in early (interstitial) oedema in isolated perfused lungs and showed that there was a reduction in the distribution of a slow inspiration to the base of the lungs. This, they concluded, was due to closure of small, peripheral airways due to peribronchiolar oedema. Increasing the lung volume was shown to increase the basal ventilation, presumably by reopening some previously closed airways. As small airways contribute only approximately 10 per cent of the total airway resistance (Macklem and Mead, 1967), any increase in peripheral airway resistance caused by airway closure would have little effect on total airway resistance. Since the regional distribution of a fast inspiration was not disturbed, in contrast to that of a slow inspiration, Iliff et al (1972) inferred that resistance to airflow through the larger airways was not changed in their preparation. Similar conclusions were reached by Hogg and his colleagues (1972). They induced pulmonary oedema in dogs under controlled vascular conditions and partitioned airway resistance by the retrograde catheter technique of Macklem and Mead (1967). Peripheral airway resistance was increased if left atrial pressure was raised though there was no consistent change in central airway resistance. Hogg et al also showed that the increase in peripheral airway resistance was reversible until left atrial pressure exceeded 15 mmHg. Their results suggested that the irreversible increase in peripheral airway resistance once left atrial pressure exceeded 15 mmHg was due to interstitial and alveolar oedema.

In man, the rapid infusion of 2 litres of saline caused an increase in the lung volume at which airway closure occurs (Muir et al, 1975), as measured by the closing volume technique of Dollfuss, Milic-Emili and Bates (1967). During the infusion period the closing volume remained within the functional residual capacity. Cardiac output and pulmonary arterial pressure increased, ventilation and perfusion were more uniformly distributed, and arterial oxygen tensions increased above control values at this time. Twenty minutes after the end of the infusion, closing volume remained high and in two of the four subjects it fell within the normal range of tidal ventilation. In these two subjects there was a significant fall in arterial oxygen tension below the control values (Muir et al, 1975).

In a group of patients with acute myocardial infarction Interiano et al (1973) were able to demonstrate frequency dependence of total pulmonary resistance which they attributed to the presence of peripheral airway oedema. However, there were abnormalities in FEV_1 and total airway resistance, suggesting that major airways were to some extent also involved. When their patients were studied again 10 weeks after infarction frequency dependence of pulmonary resistance had disappeared. Closing volume has also been measured in patients with myocardial infarction. In the acute phase, complicated by left ventricular failure, the alveolar plateau of marker gas was irregular and phase IV could not be identified, indicating that there was considerable alteration in the distribution of ventilation (Muir et al, 1975). In patients without clinical left ventricular failure, closing volume was increased and could be reduced by diuretic therapy (Hales and Kazemi, 1974). These results suggest that in man airway closure is an early feature of pulmonary oedema. If the distribution of perfusion is unaltered at this stage, then arterial hypoxaemia should also be an early feature. Further studies are required, but investigations to date suggest that tests of abnormalities of small airways function may be a useful index of early pulmonary oedema.

Treatment

Although the identification and, if possible, correction of precipitating factors must be amongst the objectives of the therapy of pulmonary oedema, the reduction of fluid accumulation and improvement of gas exchange are aims common to treating oedema of all causes.

Diuretics

The rapidly acting diuretic frusemide is now widely used in the treatment of pulmonary oedema. For some time clinicians have been puzzled that symptomatic relief appeared to occur before diuresis. This apparent paradox has been resolved by the work of Dikshit et al (1973) who showed that in patients with cardiogenic pulmonary oedema, pulmonary capillary ('wedge') pressure fell within 5 to 15 min following intravenous frusemide; at the same time there was an increase in venous capacitance of the calf. Increased urine flow only became maximal 30 to 60 min after administration of the drug. Frusemide thus appears to have a biphasic action in the treatment of pulmonary oedema; firstly, there is an extrarenal effect redistributing blood from the pulmonary vascular bed to the venous side of the systemic circulation; then there is a somewhat slower renal effect with subsequent diuresis and increase in both sodium and potassium excretion.

Morphine

Morphine remains a most valuable drug in the treatment of pulmonary oedema despite uncertainty about its mode of action. It probably produces a pharmacological phlebotomy akin to the immediate effects of frusemide (Sapru, 1966; Zelis et al, 1970). In addition, it probably acts by central depression of hyperventilation and by its ability to allay anxiety.

Digoxin

Digoxin is of value in the treatment of pulmonary oedema due to left ventricular failure. The clearest indication for its use is in the control of rapid atrial fibrillation. However, even in patients with sinus rhythm, it produces an increase in cardiac contractility, and the ventricular function curve is shifted so that, for a given left ventricular filling pressure, cardiac output is increased. Lower left ventricular filling pressures imply a reduction in pulmonary capillary hydrostatic pressures. In the failing heart the decrease in ventricular wall tension leads to a decrease in myocardial oxygen consumption. Digitalis should, of course, be used with caution in patients with acute myocardial infarction because of the risk of inducing arrhythmias and also the possibility that its use may increase the severity and extent of ischaemic injury (Maroko et al, 1971).

Oxygen

As hypoxaemia is common in all forms of pulmonary oedema, oxygen therapy is indicated. In the conscious patient, oxygen should be administered at relatively high concentrations (using an MC mask with an oxygen flow of 6 litres/min will provide an inspired oxygen concentration of approximately 60 per cent). In severe hypoxaemia, increasing the flow rate and in addition administering oxygen by nasal prongs may increase the inspired oxygen concentration.

In the seriously ill patient acid–base status should be checked, and if CO_2 retention is present consideration given to mechanical ventilation by a cuffed endotracheal tube. In a very few patients, arterial Po_2 will remain below 60 mmHg despite mechanical ventilation with 100 per cent oxygen. In these patients, ventilation with a positive end expiratory pressure (PEEP) has been advocated. Contrary to popular belief, there is no evidence that either IPPV or the application of PEEP leads to a shift of oedema out of the alveoli. Any resultant increase in arterial oxygen tension is probably due to maintenance of open airways and inflated alveoli (Staub, 1974). Care is necessary with this treatment because it may impair cardiac output and reduce net oxygen delivery to the tissues. The response of individual patients to PEEP should therefore ideally be assessed by measurement of cardiac output and arteriovenous oxygen differences.

THE LUNGS IN RENAL DISEASE

Patients with renal disease often have associated pulmonary abnormalities which at times present difficult diagnostic and therapeutic problems. With improvement in the management of patients who have renal failure, either acute or chronic, it has become increasingly important to distinguish the various pulmonary complications that may arise. It is, for instance, important to recognise oedema so that appropriate steps can be taken to reverse this; and it is vitally important to recognise infection, and to ascertain its cause, so that effective chemotherapy may be given (in optimal dosage, always bearing in mind the patient's reduced excretory capacity).

The differentiation of these various pulmonary complications is not always easy. This can be particularly perplexing in patients who have had a kidney transplant and in those receiving immunosuppressive drugs for other reasons, when there is an increased liability to infection, opportunistic and otherwise. There is, however, no reason to suppose that the so-called 'transplant lung' syndrome (Slapak, Lee and Hume, 1968) constitutes a specific syndrome; rather, this represents an illness in a post-transplant patient who has a greater or lesser degree of respiratory distress, who develops diffuse opacities on his chest radiograph, and who awaits a definitive diagnosis.

Pulmonary opacities seen on the radiograph of a patient with renal disease may be due to oedema, infection, lung damage due to immune mechanisms, haemorrhage, calcification, drug effects and pulmonary embolism. This list is not exhaustive and could be expanded to include any pulmonary or pleural pathology. Most patients with the so-called 'transplant lung' syndrome will be found to have pulmonary infection or oedema and these are the only aspect of this condition that we propose to mention further, though other pathologies may occasionally be responsible. In the wider context of the lungs in renal disease we also propose to discuss Goodpasture's syndrome, pulmonary calcification and lung function in renal failure.

Pulmonary oedema has already been dealt with in some depth though one or two additional minor points deserve mention in relationship to renal disease. Like oedema generally this may in part be due to overhydration due to a diminished excretory capacity for salt and water, as in the severely oliguric patient, and does not necessarily indicate myocardial failure though this may be present in those who have been or are severely hypertensive. That there may be increased pulmonary capillary permeability in renal failure has already been mentioned. Gibson (1966) inferred this when he found normal or only slightly elevated pulmonary arterial pressures in patients with acute pulmonary oedema due to renal failure. In 1972 Crosbie et al demonstrated increased pulmonary capillary permeability to the sodium ion when oedema of the lungs develops in patients being treated for renal failure by regular haemodialysis. To do this, they used a multiple indicator dilution method in which they measured the mean venous-arterial transit time of ^{24}Na relative to ^{125}I-labelled human serum albumin and tritiated water. A permeability factor was then derived from the three transit times. In normal individuals the dilution curve for sodium conformed more closely to that of labelled albumin rather than water, and the permeability factor was around 0.1. In patients with pulmonary oedema the transit time for sodium was prolonged and approximated more closely to the value for tritiated water so that the permeability factor approached unity. Crosbie et al went on to postulate that humoral factors were responsible for the alteration in capillary permeability.

It is thus evident that the pathogenesis of pulmonary oedema in renal failure may be multifactorial. Fortunately, in clinical practice the urgent need is to induce a diuresis or control the oedema by means of dialysis (and, rarely, by venesection) rather than to attempt to define the precise mechanism responsible.

Infection

The lungs of patients with renal disease may, of course, become infected with any pathogenic organism, including fungi as well as bacteria and viruses. However, in recent years most interest has centred on infections with what are ordinarily uncommon pathogens, especially cytomegalovirus and *Pneumocystis carinii*, to which patients on immunosuppressive therapy are prone. Nevertheless, bacterial pneumonia is, overall, much the most serious pulmonary complication facing the patient after renal transplantation. Whilst the initial response of infection to appropriate antibiotic therapy may be rapid, and Gram-positive organisms may be eradicated with apparent ease, the outcome remains uncertain, no doubt because of the tendency to develop secondary infection with mixed Gram-negative organisms and fungi.

Cytomegalovirus (CMV) infection is undoubtedly a common hazard facing the recipient of a renal transplant. Thus, Hill, Rowlands and Rifkind (1964) found evidence of CMV infection in 47 per cent of a series of 32 patients dying after renal transplantation; and it may be noted that 26, or 81 per cent, of these patients died with pulmonary infection of one form or another. Similarly, Millard et al (1973) found an incidence of 42 per cent of

CMV infection in a group of 50 adults who died after renal allotransplantation. Active CMV infection seems to be related to the transplantation procedure and the use of immunosuppressive therapy, and is probably due to reactivation of a latent infection, though other possible sources of virus are the allograft itself, transfused blood, and other patients or staff with whom the patient comes into contact.

Lopez et al (1974) carefully screened 61 immunosuppressed renal allograft recipients for the development of a virus infection. Of these, as many as 87 per cent developed a herpes virus infection, usually CMV (Fig. 3); infections due to other viruses were virtually non-existent. Altogether, 77 per cent of their patients had evidence of CMV infection, almost a quarter became infected with herpes simplex and approximately a fifth with herpes zoster; a few patients developed combined infections. Virus was isolated

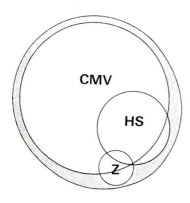

Figure 3   Frequency of herpes virus infections after renal allotransplantation. Outer ring: all transplant recipients; CMV: those who developed cytomegalovirus infection; HS: herpes simplex infection; Z: herpes zoster infection. (Data from Lopez et al, 1974)

commonly from the urine or sputum or both. It is of interest that, despite immunosuppressive therapy, most patients produced antiviral antibodies in response to infection. Lopez et al observed fever, leucopenia and episodes of graft rejection in their patients in association with these various herpes virus infections, though they were unable to establish a definite cause and effect relationship.

Pneumocystis carinii is an uncommon but serious opportunistic pulmonary pathogen and causes insidiously progressive dyspnoea, usually accompanied by a dry, unproductive cough and increasing hypoxaemia. This condition has been equated with the so-called 'transplant lung' syndrome (Doak et al, 1973). Pneumocystis infection is considerably more sinister than CMV infection and is likely to lead to death unless treated; whereas CMV causes a focal pneumonitis which may contribute to a patient's death, pneumocystis causes extensive consolidation with desquamation of alveolar lining cells and hyaline membrane formation, leading to lethal hypoxaemia. Nevertheless, both conditions may be very similar, clinically and radiographically; the x-ray shows fine micronodular opacities scattered throughout the lungs and these may produce a diffusely granular appearance. And, of course, both conditions often coexist.

Pneumocystis carinii pneumonia is very rare in the general population and is almost confined to individuals whose immune defence mechanisms are compromised. Patients undergoing renal transplantation already have a degree of immunodeficiency due to their uraemic state and this is further aggravated by the immunosuppressive drugs given postoperatively. In a review of 194 patients with confirmed *P. carinii* pneumonia in the USA during a three-year period, Walzer et al (1974) found that only three other groups of patients featured more frequently than renal transplant recipients. These were patients suffering from leukaemia, Hodgkin's disease or another lymphoma and those with a primary immune deficiency. Their data indicated that about 98 per cent of patients had an immunological defect or had received immunosuppressive or cytotoxic therapy, or both.

Diagnosis of *P. carinii* infection is not easy, especially when there is concomitant infection with other organisms, as was the case in approximately one-quarter of the patients studied by Walzer et al (1974): a high index of clinical suspicion is likely to help in this context. Walzer and his colleagues observed that open lung biopsy was both the most frequently used method of diagnosis and also the most accurate, since it produced no false negative results; unfortunately, it also proved to be the most hazardous method. Other diagnostic procedures included closed lung biopsy, needle aspiration, bronchial biopsy or aspiration, and collection of sputum or gastric aspirate. Serological testing was unfortunately not very helpful because, although frequently positive in the patients with *P. carinii* pneumonia, it was also often positive in asymptomatic immunosuppressed individuals. It remains to be seen whether endobronchial brush-biopsy maintains its early diagnostic promise (Repsher, Schroter and Hammond, 1972). However, even with good samples of tissue for histopathological study, careful staining is essential for accurate recognition of *P. carinii* and great care will clearly be necessary with the brush-biopsy technique.

Pentamidine isethionate is an effective therapeutic agent if given early in the course of *P. carinii* pneumonia. Unfortunately, it is also a toxic drug and its most serious adverse reaction is on the kidney. Walzer et al (1974) reported that 42 per cent of the patients treated with pentamidine recovered and in those treated for nine days or more, the recovery rate was 63 per cent. Side effects were observed in almost half of the patients, most commonly impaired renal function, though others were also troublesome: muscle necrosis at the site of injection, impaired liver function, hypotension, rashes and hypoglycaemia. Even so, pentamidine remains the drug of choice, though a combination of pyrimethamine and sulphadiazine may be considered as an alternative (Kirby, Kenamore and Guckian, 1971). *(Septra)* *trimethoprim + sulfamethoxazole*

Goodpasture's Syndrome

Haemoptysis may occur in patients with renal disease due to pulmonary emboli, when there is a severe haemorrhagic diathesis, as a feature of Goodpasture's syndrome, and in patients with polyarteritis nodosa or Wegener's granulomatosis. The symptom does not, therefore, have diagnostic significance, though there is often a tendency to invoke a diagnosis of Goodpasture's syndrome when pulmonary haemorrhage is associated with nephritis, especially if the patient is male. This interpretation should, strictly, be limited to patients with rapidly progressive glomerulonephritis and intra-alveolar haemorrhage. Renal injury in patients with Goodpasture's syndrome appears to be mediated by antibodies against glomerular basement membrane (GBM) (Sissons et al, 1974). Unfortunately, the capability of demonstrating such antibodies is not generally available and for most clinicians the diagnosis must, for the present, remain essentially clinical. It remains to be seen whether the widespread alveolar bleeding is also due to damage by antibodies directed at the alveolar basement membrane, though this seems possible (McPhaul and Dixon, 1970).

It is logical to treat patients with corticosteroids and immunosuppressive drugs when immune mechanisms are implicated as a cause of tissue damage. Although postulated rather than proved, this is the case with polyarteritis nodosa and Wegener's granulomatosis as well as Goodpasture's syndrome. Unfortunately, such treatment is generally ineffective in Goodpasture's syndrome (though the response can be impressive in the other disorders).

Whereas renal failure can be controlled by dialysis, this does nothing to alleviate the pulmonary haemorrhage of Goodpasture's syndrome which therefore becomes the greater threat to life. Bilateral nephrectomy has even been performed so as to remove GBM antigenic sites, in the hope that there will be a consequent reduction in anti-GBM antibody production; this assumes that such antibodies are cross-reacting with the lungs and are responsible for the bleeding. Even this may be ineffective (Sissons et al, 1974). Lockwood et al (1975) therefore treated a patient by plasmapheresis in addition to immunosuppressive drugs and dialysis, in an apparently successful attempt to reduce the level of circulating antibody and prevent further renal damage.

Pulmonary Calcification

It is customary to divide soft tissue calcification into *dystrophic*, in which calcification takes place in tissues already damaged by disease, and *metastatic*, where calcium salts are deposited in previously normal tissue. The latter is attributed to saturation of extracellular fluid with calcium phosphate. It is liable to occur when the $Ca \times PO_4$ product is in excess of 70 to 75 (both ions being measured in mg/100 ml).

Whereas dystrophic calcification of the lungs is common, being seen for instance in tuberculosis, histoplasmosis and varicella pneumonia, metastatic calcification is rare as a clinical entity. Pathologists, however, have recognised metastatic calcification of the lungs for many years. In 1947 Mulligan reviewed the literature on metastatic calcification from the time of Virchow onwards and showed how frequently the lungs were a site of calcium deposition.

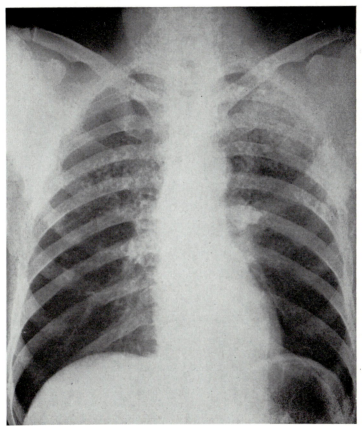

Figure 4 Alveolar metastatic calcification in a middle-aged male patient with chronic renal failure

He subdivided the published cases into those due to widespread bone disease, renal disease, hyperparathyroidism, vitamin D administration and a group where the aetiology was uncertain.

Mulligan (1947) described clearly the pathology of metastatic pulmonary calcification in renal disease and observed that this most often involved the alveolar walls and the intima and media of arteries and veins. He noted that the lungs were involved in almost half of the renal cases of metastatic calcification.

Although the density of the pulmonary calcium deposit is usually insufficient to be evident on the plain chest radiograph, it can at times be extensive (McLachlan, Wallace and Seneviratne, 1968; Neff et al, 1974). The x-ray appearances may be confused with pulmonary oedema or be confused by its presence. However, careful inspection of good quality radiographs may reveal the characteristic finely punctate stippling (Fig. 4).

Metastatic calcification in patients with renal failure may be due to injudicious vitamin D therapy aimed at correcting renal rickets, or to secondary hyperparathyroidism, and it may be more common in those treated by haemodialysis. In some patients, however, there is no ready explanation.

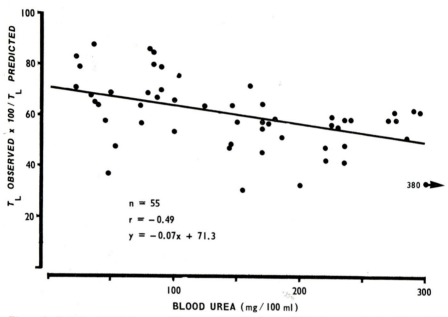

Figure 5   Relationship between pulmonary transfer factor (diffusing capacity) and level of blood urea in renal failure patients (from Lee and Stretton (1975) by permission of the Editor of *Thorax*)

The nature of soft tissue calcification in uraemia was studied by Contiguglia et al (1973). They showed that visceral calcification did not have the expected x-ray diffraction pattern of hydroxyapatite. The latter was found in the discrete metastatic calcium deposits that occur in subcutaneous tissue; but in the lungs, heart and skeletal muscle the x-ray diffraction pattern was amorphous and the ratios of Ca:Mg:P were different.

Pulmonary Function in Uraemia

Impairment of lung function is to be expected in the face of pulmonary oedema, infection, haemorrhage (with or without damage due to immune mechanisms) or alveolar wall calcification. However, it is now well recognised that pulmonary function is disturbed in patients with uraemia who have no evidence of such problems. Lee and Stretton (1975) examined 55 patients with renal failure who had neither clinical nor radiographic evidence of lung disease. In these patients they noted a small restrictive ventilatory defect, more marked in male patients than in females, which was statistically signi-ficant though of little or no biological importance. They also invariably found a defect in gas transfer which showed a significant negative correlation with the level of blood urea (Fig. 5) ($r = -0.49$; $P < 0.001$); this could not be accounted for by the presence of anaemia and was shown to be due to a reduction in the diffusing capacity across the alveolar capillary membrane (D_m).

Whilst Lee and Stretton (1975) were unable to present confirmatory pathological data, their physiological observations led them to conclude that pulmonary oedema was not present at the time of investigation though previous episodes of oedema, due to abnormal capillary leakage, could have led to persistent structural changes in the alveolar walls which could explain their findings (see Fig. 3, Chapter 7).

SHOCK LUNG

The increase in road traffic accidents and the recent conflict in Vietnam have drawn attention to the syndrome of progressive hypoxaemia following non-thoracic trauma. Collins and colleagues (1968) reported that 14 out of 69 battle casualties had an arterial Po_2 below 80 mmHg on admission. All had arterial Pco_2 levels below 40 mmHg so that hypoventilation was excluded and they could not relate their findings to the duration of recumbency, transfusion of stored blood or degree of haemorrhagic shock. One hypoxaemic patient died and autopsy demonstrated severe fat embolism, and they specu-lated that the hypoxaemia in the other casualties was also due to fat embolism. In the following year Lowery, Cloutier and Carey (1969) examined sequential changes in the blood gases of 66 badly injured battle casualties at Da Nang. They reported normal P_ao_2 levels on admission but 12 h later most cases had hypoxaemia, some of which was progressively refractory to increasing oxygen concentrations. Since almost all patients showed biochemical evidence of fat emboli whether or not they developed hypoxaemia, it was felt that fat embolism alone was not a sufficient explanation. Similar observations have been made following civilian trauma (Olcott, Barber and Blaisdell, 1971). Progressive respiratory failure following trauma or shock has been variously termed 'shock lung', 'wet lung' and 'Da Nang lung'. But is there a specific lesion in the lungs following shock?

A characteristic clinical syndrome has begun to emerge. After a period of shock followed by successful resuscitation, there is an interval during which all appears to be well. The patient then insidiously develops rapid, shallow breathing followed by breathlessness and cough; on auscultation of the lungs both crepitations and rhonchi are audible, and refractory cyanosis becomes evident on inspection. The radiological appearance is of increasing alveolar infiltrates which continue to extend until the entire lung is enveloped in a diffuse haze (Fishman, 1973). Despite assisted ventilation with high concentrations of oxygen there is progressive hypoxaemia. At autopsy the lungs show oedema, perialveolar haemorrhage and alveolar collapse. Lungs from patients who have survived longer show, in addition, diffuse bronchopneumonia and hyaline membrane formation. Vascular thrombi, fat emboli and fibrin deposits are often seen but are not consistently present.

In an attempt to define the syndrome more precisely, Ratliff et al (1972) investigated the nature of the 'lung lesion' in battle casualties. They studied the central haemodynamics and gas exchange in five soldiers with haemorrhagic shock, five soldiers with septic shock, and in six wounded but non-shocked soldiers. Those with haemorrhagic shock had no increased shunt in their lungs and, apart from a slightly greater pulmonary vascular resistance, they were no different from the non-shocked controls. Those with septic shock had a high cardiac output, a high oxygen consumption, low central venous pressure and low peripheral vascular resistance, but an increased mean pulmonary arterial pressure. There was an increased $A - a\, D_{O_2}$ and transpulmonary shunting was increased. These patients had at autopsy a haematogenous pneumonia with protein-rich pulmonary oedema despite normal pulmonary arterial wedge pressures. In their hospital, during an eight month period 20 patients died of pulmonary insufficiency, half dying from progressive pneumonia and sepsis, and the remainder from aspiration, fat embolism, blast injury or massive overload of infused crystalloid.

Progressive hypoxaemia also follows shock in acute myocardial infarction (MacKenzie et al, 1964). Here, left atrial pressures are high despite low pulmonary blood flow, and 'shock lung' represents pulmonary oedema due to left ventricular failure. In septic shock, endotoxins may modify pulmonary capillary permeability, causing oedema, whilst in other forms of shock leucocyte and platelet aggregates may modify vascular permeability to cause increased fluid accumulation in the lung or lead to defective surfactant synthesis.

There is evidence from canine experiments that a period of hypotension alters the distribution of blood flow within the lung (Martin et al, 1971; Tiefenbrun and Shoemaker, 1971), but whether this is due to microthrombi, platelet aggregates, sequestration of polymorphonuclear leucocytes, vasoactive substances, fat embolism or overtransfusion remains unresolved. Pulmonary oxygen toxicity has also been implicated in shock lung, but the syndrome has developed even in the presence of low oxygen concentrations. It is of note that in canine experiments, when the circulation was excluded from one lung during haemorrhagic shock, that lung did not develop changes of oedema and atelectasis (Willwerth et al, 1967). However, Buckberg and colleagues (1970) have questioned the relevance of canine studies since in experiments with baboons they were unable to produce any pulmonary lesion.

As the precise pathogenesis of 'shock lung' remains to be elucidated, a rational therapeutic approach should be to try to identify and treat possible precipitating factors such as overtransfusion, hypoalbuminaemia, disseminated intravascular coagulation and sepsis. Gas exchange can be improved by diuretics and the judicious use of oxygen. Ventilator therapy by cuffed endotracheal tube may be required and in some cases positive end-expiratory pressure (PEEP) may be used. This will increase arterial oxygen tensions, but may diminish tissue oxygen delivery by decreasing cardiac output. The use of PEEP increases the hazard of producing a tension pneumothorax. The place of steroids (Wilson, 1972) will depend on more precise identification of the pathogenesis of the progressive hypoxaemia. With improved resuscitation from road accidents and other trauma, it is likely that the syndrome of 'shock lung' will become an increasing problem in intensive care units. It is only hoped that the use of the term will not divert clinicians from attempting to elucidate the mechanisms of progressive hypoxaemia in individual patients.

REFERENCES

Anthonisen, N. R. & Smith, H. J. (1965) Respiratory acidosis as a consequence of pulmonary edema. *Annals of Internal Medicine*, **62**, 991–999.

Avery, W. G., Samet, P. & Sackner, M. A. (1970) The acidosis of pulmonary edema. *American Journal of Medicine*, **48**, 320–324.

Ball, I. M., Dundee, J. W. & Stevenson, H. M. (1973) Ventilation during bronchoscopy with an injector. *British Journal of Anaesthesia*, **45**, 1063–1066.

Bø, G., Hauge, A. & Waaler, B. A. (1973) Does interstitial lung edema cause change in lung compliance? *New England Journal of Medicine*, **288**, 471.

British Medical Journal (1974) Safety and fibreoptic bronchoscopy. **3**, 542–543.

Buckberg, G. D., Lipman, C. A., Hahn, J. A., Smith, M. J. & Hennessen, J. A. (1970) Pulmonary changes following hemorrhagic shock and resuscitation in baboons. *Journal of Thoracic and Cardiovascular Surgery*, **59**, 450–460.

Chinard, F. P. & Enns, T. (1954) Transcapillary pulmonary exchange of water in the dog. *American Journal of Physiology*, **178**, 197–202.

Collins, J. A., Gordon, W. C., Hudson, T. L., Irvin, R. W., Kelly, T. & Hardaway, R. M. (1968) Inapparent hypoxemia in casualties with wounded limbs: pulmonary fat embolism? *Annals of Surgery*, **167**, 511–520.

Contiguglia, S. R., Alfrey, A. C., Miller, N. L., Runnells, D. E. & Le Geros, R. Z. (1973) Nature of soft tissue calcification in uremia. *Kidney International*, **4**, 229–235.

Cook, C. D., Mead, J., Schreiner, G. L., Frank, N. R. & Craig, J. M. (1959) Pulmonary mechanics during induced pulmonary edema in anesthetised dogs. *Journal of Applied Physiology*, **14**, 177–186.

Cottrell, T. S., Levine, O. R., Senior, R. M., Wiener, J., Spiro, D. & Fishman, A. P. (1967) Electron microscopic alterations at the alveolar level in pulmonary edema. *Circulation Research*, **21**, 783–797.

Credle, W. F. Jr, Smiddy, J. F. & Elliott, R. C. (1974) Complications of fiberoptic bronchoscopy. *American Review of Respiratory Disease*, **109**, 67–72.

Crosbie, W. A., Snowden, S. & Parsons, V. (1972) Changes in lung capillary permeability in renal failure. *British Medical Journal*, **4**, 388–390.

Dikshit, K., Vyden, J. K., Forrester, J. S., Chatterjee, K., Prakash, R. & Swan, H. J. C. (1973) Renal and extrarenal hemodynamic effects of furosemide in congestive heart failure after acute myocardial infarction. *New England Journal of Medicine*, **288**, 1087–1080.

Doak, P. B., Becroft, D. M. O., Harris, E. A., Hitchcock, G. C., Leeming, B. W. A., North, J. D. K., Montgomerie, J. Z. & Whitlock, R. M. L. (1973) *Pneumocystis carinii* pneumonia-transplant lung. *Quarterly Journal of Medicine*, **42**, 59–71.

Dollfuss, R. E., Milic-Emili, J. & Bates, D. V. (1967) Regional ventilation of the lung studied with boluses of ^{133}Xenon. *Respiration Physiology*, **2**, 234–246.

Fishman, A. P. (1973) Shock lung: a distinctive nonentity. *Circulation*, **47**, 921–923.

Földi, M. (1969) *Diseases of Lymphatics and Lymph Circulation*. Springfield, Illinois: Charles C. Thomas.

Fraser, R. G. & Paré, J. A. P. (1970) *Diagnosis of Diseases of the Chest*. Philadelphia: W. B. Saunders.

Gibson, D. G. (1966) Haemodynamic factors in the development of acute pulmonary oedema in renal failure. *Lancet*, **2**, 1217–1220.

Goresky, C. A., Cronin, F. P. & Wangel, B. E. (1969) Indicator dilution measurements of extravascular water in the lungs. *Journal of Clinical Investigation*, **48**, 487–501.

Guyton, A. C. & Lindsey, A. W. (1959) Effect of elevated left atrial pressure and decreased plasma protein concentrations on the development of pulmonary edema. *Circulation Research*, **7**, 649–657.

Hales, C. A. & Kazemi, H. (1974) Small-airways function in myocardial infarction. *New England Journal of Medicine*, **290**, 761–765.

Hill, R. B. Jr, Rowlands, D. T. Jr & Rifkind, D. (1964) Infectious pulmonary disease in patients receiving immunosuppressive therapy for organ transplantation. *New England Journal of Medicine*, **271**, 1021–1027.

Hogg, J. C., Agarawal, J. B., Gardiner, A. J. S., Palmer, W. H. & Macklem, P. T. (1972) The distribution of airway resistance with developing pulmonary edema in dogs. *Journal of Applied Physiology*, **32**, 20–24.

Hugh-Jones, P. (1967) Localisation of disordered function. *Bulletin de Physiopathologie Respiratoire*, **3**, 419.

Ikeda, S. (1974) *Atlas of Flexible Bronchofiberscopy*. Baltimore: University Park Press.

Ikeda, S., Yanai, N. & Ishikawa, S. (1968) Flexible bronchofiberscope. *Keio Journal of Medicine*, **17**, 1–18.

Iliff, L. D., Greene, R. E. & Hughes, J. M. B. (1972) Effect of interstitial edema on distribution of ventilation and perfusion in isolated lung. *Journal of Applied Physiology*, **33**, 462–467.

Interiano, B., Hyde, R. W., Hodges, M. & Yu, P. N. (1973) Interrelation between alterations in pulmonary mechanics and hemodynamics in acute myocardial infarction. *Journal of Clinical Investigation*, **52**, 1994–2006.

Kirby, H. B., Kenamore, B. & Guckian, J. C. (1971) *Pneumocystis carinii* pneumonia treated with pyrimethamine and sulfadiazine. *Annals of Internal Medicine*, **75**, 505–509.

Lee, H. Y. & Stretton, T. B. (1975) The lungs in renal failure. *Thorax*, **30**, 46–53.

Levine, O. R., Mellins, R. B. & Fishman, A. P. (1965) Quantitative assessment of pulmonary edema. *Circulation Research*, **17**, 414–426.

Lockwood, C. M., Boulton-Jones, J. M., Lowenthal, R. M., Simpson, I. J., Peters, D. K. & Wilson, C. B. (1975) Recovery from Goodpasture's syndrome after immunosuppressive treatment and plasmapheresis. *British Medical Journal*, **2**, 252–254.

Lopez, C., Simmons, R. L., Mauer, S. M., Najarian, J. S. & Good, R. A. (1974) Association of renal allograft rejection with virus infections. *American Journal of Medicine*, **56**, 280–289.

Lowery, B. D., Cloutier, C. T. & Carey, L. C. (1969) Blood gas determinations in the severely wounded in hemorrhagic shock. *Archives of Surgery*, **99**, 330–338.

McHugh, T. J., Forrester, J. S., Adler, L., Zion, D. & Swan, H. J. C. (1972) Pulmonary vascular congestion in acute myocardial infarction: hemodynamic and radiologic correlations. *Annals of Internal Medicine*, **76**, 29–33.

MacKenzie, G. J., Taylor, S. H., Flenley, D. C., McDonald, A. H., Staunton, H. P. & Donald, K. W. (1964) Circulatory and respiratory studies in myocardial infarction and cardiogenic shock. *Lancet*, **2**, 825–832.

Macklem, P. T. & Mead, J. (1967) Resistance of central and peripheral airways measured by a retrograde catheter. *Journal of Applied Physiology*, **22**, 395–401.

McLachlan, M. S. F., Wallace, M. & Seneviratne, C. (1968) Pulmonary calcification in renal failure. Report of three cases. *British Journal of Radiology*, **41**, 99–106.

McPhaul, J. J. Jr & Dixon, F. J. (1970) Characterisation of human antiglomerular basement membrane antibodies eluted from glomerulonephritic kidneys. *Journal of Clinical Investigation*, **49**, 308–317.

Maroko, P. R., Kjekshus, J. K., Sobel, B. E., Watanabe, T., Covell, J. W., Ross, J. & Braunwald, E. (1971) Factors influencing infarct size following experimental coronary artery occlusions. *Circulation*, **43**, 67–82.

Martin, R. R., Lowery, B. D., Sugg, J. H. & Anthonisen, N. R. (1971) Regional ventilation and perfusion distribution in experimental 'shock lung'. *Clinical Research*, **19**, 803.

Merrill, J. P. & Hampers, C. L. (1970) Uremia. *New England Journal of Medicine*, **282**, 953–961.

Meyer, B. J., Meyer, A. & Guyton, A. C. (1968) Interstitial fluid pressure v. negative pressure in the lungs. *Circulation Research*, **22**, 263–271.

Millard, P. R., Herbertson, B. M., Nagington, J. & Evans, D. B. (1973) The morphological consequences and the significance of cytomegalovirus infection in renal transplant patients. *Quarterly Journal of Medicine*, **42**, 585–596.

Muir, A. L. (1970) M.D. Thesis, University of Edinburgh.

Muir, A. L., Hall, D. L., Despas, P. & Hogg, J. C. (1972) Distribution of blood flow in the lungs in acute pulmonary edema in dogs. *Journal of Applied Physiology*, **33**, 763–769.

Muir, A. L., Hall, D. L. & Hogg, J. C. (1972) The site of increased vascular resistance in the lung in pulmonary edema. *Federation Proceedings*, **31**, Abstract 525, p. 308.

Muir, A. L., Flenley, D. C., Kirby, B. J., Sudlow, M. F., Guyatt, A. R. & Brash, H. M. (1975) Cardiorespiratory effects of rapid saline infusion in normal man. *Journal of Applied Physiology*, **38**, 786–793.

Mulligan, R. M. (1947) Metastatic calcification. *Archives of Pathology*, **43**, 177–230.

Naimark, A., Kirk, B. W. & Chernecki, W. (1971) Regional water volume, blood volume and perfusion in the lung. *Central Hemodynamics and Gas Exchange*. Torino: Minerva Medica.

Neff, M., Yalcin, S., Gupta, S. & Berger, H. (1974) Extensive metastatic calcification of the lung in an azotemic patient. *American Journal of Medicine*, **56**, 103–109.

Noble, W. H. & Severinghaus, J. W. (1972) Thermal and conductivity dilution curves for rapid quantitation of pulmonary edema. *Journal of Applied Physiology*, **32**, 770–775.

Olcott, C. IV, Barber, R. E. & Blaisdell, F. W. (1971) Diagnosis and treatment of respiratory failure after civilian trauma. *American Journal of Surgery*, **122**, 260–266.

Pain, M. C. F., Stannard, M. & Sloman, G. (1967) Disturbances of pulmonary function after acute myocardial infarction. *British Medical Journal*, **2**, 591.

Pattle, R. E. (1965) Surface lining of lung alveoli. *Physiological Reviews*, **45**, 48–79.

Pietra, G. G., Szidon, J. P., Leventhal, M. M. & Fishman, A. P. (1969) Hemoglobin as a tracer in hemodynamic pulmonary edema. *Science*, **166**, 1643–1646.

Pietra, G. G., Szidon, J. P., Leventhal, M. M. & Fishman, A. P. (1971) Histamine and interstitial pulmonary edema in the dog. *Circulation Research*, **29**, 323–337.

Ratliff, J. L., Fletcher, J. R., Hirsch, E. F. & Kopriva, C. J. (1972) The mechanism of the 'lung lesion' in shock. In *The Fundamental Mechanisms of Shock*, ed. Hirshaw, L. B. & Cox, B. G., pp. 203–214. London: Plenum Press.

Reichert, W. W., Hall, W. J. & Hyde, R. W. (1974) A simple disposable device for performing fiberoptic bronchoscopy on patients requiring continuous artificial ventilation. *American Review of Respiratory Disease*, **109**, 394–396.

Repsher, L. H., Schroter, G. & Hammond, W. S. (1972) Diagnosis of *Pneumocystis carinii* by means of endobronchial brush biopsy. *New England Journal of Medicine*, **287**, 340–341.

Robin, E. D., Cross, C. E. & Zelis, R. (1973) Pulmonary edema. *New England Journal of Medicine*, **288**, 239–246, 292–304.

Sackner, M. A. (1975) Bronchofiberscopy. *American Review of Respiratory Disease*, **111**, 62–88.

Said, S. I., Longacher, J. W., Davis, R. K., Banerjee, C. M., Davis, W. M. & Woodell, W. J. (1964) Pulmonary gas exchange during induction of pulmonary edema in anesthetised dogs. *Journal of Applied Physiology*, **19**, 403–407.

Sanders, R. D. (1967) Two ventilating attachments for bronchoscopes. *Delaware Medical Journal*, **39**, 170–175, 192.

Sapru, R. P. (1966) Ph.D. Thesis, University of Edinburgh.

Severinghaus, J. W. (1971) Electrical measurement of pulmonary oedema with a focusing conductivity bridge. *Journal of Physiology*, **215**, 53P–55P.

Sharp, J. T., Griffith, G. T., Bunnell, I. L. & Greene, D. G. (1958) Ventilatory mechanics in pulmonary edema in man. *Journal of Clinical Investigation*, **37**, 111–117.

Sharp, J. T., Bunnell, I. L., Griffith, G. T. & Greene, D. G. (1961) The effects of therapy on pulmonary mechanics in human pulmonary edema. *Journal of Clinical Investigation*, **40**, 665–672.

Sissons, J. G. P., Evans, D. J., Peters, D. K., Eisinger, A. J., Boulton-Jones, J. M., Simpson, I. J. & Macanovic, M. (1974) Glomerulonephritis associated with antibody to glomerular basement membrane. *British Medical Journal*, **4**, 11–14.

Slapak, M., Lee, H. M. & Hume, D. M. (1968) Transplant lung—a new syndrome. *British Medical Journal*, **1**, 80–84.

Starling, E. H. (1896) On the absorption of fluids from the connective tissue spaces. *Journal of Physiology*, **19**, 312–326.

Staub, N. C. (1971) Steady state pulmonary transvascular water filtration in unanesthetised sheep. *Circulation Research*, **28**, Suppl. 1, 135–139.

Staub, N. C. (1974) Pulmonary edema. *Physiological Reviews*, **54**, 678–811.

Staub, N. C., Nagano, H. & Pearce, M. L. (1967) Pulmonary edema in dogs, especially the sequence of fluid accumulation in lungs. *Journal of Applied Physiology*, **22**, 227–240.

Taylor, A. E. & Gaar, K. A. Jr (1970) Estimation of equivalent pore radii of pulmonary capillary and alveolar membranes. *American Journal of Physiology*, **218**, 1133–1140.

Tiefenbrun, J. & Shoemaker, W. C. (1971) Sequential changes in pulmonary blood flow distribution in hemorrhagic shock. *Annals of Surgery*, **174**, 727–733.

Van de Water, J. M., Miller, I. T. & Milne, E. N. C. (1970) Impedance plethysmography: a non-invasive means of monitoring the thoracic surgery patient. *Journal of Thoracic and Cardiovascular Surgery*, **60**, 641–647.

Walzer, P. D., Perl, D. P., Krogstad, D. J., Rawson, P. G. & Schultz, M. G. (1974) *Pneumocystis carinii* pneumonia in the United States. Epidemiologic, diagnostic and clinical features. *Annals of Internal Medicine*, **80**, 83–93.

West, J. B., Dollery, C. T. & Heard, B. E. (1965) Increased pulmonary vascular resistance in the dependent zone of the isolated dog lung caused by perivascular edema. *Circulation Research*, **17**, 191–206.

Willwerth, B. M., Crawford, F. A., Young, W. G. Jr & Sealy, W. C. (1967) The role of functional demand on the development of pulmonary lesions during hemorrhagic shock. *Journal of Thoracic and Cardiovascular Surgery*, **54**, 658–665.

Wilson, J. W. (1972) Treatment or prevention of pulmonary cellular damage with pharmacologic doses of corticosteroid. *Surgery, Gynaecology and Obstetrics*, **134**, 675–681.

Zelis, R. F., Mason, D. T., Spann, J. F. & Amsterdam, E. A. (1970) The effects of morphine on the venous bed in man: demonstration of a biphase response. *American Journal of Cardiology*, **25**, 136, Abstract.

Ziskind, M. M., Weill, H. & George, R. A. (1965) Acute pulmonary edema following the treatment of spontaneous pneumothorax with excessive negative intrapleural pressure. *American Review of Respiratory Disease*, **92**, 632–636.

INDEX

Printed by Adlard and Son Ltd, Bartholomew Press, Dorking